MEDICAL RADIOLOGY

Diagnostic Imaging

Editors:
A. L. Baert, Leuven
K. Sartor, Heidelberg

Springer
Berlin
Heidelberg
New York
Hong Kong
London
Milan
Paris
Tokyo

S. Peer · G. Bodner (Eds.)

High-Resolution Sonography of the Peripheral Nervous System

With Contributions by

G. Bodner · H. Gruber · S. Kiechl · P. Kovacs · S. Peer · H. Piza-Katzer

Foreword by

A. L. Baert

With 141 Figures in 237 Separate Illustrations, 7 in Color and 6 Tables

Springer

Siegfried Peer, MD
Gerd Bodner, MD
Department of Radiology
Section for Diagnostic and Interventional Sonography
University Hospital Innsbruck
Anichstrasse 35
6020 Innsbruck
Austria

Medical Radiology · Diagnostic Imaging and Radiation Oncology
Series Editors: A. L. Baert · L. W. Brady · H.-P. Heilmann · M. Molls · K. Sartor

Continuation of Handbuch der medizinischen Radiologie
Encyclopedia of Medical Radiology

ISBN 3-540-43260-4 Springer-Verlag Berlin Heidelberg New York

Library of Congress Cataloging-in-Publication Data

High-resolution sonography of the peripheral nervous system / S. Peer, G. Bodner, eds. ;
with contributions by G. Bodner ... [et al.] ; foreword by A. L. Baert.
p. ; cm. -- (Medical radiology)
Includes bibliographical references and index.
ISBN 3540432604 (alk. paper)
1. Nerves, Peripheral--Ultrasonic imaging. I. Peer, S. (Siegfried), 1962- II. Bodner G. (Gerd), 1960- III: Series.
[DNLM: 1. Peripheral Nervous System--ultrasonography. 2. Peripheral Nervous System Diseases--ultrasonography. 3. Ultrasonography--methods. WL 500 H638 2003]
RC409 .H.547 2003
616.8'7--dc21 2002036598

Springer-Verlag Berlin Heidelberg New York
a member of BertelsmannSpringer Science+Business Media GmbH

http//www. springer.de

Printed in Germany

Cover-Design and Typesetting: Verlagsservice Teichmann, 69256 Mauer

21/3150 – 5 4 3 2 1 0 – Printed on acid-free paper

Foreword

Progress in hardware and software for clinical ultrasound equipment has been tremendous during the past few years.

Exquisite morphological visualisation of soft tissues and related pathology is now possible in clinical daily routine work. Periarticular anatomy and pathology of ligaments, bursae or tendons can now be depicted with unprecedented precision by sonography, and this technique provides important support for better management of patients affected by trauma or diseases of the locomotor system.

The important role of high-resolution sonography in the visualisation and management of traumatic or tumoral conditions of the peripheral nervous system is less well known. This volume provides an excellent and comprehensive overview of our knowledge in this emerging field of radiological imaging. It is the result of considerable original sonographic research by the authors in close collaboration with colleagues from several other disciplines, including anatomists, neurologists and surgeons.

Dr. S. Peer and Dr. G. Bodner are internationally renowned pioneers in the new area of peripheral nerve sonography, and their book is based on extensive personal experience and exhaustive study of the existing literature on the topic. I would like to congratulate them on this outstanding work.

I am confident that this superiorly illustrated volume is a timely and well-needed work and that it will meet with great interest from radiologists, neurologists and specialists in reconstructive and plastic surgery, as well as from trauma surgeons and all those involved in rehabilitation medicine. I sincerely wish it the same success with readers as encountered by the previous volumes published in this series.

Leuven

Albert L. Baert

Preface

Scientific progress is always based on knowledge, which is acquired from interaction with other people (our teachers, clinical partners), from the industry, from the expertise expressed by colleagues in scientific publications, from meetings, from personal communications and, as far as the imaging disciplines are concerned, even more from the daily interdisciplinary collaboration in the quest for the optimum diagnosis and therapy for a given patient. With this in mind, we would like to express our thanks to all those who supported our efforts in the institution of peripheral nerve sonography at our hospital, its further development and scientific evaluation, especially our partners at the Departments of Neurology, Plastic and Reconstructive Surgery and Traumatology.

This book is intended to provide the reader with the state of the art in peripheral nerve sonography, based on several years of personal experience and an overview of the current literature. It would not have been possible without the help of several people who may not go unmentioned. We are especially grateful for the support we received from Prof. Helga Fritsch and Prof. Othmar Gaber of the Innsbruck University Institute of Anatomy for their expert advice and provision of specimens for the anatomic/sonographic correlations. In this regard special thanks are also due to Dr. Felix Aigner as well as Gottfried and Rupert Gstrein of the Institute of Anatomy for their help in production of the anatomic cryosections and plastinated specimens.

We would like to express our thanks to the editorial staff of Springer Verlag (especially Mrs. Ursula Davis) for their contribution with editing and production of this volume. Last but not least, thanks are also due to Prof. Albert Baert, the series editor, for his trust and encouragement which enabled us to share our knowledge with a larger public in this volume of an already well-acclaimed radiologic imaging series.

Innsbruck

Siegfried Peer
Gerd Bodner

Contents

1 General Considerations and Technical Concepts
S. Peer ... 1

2 Sonographic Anatomy of the Peripheral Nervous System
H. Gruber and P. Kovacs ... 13

3 Nerve Compression Syndromes
S. Peer, S. Kiechl, and G. Bodner ... 37

4 Traumatic Nerve Lesions
G. Bodner and S. Peer ... 61

5 Tumors and Tumor-Like Lesions
S. Peer and G. Bodner ... 83

6 Interventional Techniques
P. Kovacs, H. Gruber, and G. Bodner ... 95

7 Clinical Considerations: The Surgeon's Perspective
H. Piza-Katzer ... 107

8 An Introduction to Electrodiagnostic Testing
S. Kiechl ... 121

Subject Index ... 135

List of Contributors ... 137

1 High-Resolution Sonography of the Peripheral Nervous System: General Considerations and Technical Concepts

S. Peer

CONTENTS

1.1 Introduction to High-Resolution Sonography of the Peripheral Nervous System 1
1.1.1 Historical Development of Peripheral Nerve Sonography 1
1.1.2 Why Sonography of the Peripheral Nervous System? 3
1.2 Ultrasound Scanner Hardware and Software Requirements 4
1.2.1 Hardware Requirements 4
1.2.2 Software Requirements 5
1.3 General Technique of Sonographic Nerve Examination 8
1.3.1 Anatomic Considerations 8
1.3.2 Nerve Examination 9
References 10

1.1 Introduction to High-Resolution Sonography of the Peripheral Nervous System

Since the first report on the feasibility of sonographic imaging of peripheral nerves (Fornage 1988), we have experienced profound technical developments in sonography. High-resolution linear scanheads with superior near-field resolution, software applications such as compound imaging, extended field of view imaging and tissue harmonic imaging together with improved scanner hardware have changed the role of sonography in musculoskeletal diagnosis in general. For inspection of the peripheral nerve sonography may be regarded as the number one imaging modality. Peripheral nerves are in most cases superficially lying structures easily accessible with sonography, they show a typical and quite distinct sonographic texture and recent studies have revealed characteristic findings in various disease entities. Besides being cheap and commonly available, sonography spares the patient from ionizing radiation and is an interactive and non-discomforting method, which makes it the first choice from a patient's view-point. In this chapter a short overview of the historical development of sonography of the peripheral nervous system, the rationale for the widespread use of sonography in the work-up of patients with peripheral nerve disease, the technical requirements for performance of nerve sonography and an overview of the basic image features of peripheral nerves on sonography are presented.

S. Peer, MD
Professor, Department of Radiology, Section for Diagnostic and Interventional Sonography, University Hospital Innsbruck, Anichstrasse 35, 6020 Innsbruck, Austria

1.1.1 Historical Development of Peripheral Nerve Sonography

The first report on the feasibility of peripheral nerve sonography was presented by Fornage in 1988 (Fornage 1988). In this report the appearance of nerves on sonograms was for the first time reported to be of a tubular structure with a speckled internal appearance. Fornage also stated that the identification of a nerve is facilitated by identification of surrounding anatomic landmarks. Besides this, Fornage focused more on the identification and differential diagnosis of peripheral nerve tumors. How technical aspects hampered the more widespread introduction of this newly presented method into clinical routine may be realized if we imagine that it took three more years for the first report to appear in the literature concerned with direct evaluation of a single peripheral nerve (the sciatic nerve, which is the largest peripheral nerve in the body) and an attempt at sonographic diagnosis of various disease entities such as nerve compression and trauma as well as a first report on the appearance of a surgically reconstructed nerve (Graif et al. 1991). One of the first evaluations of special disease entities in the peripheral nervous system with sonography was published shortly thereafter, and concentrated on the median nerve compression syndrome in the carpal tunnel (Buchberger et al. 1991). While Buchberger and coworkers were able to show the potential of sonography for the differential diagnosis of this common disease entity, sonography did not gain wide acceptance. In their work they correlated the presence of carpal tunnel disease with flattening of the median nerve on sonography (Fig. 1.1), but to go deeper into the ultrastructure of the impaired nerve was beyond the abilities of their equipment.

In 1995 Silvestri et al. presented a basic report on the ultrastructural sonographic/histological correlation of peripheral nerves and for the first time reported the now commonly known criteria which aid in the differentiation of nerves and tendons (Silvestri et al. 1995). While nerves consist of multiple hypoechoic nodular (transverse scan plane) or continuous longitudinal structures (sagittal scan plane) with a thin echoic stroma (Fig. 1.2), small discontinuous hyperechoic speckles interspersed with hypoechoic elements represent the typical appearance of tendons (Fig. 1.2). With angulation of the scanhead, a tendon changes markedly from hyperechoic to a more hypoechoic appearance, while the echotexture of a peripheral nerve is influenced to a much lesser extent (Fig. 1.3).

Since then various reports in the literature have shown the high potential of sonography for imaging of peripheral nerve diseases (Martinoli et al. 1996; Chiou et al. 1998; Bodner et al. 1999; Peer et al. 2001, 2002). Nevertheless, the application of sonography to the diagnosis of peripheral nerve diseases is still limited to only a few centers around the world and is not widely known in the medical community. This may

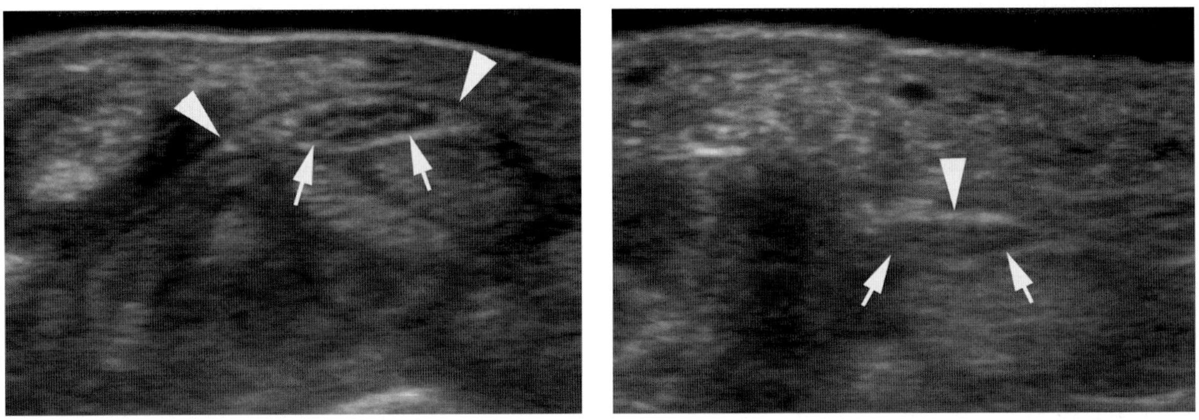

Fig. 1.1. Transverse sonograms through proximal (*left image*; *arrowheads* flexor retinaculum) and distal (*right image*) carpal tunnel in a patient with carpal tunnel disease. In the distal carpal tunnel the median nerve (*small arrows*) is flattened with loss of fascicular echotexture. There is a small indentation of the nerve by the thickened retinaculum (*arrowhead in right image*)

a 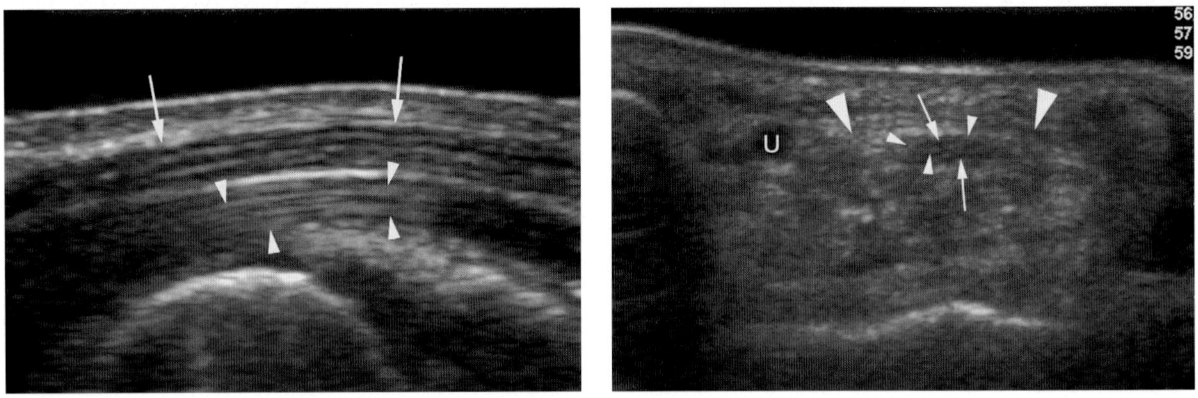

b

Fig. 1.2. **a** Longitudinal sonogram of the wrist in a healthy volunteer demonstrating typical appearance of peripheral nerve (*arrows* median nerve) with continuous hypoechoic longitudinal elements (fascicle groups) interspersed with echoic perineurium and epineurium and tendons (discontinuous hyperechoic speckles, *arrowheads*). **b** Transverse sonogram showing dotted appearance of normal nerve with multiple rounded hypoechoic fascicle groups (*arrows*) surrounded by hyperechoic perineurium and epineurium (*small arrowheads*) (*U* ulnar artery, *large arrowheads* flexor retinaculum)

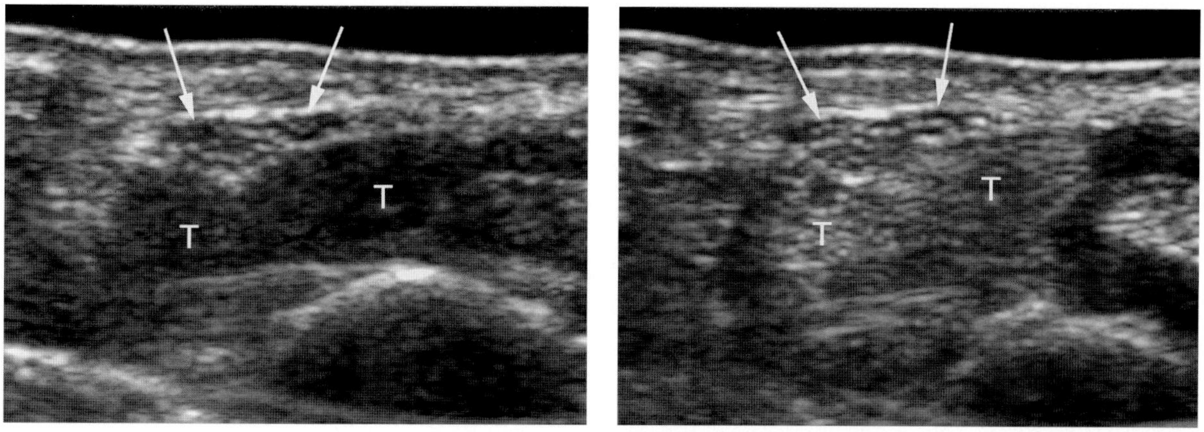

Fig. 1.3. Transverse sonogram through median nerve at level of the wrist with different angulation of scanhead in left half and right half of image. Note the markedly changing echotexture of tendons (*T*) with rather consistent echotexture of nerve (*arrows*)

have several reasons. The value of sonography especially for diagnosis of nerve diseases is highly user-dependent. A profound knowledge of the regional anatomy, the course of a nerve and its accompanying structures, a basic knowledge of neurological signs and symptoms as well as underlying pathological processes in typical disease entities and a certain amount of skill are mandatory to be able to identify and analyze peripheral nerves with sonography.

1.1.2 Why Sonography of the Peripheral Nervous System?

If sonography is user-dependent, difficult to perform and not widely accepted – why should we do it?

From an imaging point of view this question is in our opinion easily answered: there is no real alternative! The only possible alternative we might think of is MRI, but the reader who has already been involved with MRI of peripheral nerve disease will agree that MRI of peripheral nerves – despite its high soft-tissue contrast and multiplanar capabilities – is often unsatisfactory. The basic problem with MRI lies in the only subtle contrast differences of nerves and surrounding tissues (Fig. 1.4) and besides this the resolution of MRI is still far below that of sonography. While in bigger nerves surrounded by fat the nerve and its ultrastructure may be accessible to MRI (Filler et al. 1996), the visualization of small nerves is limited. Only with small high-resolution surface coils and special imaging sequences can the fascicular pattern of a small peripheral nerve be visualized

a

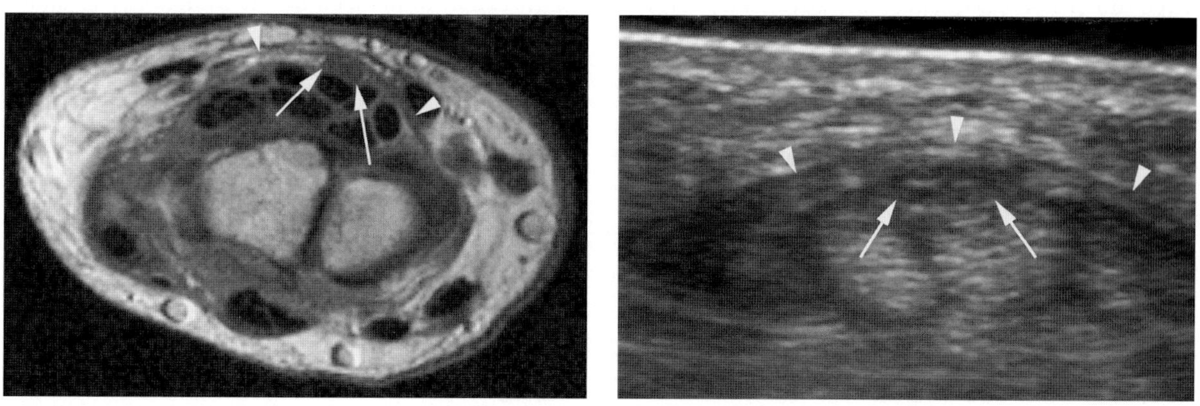

b

Fig. 1.4a, b. Transverse T1-weighted MR image (**a**) and sonogram (**b**) through median nerve (*arrows*) at level of the carpal tunnel. Note the slight flattening of the median nerve (*arrows*) underneath the flexor retinaculum (*arrowheads*). While the median nerve is only faintly visible in the MR image acquired with a normal surface coil, the outer margin of the nerve and its inner structure are readily visualized in the sonogram – thickening of the flexor retinaculum (*arrowheads*) is easily assessed in the sonogram, but hardly identified in the MR image

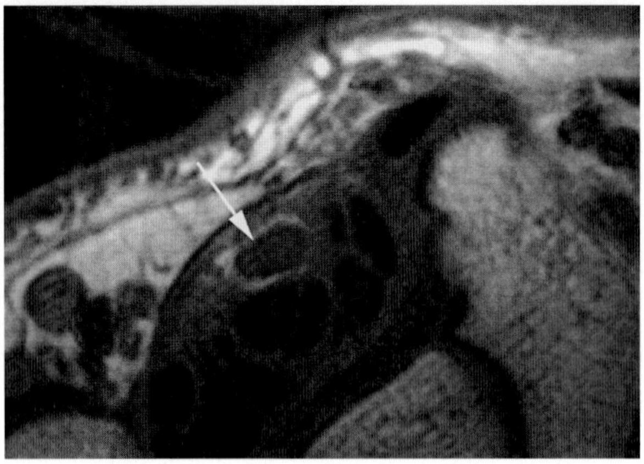

Fig. 1.5. Transverse high-resolution MR image of the median nerve at wrist level (*arrow*) with small loop-type surface coil. Note the visibility of nerve fascicles inside the median nerve but at the expense of increased noise

with MRI (Fig. 1.5), but at the expense of a small field of view and only for nerves lying close to the skin surface.

Therefore besides the lower resolution which limits MRI to imaging of bigger nerves only, above all the ultrastructure of nerves is not as easily accessible to MRI as it is to sonography. Whether this will change with the advent of new ultra-high-field 3.0 T clinical MR scanners remains to be proven with correlative studies, but today MRI is second in line regarding anatomic analysis of peripheral nerves. Another reason for the low impact of MRI for diagnosis of peripheral nerve disease is the oblique course of nerves in the extremities – while it is easy to follow a nerve with a longitudinal sonographic scan, this is hardly accomplished with MRI. The use of three-dimensional sequences and advanced postprocessing may be a choice with MRI, but this is highly time consuming. In this regard the only region where MRI may challenge sonography is the examination of the brachial or sacral plexus (Hayes 1997; Gierada et al. 1993; Gierada and Erickson 1993; Blake et al. 1996), and if we look at the MRI literature concerned with imaging of peripheral nerves, this is the main topic of interest (besides the differential diagnosis of peripheral nerve tumors). However, despite limitations in the diagnosis of radicular avulsions, the peripheral parts of the plexus are also much more easily assessed with sonography than with MRI.

An important asset of MRI in the evaluation of peripheral nerves is the possibility of acquiring images after intravenous administration of gadolinium contrast agents, which may add some information regarding nerve inflammation or hyperperfusion and inflammatory edema in neuritis and chronic nerve compression. The same information may probably be gained with color Doppler and power Doppler sonography of peripheral nerves, but there are no data in the literature on the value of Doppler techniques for diagnosis. Nevertheless with modern equipment the evaluation of perineural vasculature is certainly within reach.

There are other reasons for advocating sonography of peripheral nerves, and one lies in the limitations of electrodiagnostic methods, which are discussed in more detail in Chapter 8 of this book. While electrodiagnosis is able to definitely confirm and in many cases localize a nerve lesion, to define the nature of the underlying pathology is often beyond its reach. The latter, however, is important information for the planning of treatment. Another favorable aspect of sonography lies in the interactive nature of the examination. The examination is easily tailored to the exact location of a patient's pain sensations, or areas of possible coexisting trauma, it is quick and lacks the discomfort caused by pricking with needles during electrodiagnostic studies or by positioning in MRI. The possible interaction between the examiner and the patient with the ability to react to clues in a patient's history is a further important advantage.

1.2 Ultrasound Scanner Hardware and Software Requirements

The results which may be obtained in the diagnosis of peripheral nerve disease with sonography are to a high extent influenced by the availability of state-of-the-art equipment. We will not touch on the basic physical principals of sonographic imaging but only on some of the aspects which are especially critical for nerve examinations. In addition, some of the newer developments which are likely to influence clinical practice are discussed in the next paragraphs.

1.2.1 Hardware Requirements

Imaging with ultrasound depends on both contrast and resolution. With current clinically available transducers imaging of superficial structures is possible at frequencies of up to 15 MHz, which results in an axial resolution of 250 to 500 μm. Spatial detail in a sonogram, however, is not only dependent on axial resolution, but also on resolution within the scan plane (lateral resolution) and the slice thickness (elevation). High frequency broad-band linear array transducers are state of the art for small-parts sonography and a *sine qua non* as far as imaging of peripheral nerves is concerned. Future scanhead development will supply us with multidimensional arrays, which will further enhance resolution in the elevation plane with reduction of clutter (Wildes et al. 1997). For peripheral nerve sonography the choice of transducer depends on the anatomical region to be examined, but generally a high-frequency scanhead is preferred wherever possible. For superficially lying nerves therefore a 12 to 15 MHz transducer is highly recommended, while for deep lying nerves such as the sciatic nerve a 10 or even 7.5 MHz transducer may be more feasible.

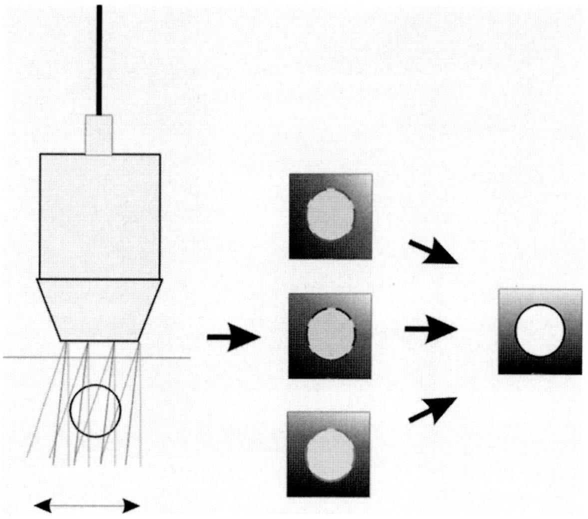

Fig. 1.6. Schematic drawing of compound imaging technology. A structure is scanned from different view angles by the use of beam steering, which results in single images with somewhat different representations of the structure and different artifact patterns. The latter are added in real time format and a "compound image" is constructed

1.2.2 Software Requirements

1.2.2.1 Compound Imaging

While real-time compound imaging is common in modalities such as CT and MR, ultrasound systems have traditionally lacked the power needed for acquisition and processing of such images in real time. New developments in the processing speed of ultrasound scanners made this technique available. Computed beam-steering software is used to steer the ultrasound beam "off axis", which results in several lines of sight to a sonographic target within a single scan. With powerful signal processing software, the single image frames are accurately rendered according to the visualized geometry and updated in real time. A schematic illustration of compound imaging technology is given in Fig. 1.6.

The clinical value of compound imaging lies in the reduction of sonographic artifacts (Piccoli et al. 2000). By scanning from different view angles, different artifact patterns are produced in the single views. By averaging these single frames into a compound image, artifacts such as speckle, noise, dropout or refractive shadowing are suppressed. This results in a sharper delineation of tissue interfaces and better discrimination of lesions against their background, as well as improvement of image contrast and detail resolution (Fig. 1.7).

In addition, the mode of compound technology applied can be changed by the examiner to either target the beam to an enhanced resolution of regions of interest or to a quicker overview mode.

1.2.2.2 Tissue Harmonic Imaging

Tissue harmonic imaging is another sonographic technology which improves image quality of sonograms in state-of-the-art scanners (Burns et al. 1996). The fundamental ultrasound signal transmitted to the tissue consists of a broad band of low frequencies. The transmitted signal resonates off tissue in the body at a frequency twice the transmitted signal and only these high-frequency resonant signals are detected by the scanhead. In a normal scan the signal travels into the body and back to the scanhead again, which means the ultrasound beam passes tissue interfaces twice and therefore artifacts increase. With tissue harmonic imaging the detected signal (which is produced by resonance inside the tissue) travels only one way towards the scanhead, which means it is not attenuated by round-trip travel through tissue and therefore we experience a reduction of artifacts. In addition resonance at object margins (the main source of artifacts in a normal scan) is of very low energy and therefore does not contribute to the image to the same extent as it does in conventional imaging. The value of tissue harmonic imaging for sonography of the peripheral nerves, however, is limited, since it only slightly improves the image quality (Fig. 1.8).

We might add that somehow the value of this technology for B-mode imaging has in our opinion been

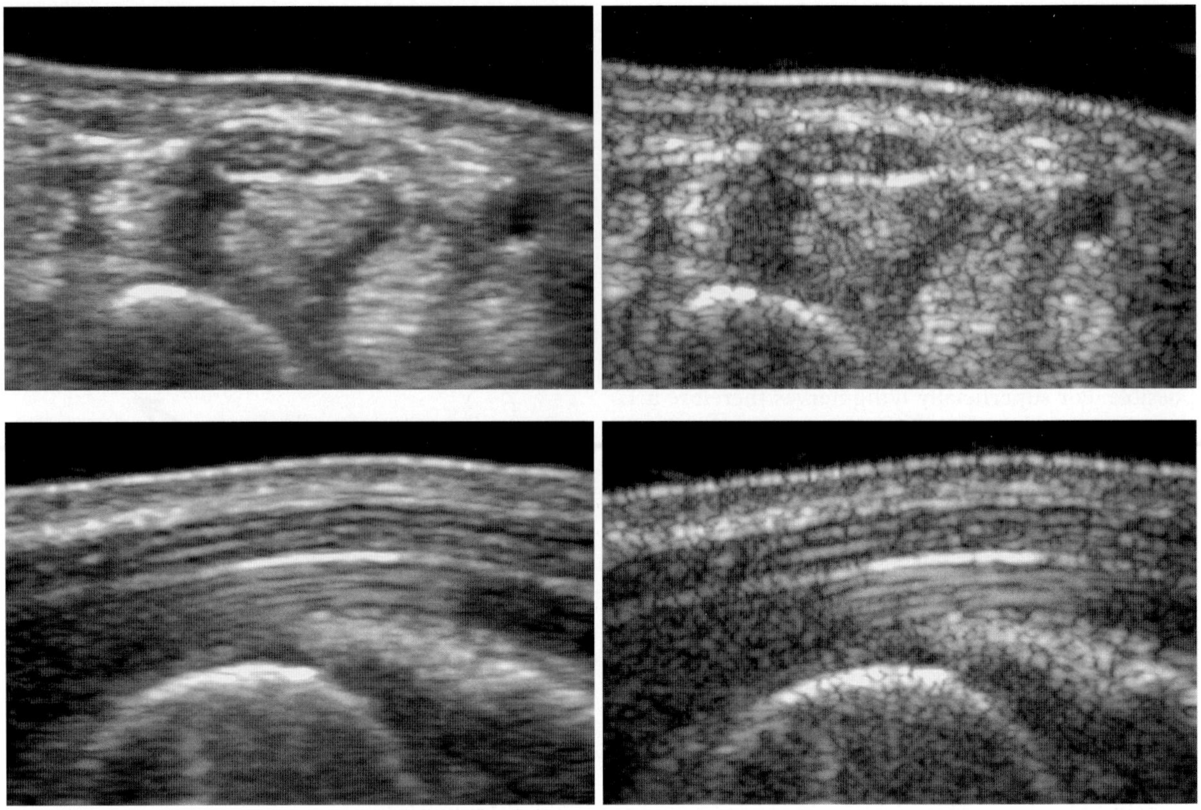

a

b

Fig. 1.7a, b. Transverse (**a**) and longitudinal (**b**) sonograms through the median nerve at wrist level with (*left half of images*) and without (*right half of images*) compound imaging technology. Note the marked improvement of image sharpness, with better definition of tissue borders and an overall reduction of image noise in images acquired in compound mode

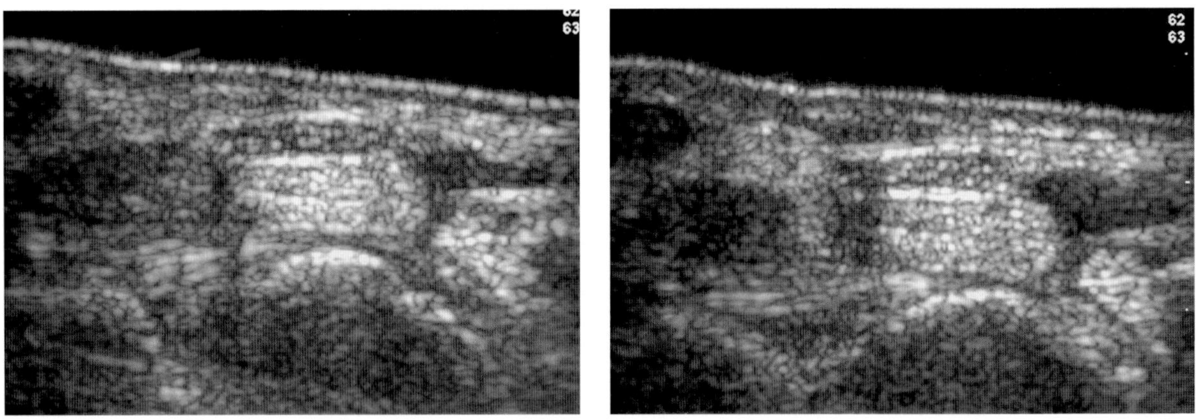

Fig. 1.8. Transverse sonograms through the median nerve at wrist level acquired in normal mode (*left half of image*) and with tissue harmonic imaging (*right half of image*). Note that there is only a subtle difference in tissue contrast and only a subtle improvement in discrimination of structures in the tissue harmonic mode

surpassed by compound imaging, which is certainly the better choice for imaging of peripheral nerves.

1.2.2.3
Extended Field of View Imaging

With extended field of view imaging (also called panoramic imaging by some manufacturers) the potential for sonography to display longitudinal structures is enhanced. With this technique the scanhead is swept longitudinally along a structure of interest and dedicated software reconstructs an image out of single scans along the course of the sweep (Fig. 1.9).

Newer technology not only uses pixel information at the edge of the scan for reconstruction of the panoramic image, but by application of a pattern recognition algorithm extracts information from every entire single scan and adds it to the final panoramic view. This technique not only yields better image quality in panoramic scans but also enables the user to easily redirect the sweep by moving back and forth with a continuous update of the panoramic view and without having to restart the sweep. Once the panoramic image has been acquired, dedicated software allows the image to be further refined by the application of various postprocessing tools such as magnification, rotation, etc. With high-end ultrasound scanners, panoramic imaging is also possible in compound mode, which adds the benefit of improved resolution (Fig. 1.10).

From a clinical point of view, panoramic imaging is mainly a tool for documentation or presentation of results, which – as far as the peripheral nerves are concerned – may add valuable information for the planning of surgical interventions.

1.2.2.4
High-resolution Imaging

During recent years different ultrasound companies have tried to enhance the quality of sonographic images with the introduction of various image processing tools. One of these tools, which was recently introduced into clinical practice by ATL/Philips is XRES. This pattern analysis tool works at the pixel level. It looks at the predominant patterns within groups of pixels and brings them into order. By emphasizing patterns and de-emphasizing speckle, noise and clutter, XRES imaging enhances diagnostic features by reducing artifacts, improving visibility of existing tissue texture patterns and bringing margins and borders into greater definition. One of the special

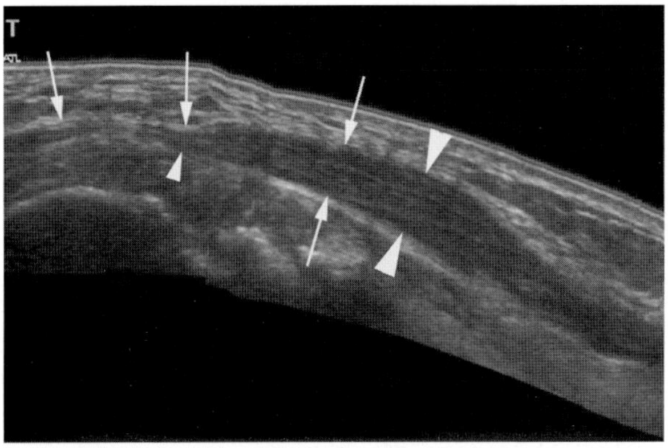

Fig. 1.10. Panoramic image in compound mode of the ulnar nerve (*arrows*) at the level of the elbow in a patient with a stricture narrowing the nerve diameter. The site of the stricture (*small arrowhead*) and the extent of edematous swelling of the nerve proximal to this level (*large arrowheads*) are nicely demonstrated over a substantial distance

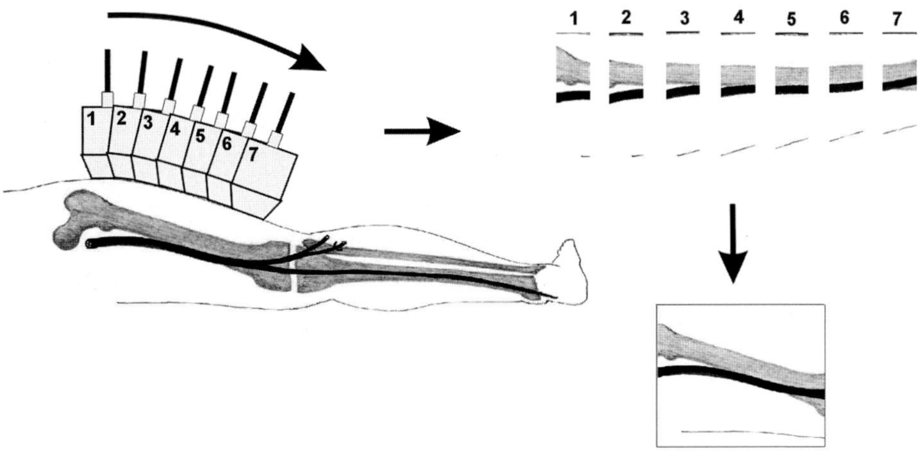

Fig. 1.9. Schematic drawing of panoramic imaging technology. Continuous single images (as wide as the width of the scanhead allows) acquired at a fixed distance during a longitudinal sweep along an anatomic structure are summed and reconstructed as a "panoramic view" of the structures along the whole sweep

aspects of XRES imaging is the ability to combine this tool with image compounding thus adding further to image improvement by significantly improving the visibility of the tissue patterns that are detected in SonoCT mode, so that the patterns are more vivid and clearly evident. Images take on a significant depth they did not have before. There is also an overall sharpening of margins, borders and tissue interfaces. A comparison of XRES imaging and simple compound imaging is given in Fig. 1.11.

1.3 General Technique of Sonographic Nerve Examination

In this section we focus briefly on some general recommendations for examination of peripheral nerves and documentation of results.

1.3.1 Anatomic Considerations

Nerves are round or ovoid structures with a complex internal architecture resembling a cable. The single nerve fibers are composed of axons, myelin sheaths and Schwann cells. Several fibers form a single fascicle and a variable number of such fascicles combine into an individual nerve. The size of a single fascicle and the numbers of fascicles included in a nerve depend on the size of the nerve and its location (distance from its origin, type and tightness of surrounding tissue). The single nerve fascicles and the nerve as a whole are interwoven and surrounded by supportive tissue, the interfascicular and superficial epineurium. The latter may be identified to a certain extent with sonography, while the connective tissue comprising the endoneurium, which surrounds a single nerve fiber and the perineurium surrounding a fascicle are very thin membranes and below sonographic resolution. Sonographic histological correlations first presented by Silvestri and coworkers (Silvestri et al. 1995) confirmed the ability of sonography to identify the fascicular architecture of a peripheral nerve. On transverse sonograms a normal nerve shows an echotexture of tiny hypoechogenic dots – the fascicles (or fascicle groups) – embedded in a hyperechoic meshwork of connective tissue – the interfascicular and superficial epineurium (Fig. 1.12).

However, we must note that the overall number of fascicles visualized on sonograms does not correspond exactly with the real number of fascicles in a nerve, probably due to coalescence of some adjacent fascicles in a single image. Another reason for this lies in the somewhat intertwined course of nerve fascicles, and this is also why the analysis of the continuity of single fascicles in traumatic lesions or after nerve repair has to be done with caution. We must also be aware that a reduction in transducer frequency leads to a diminishing number of individual fascicles, which may be visualized in the image.

In contrast to tendons, nerves are highly vascularized structures with small vessels running along the perineurium and supplying a tight microvascular plexus. These vessels may sometimes be seen with color or power Doppler sonography (Fig. 1.13).

In our experience an increase of vessels inside and along the surface of a nerve may be suspicious for a hypervascular state in a postoperative nerve

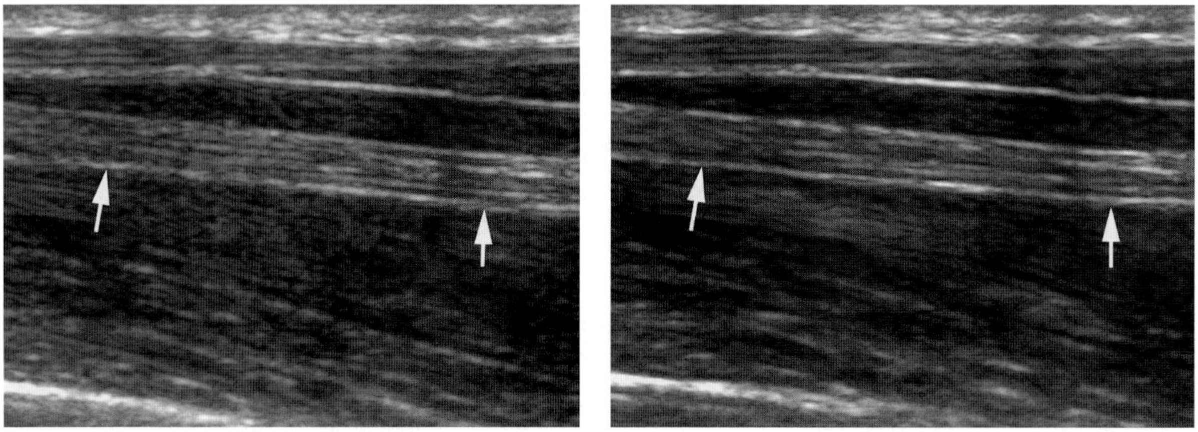

Fig. 1.11. Longitudinal sonograms through the median nerve in the forearm in compound mode (*left half of image*) and compound plus XRES mode (*right half of image*). Note the further improvement of image sharpness especially on the surface of structures (*arrows* on bottom surface of median nerve) and of the internal structure of nerve

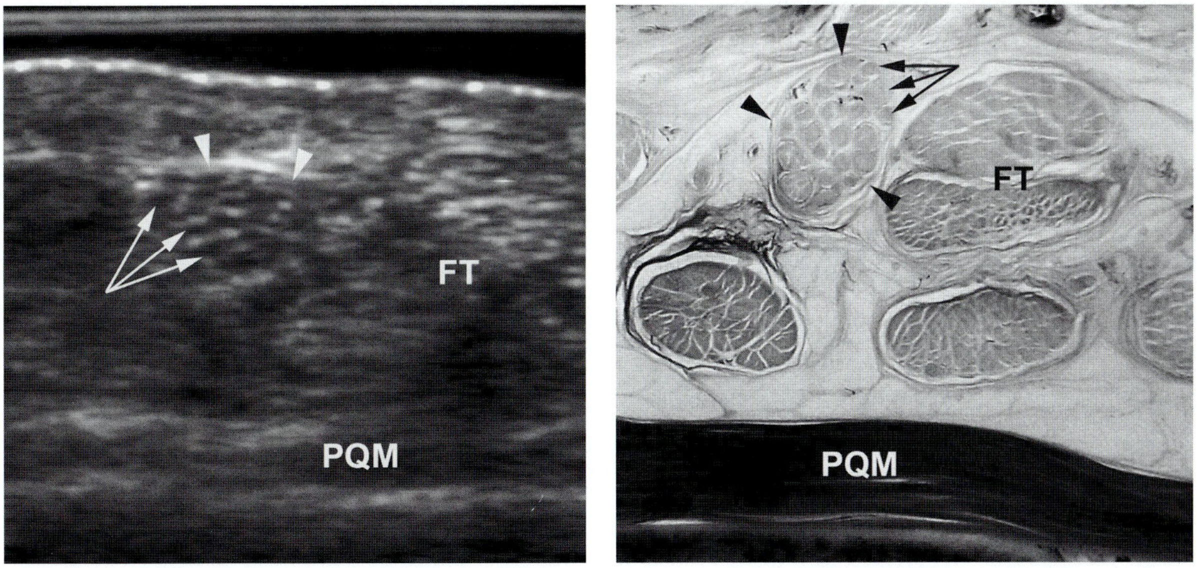

Fig. 1.12. Corresponding transverse sonogram (*left half of image*) and plastinated anatomic section (*right half of image*) of cadaver specimen acquired at the distal forearm. The median nerve fascicles (*arrows*) are clearly visualized as hypoechoic nodular structures in the sonogram. Note also visualization of superficial epineurium (*arrowheads*) with tiny extensions between the nerve fascicles (*PQM* pronator quadratus muscle, *FT* flexor tendons)

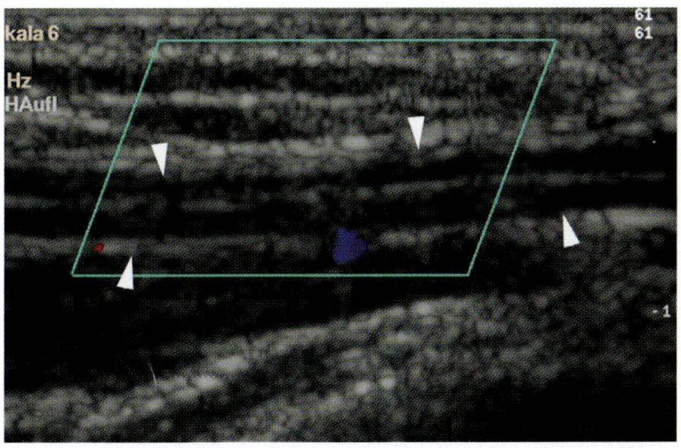

Fig. 1.13. Longitudinal sonogram along ulnar nerve (*arrowheads*) in a healthy volunteer. Only a single small vessel is identified along the surface of this normal nerve

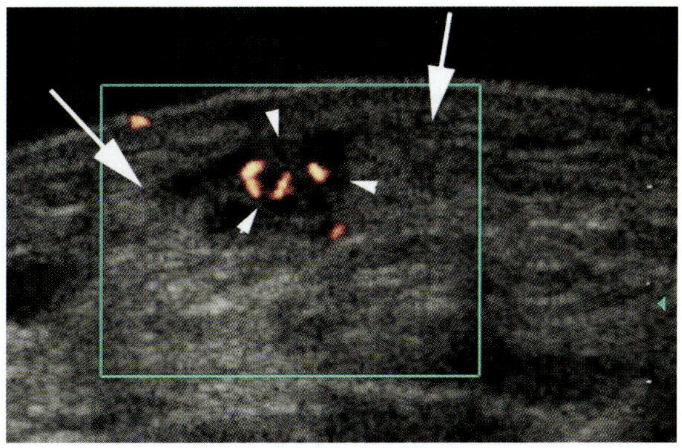

Fig. 1.14. Transverse power Doppler sonogram through the ulnar nerve in a patient who had undergone decompression because of ulnar tunnel syndrome. Note the marked hypervascularization of the swollen postoperative nerve (*arrowheads*) due to compression by hypertrophic scar (*arrows*)

(Fig. 1.14), in perineuritis or in a nerve proximal to a compression. However, this is preliminary experience with lack of confirmation in larger statistically controlled clinical trials.

Variations of the course or shape of peripheral nerves are known and may be studied with sonography. Not uncommonly variations of the median nerve may be found in the carpal tunnel, for example, which should be known to the examiner as they may be important in a preoperative setting. In 16% of asymptomatic volunteers a unilateral persistent median artery and in 6% a bilateral persistent median artery is detectable with sonography (Gassner et al. 2002), which is associated with a high division or a bifid median nerve (Fig. 1.15).

1.3.2 Nerve Examination

The examination of a peripheral nerve should include transverse and longitudinal scanning. For superficially

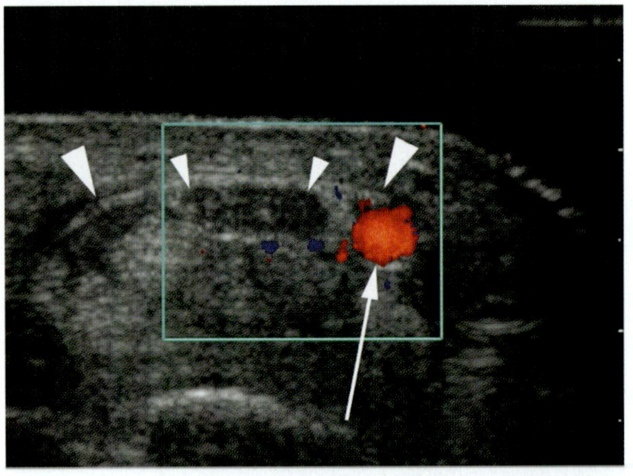

Fig. 1.15. Transverse color Doppler sonogram through the carpal tunnel in a patient with suspected carpal tunnel disease. Single median nerve stem with normal configuration (*small arrowheads*) is accompanied by a large median artery (*arrow*). Both structures run underneath the flexor retinaculum (*large arrowheads*)

lying nerves (median nerve) or nerves coursing along bony ridges, we generally recommend the use of a stand-off gel pad which improves the contact of the transducer with the skin surface and results in substantial improvement of image quality. The identification of a nerve inside an image scan is easily accomplished if common anatomical landmarks are observed (i.e. the peroneal nerve at the fibular neck, or the tibialis nerve following the course of the posterior tibial artery and veins, etc.), and Chapter 2 focuses extensively on these relationships.

For the evaluation of nerve compression syndromes, the recommendation is straightforward, as they typically occur in distinct locations along the course of a nerve, i.e. the carpal tunnel, the ulnar sulcus etc.! If a patient's history and/or clinical examination is typical for one of these compressive lesions, the sonographic examination will be tailored to evaluation of the site where the nerve lies close to ligaments, bony ridges or spurs or tight to a bony surface and is followed for 5 to 10 cm proximal and distal to this area. While transverse scanning is better suited to identifying edematous swelling of nerve fascicles proximal to a compressive lesion, longitudinal scans or panoramic views are better suited to revealing a sudden change in the diameter of a nerve traversing underneath a ligament, for example. In cases of unclear or atypical symptoms, an attempt to scan the whole course of a nerve, searching for pathology, is to be made, and sometimes it will be necessary to scan even the brachial plexus of the affected side. In these cases we often prefer to identify the nerve at a site where it lies close to the surface or near distinct anatomical landmarks and follow it from there to the level of suspected pathology. This type of examination is highly recommended in cases where the nerve lies inside scar tissue or close to hematomas, as the nerve itself is often rather difficult to distinguish at the level of the lesion in such situations.

Another general recommendation concerns the examination of the nerve at the unaffected side. The diagnosis of nerve pathology is often achieved with identification of subtle changes in nerve diameter or echotexture, which is why we always confirm our local findings by comparison with the contralateral unaffected side. The latter is of utmost importance if measurements of nerve diameters or cross-sectional area are used for the identification of a compression syndrome. High interindividual variations in these measurements exist and a reliable diagnosis of pathology is only possible in correlation with the measurement of the normal contralateral nerve.

Positioning of the patient is another important aspect in sonographic nerve examinations. In some cases the examination will be time consuming, which is why a position that is comfortable to sustain for the patient and at the same time allows easy access to the region of interest for the sonographer should be sought. In many cases we use supportive cushions or pillows to put a patient's extremity in a position that allows easier access to a nerve.

While peripheral nerves may be scanned with normal B-mode sonography, we always use compound imaging because of the resulting gain in soft-tissue resolution (see above). We further use color or power Doppler in general nerve examinations because of our interest in the vascular situation of a nerve. We highly recommend this for all cases of inflammatory lesions, tumors or postoperative nerves, as the demonstration of increased vascular supply to a nerve (correlation with contralateral nerve!) may have important implications for diagnosis and treatment. Color Doppler is mandatory for the examination of nerve tumors. In contrast to neurofibromas, Schwannomas for example are generally hypervascular lesions, which helps in the differential diagnosis of neurogenic tumors.

References

Blake LC, Robertson WD, Hayes CE (1996) Sacral plexus: optimal imaging planes for MR assessment. Radiology 199:767–772

Bodner G, Huber B, Schwabegger A, et al (1999) Sonographic

detection of radial nerve entrapment within a humerus fracture. J Ultrasound Med 18:703–706

Buchberger W, Schoen G, Strasser, et al (1991) High resolution ultrasonography of the carpal tunnel. J Ultrasound Med 101:531–537

Burns PN, Powers JE, Hope SD, et al (1996) Harmonic imaging: Principles and preliminary results. Angiology 47:63–69

Chiou HJ, Chou YH, Cheng SP, et al (1998) Cubital tunnel syndrome: diagnosis by high resolution ultrasonography. J Ultrasound Med 17:643–648

Filler AG, Kliot M, Howe FA, et al (1996) Application of magnetic resonance neurography in the evaluation of patients with peripheral nerve pathology. J Neurosurg 85:299–309

Fornage BD (1988) Peripheral nerves of the extremities: imaging with ultrasound. Radiology 167:179–182

Gassner E, Schocke M, Peer S, et al (2002) Persistent median artery in the carpal tunnel – color Doppler ultrasonographic findings. J Ultrasound Med 21:455–461

Gierada DS, Erickson SJ (1993) MR imaging of the sacral plexus: abnormal findings. AJR Am J Roentgenol 160: 1067–1071

Gierada DS, Erickson SJ, Haughton WM, et al (1993) MR imaging of the sacral plexus: normal findings. AJR Am J Roentgenol 160:1059–1065

Graif M, Seton A, Nerubali J, et al (1991) Sciatic nerve: sonographic evaluation and anatomic pathologic considerations. Radiology 181:405–408

Hayes CE, Tsuruda JS, Mathis CM, et al (1997) Brachial plexus: MR imaging with a dedicated phased array of surface coils. Radiology 203:286–289

Martinoli C, Serafini G, Bianchi S, et al (1996) Ultrasonography of peripheral nerves. J Peripher Nerv Syst 1:169–174

Peer S, Bodner G, Meirer R, et al (2001) Evaluation of postoperative peripheral nerve lesions with high resolution ultrasound. AJR Am J Roentgenol 177:415–419

Peer S, Kovacs P, Harpf C, et al (2002) High resolution sonography of lower extremity peripheral nerves: anatomic correlation and spectrum of pathology. J Ultrasound Med 21: 315–322

Piccoli C, Merrit CRB, Forsberg F, et al (2000) Real-time compound imaging of the breast. Presented at the Annual Meeting of the American Institute of Ultrasound in Medicine, San Francisco, Apr 2000

Silvestri E, Martinoli C, Derchi LE, et al (1995) Echotexture of peripheral nerves: correlation between US and histologic findings and criteria to differentiate tendons. Radiology 197:291–296

Wildes DG, Chiao RY, Daft CMW, et al (1997) Elevation performance of 1.25D and 1.5D transducer arrays. IEEE Trans Ultrasonics Ferroelectrics Frequency Control 44:1027–1031

2 Sonographic Anatomy of the Peripheral Nervous System

H. GRUBER and P. KOVACS

CONTENTS

2.1 Introduction 13
2.2 Cranial Nerves 13
2.3 The Upper Extremity 15
2.3.1 Cervical and Brachial Plexus 15
2.3.2 Nerves of the Upper Arm 17
2.3.3 Nerves of the Forearm 22
2.3.4 Nerves of the Hand 25
2.4 The Lower Extremity 28
2.4.1 Nerves of the Groin and the Thigh 29
2.4.2 Nerves of the Lower Leg 32
2.4.3 Nerves of the Foot 32
2.5 The Trunk 35
References 35

2.1 Introduction

One of the major advantages of sonography compared to other imaging modalities, such as MRI for example, is its ability to acquire images in virtually every orientation along the course of a peripheral nerve. This, however, results in a very complex regional topographic anatomy. Therefore, a well-founded knowledge of regional anatomy and topography is an indispensable prerequisite for the sonographic assessment of peripheral nerves. The typical sonographic appearance of nerves must be distinguished from other soft-tissue structures and may change substantially depending on the type of surrounding tissue elements. Usually nerves present as longitudinal bands with a mixture of hyperechoic (epineurium) and hypoechoic elements (fascicle groups) in longitudinal sonograms. In the transverse plane a variable number of hypoechoic dots (fascicle groups) are surrounded by hyperechoic epineurium with hyperechoic septa between the fascicles (SILVESTRI 1995).

H. GRUBER, MD; P. KOVACS, MD
Department of Radiology, University Hospital Innsbruck, Anichstrasse 35, 6020 Innsbruck, Austria

In the following paragraphs the regional anatomy of nerves, which may be assessed with state-of-the-art sonographic equipment, is demonstrated with anatomic cryosections in correlation with representative sonograms. Transverse and longitudinal sonograms in typical locations for peripheral nerve disease were acquired in cadaver specimens. The sonographic scan planes were marked on the cadaver surface and correlative anatomic cryosections were produced along the skin markings with a fine needle-tooth band saw. In this way an exact correlation of paired sonograms and cross-sections was achieved in order to recapitulate topographic relations and to present the normal topographic anatomy of the peripheral nerves. The figures demonstrate sonograms of peripheral nerves being visualized clearly and found easily according to the given landmarks. That is why cutaneous nerves and terminal nerve branches were excluded *ex ante* as their detection is very tricky and can sometimes only be achieved if pathologically altered.

2.2 Cranial Nerves

The 12 cranial nerve pairs originate from the brain stem to the mesencephalon and course mainly within the bony parts of the neurocranium and/or viscerocranium, which is why they are only poorly accessible by sonography. The facial, the accessory and the vagal nerves, however, may be visualized to a certain extent along their extracranial course. Sonographic imaging, however, is limited by the caliber of the nerves and by the effects of surrounding soft tissues, which sometimes impair direct visualization.

The *facial nerve* (cranial nerve number seven) enters the facial soft tissues at its emission through the stylomastoid foramen of the temporal bone. It consists completely of motor fibers for viscerocranial muscles (mimic muscles and parts of the chew musculature). It enters directly into the parotid gland, where it usually spreads into two or three main branches. The latter are interconnected by thin nerve fibers forming the so-called parotid plexus. From here the nerve distributes into five nerve branch groups (each with one to four branches): the temporal, the zygomatic, the buccal and the marginal mandibular branches, and one cervical branch (usually anastomosing with branches of the cervical plexus in the superficial cervical ansa).

Sonographic identification of the facial nerve is easiest after its emission from the temporal bone posterior to the perpendicular mandibular branch. Its visualization gets difficult after it enters the parotid gland, where the two or three main branches may only occasionally be visualized with very high-frequency transducers (more than 15 MHz). Within the more ventral parts of the parotid gland nerve branches must be distinguished clearly from the equally hypoechoic minor and major exocrine parotid duct (Fig. 2.1). The latter are always oriented towards the mouth, where they usually end in the region of the premolar teeth of the upper jaw. The terminal peripheral branches of the facial nerve inside the mimic musculature cannot be discerned sufficiently even with state-of-the-art sonographic equipment.

The *vagal nerve* (cranial nerve number ten) represents the strongest parasympathetic nerve and exits from the jugular foramen where it forms its two ganglia: the superior ganglion (ganglion jugulare) and the larger inferior ganglion (ganglion nodosum). Releasing several branches with several different neuronal qualities, it descends inside a common soft-tissue sheath together with the internal jugular vein, the internal carotid artery and more caudal with the common carotid artery.

The vagal nerve is best assessed at the level of the carotid sinus (division of the common carotid artery), where it lies in the posterior triangular space between the slightly offset venous and arterial lumen (Fig. 2.2). The vessels and the nerve altogether lie directly ventral to the sloping anterior scalene muscle in their superior cervical sections. More inferiorly the vagal nerve directly abuts the cervical prevertebral fascia. Its main stem can be followed with sonography from inframandibular (along a short individual stretch cranial to the hyoid bone) down to the division of the brachiocephalic trunk on the right side and to the origin of the common carotid artery from the aortic arch on the left side. Within the inferior cervical space the detection of the nerve becomes difficult because of interposed fat impairing sonographic contrast.

The two major branches of the vagal nerve (the superior laryngeal and the recurrent laryngeal nerves) may not be clearly visualized with sonography due to their complex course and limited sonographic depth resolution.

The *accessory nerve* (cranial nerve number eleven) being a mere motor nerve also exits from the jugular foramen and hands its internal branch over to the neighboring vagal nerve. The residual external branch (forming the proper accessory

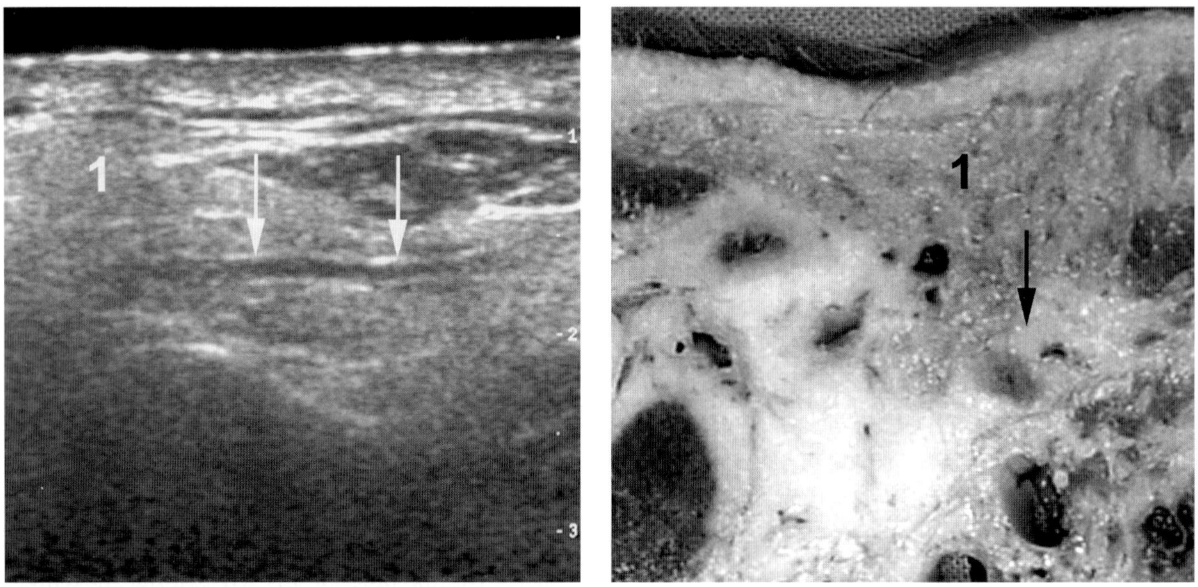

Fig. 2.1a, b. Longitudinal US scan and the corresponding cryosection of facial nerve (*arrows*) in its course within the parotid gland (*1*) with high contrast of the fascicular parts of the nerve in relation to the surrounding glandular tissue

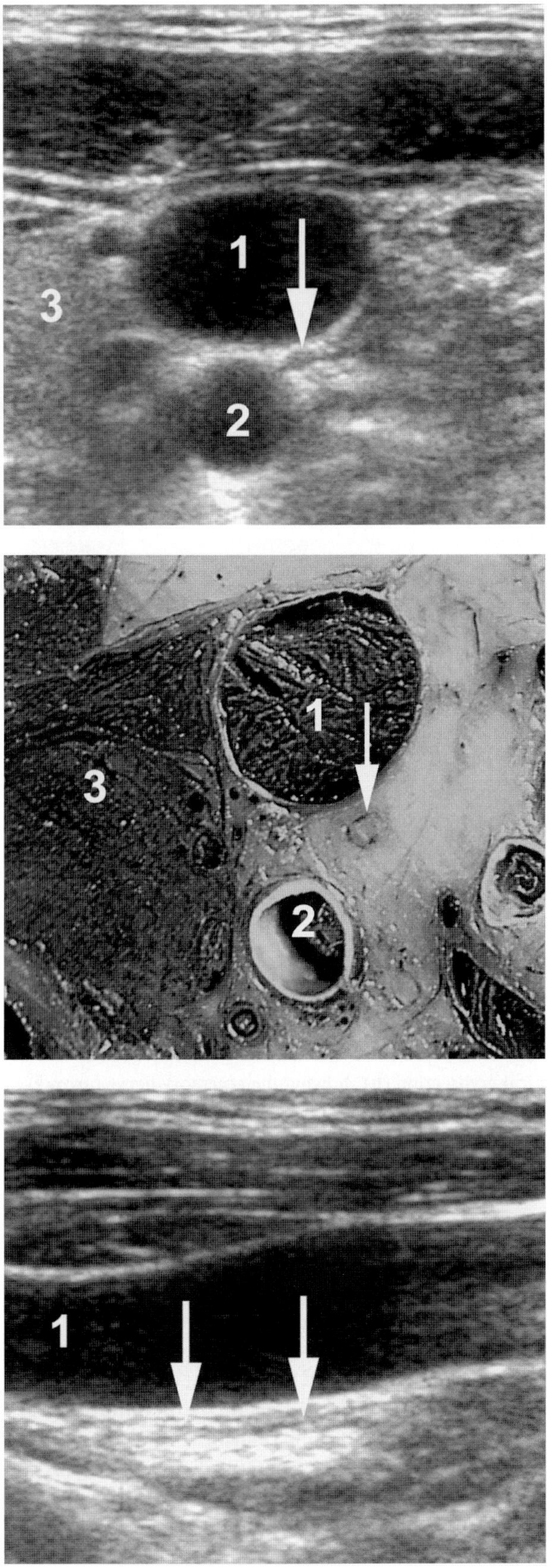

a
b
c

Fig. 2.2a–c. Transverse US scan (**a**) and the corresponding cryosection (**b**) showing the vagal nerve (*arrow*) in its typical position between the internal jugular vein (*1*) and the common carotid artery (*2*) (*3* thyroid gland). **c** Longitudinal US scan of the vagal nerve (*arrow*) lying adjacent to the internal jugular vein (*1*)

nerve) is responsible for the innervation of the sternocleidomastoid and trapezius muscle (Fig. 2.3). In its superior part it lies ventral to the cervical splenius muscle turning onto the lateral surface of the internal jugular vein, usually perforating the superior third of the sternocleidomastoid muscle at a variable height. Its further course follows the medial part of the superior margin of the trapezius muscle, where it may be detected most easily by sonography, before its entrance into the muscle. The loose fatty and connective tissue in the lateral cervical region results in artifacts hampering the nerve's detection in some cases (Bodner et al. 2002).

2.3 The Upper Extremity

The upper extremity forms paddle-like during the fetal period being supplied by the corresponding neural segments of the rump wall (metameric segmentation of the vertebrate rump). In later life this ontological specialization finds its expression in the distribution of the sensory dermatomes in relation to the spinal nerves. The annular organization of the dermatomes on the rump wall is continued in a longish fashion in the extremities (segments C3 to Th1 for the upper extremity). The order of the axons of the corresponding spinal segments passes through rather complicated combinations and reorganizations compared to the simple distribution of the nerves in the rump wall. This redistribution of the segmental axons mainly takes place at the level of the cervical and brachial plexus, where the individual peripheral nerves of the extremity are formed (Kahle 1991).

2.3.1 Cervical and Brachial Plexus

The *cervical plexus* forms out of the ventral roots of the first four spinal nerves (C1-C4). The recombination of the involved axons takes place in the intermuscular soft tissue resulting in several sensible cutaneous nerves,

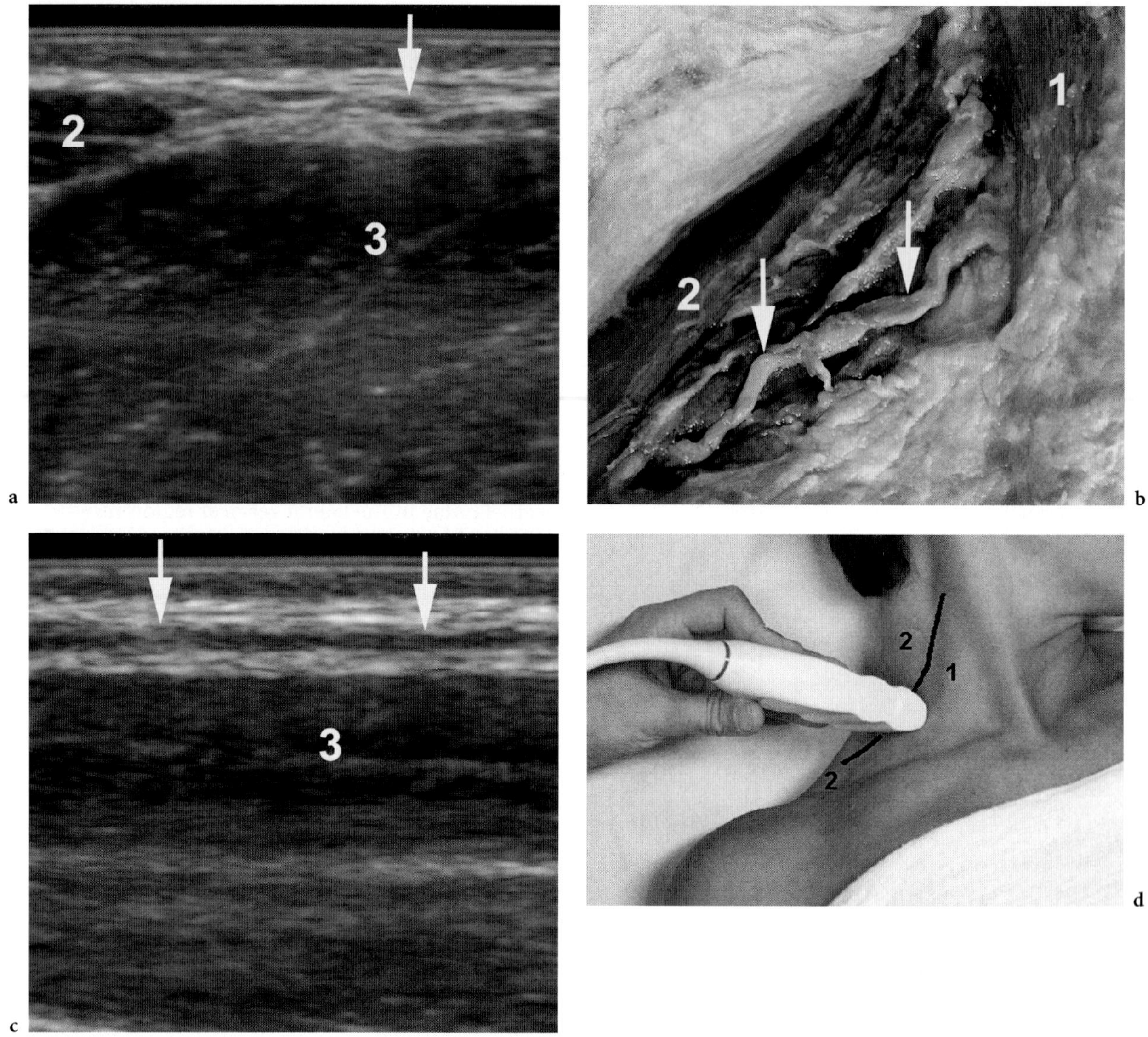

Fig. 2.3a–d. Transverse US scan (**a**) and the corresponding anatomical cryosection (**b**) showing the accessory nerve (*arrows*) in its typical topographic situation lying on the scalene muscles (*3*) ventral to the anterior border of the trapezius muscle (*2*) (*1* sternocleidomastoid muscle). **c** Longitudinal US scan corresponding to the course of the accessory nerve (*arrows*) lying on a scalene muscle (*3*). **d** Scheme with the projection of the accessory nerve (*line*) onto the skin surface. Landmarks for identification of scanhead position are the sternocleidomastoid muscle (*1*) and the trapezius muscle (*2*)

which all perforate the lateral superficial cervical fascia at the posterior margin of the sternocleidomastoid muscle to run onward subcutaneously.

The most important nerve of this plexus is the *phrenic nerve*, which innervates the ipsilateral hemidiaphragm. It is formed by axons from C3 and C4 and runs, lying ventral on the anterior scalene muscle, downward to the upper chest aperture (Fig. 2.4).

The *brachial plexus* forms out of the ventral roots of the spinal nerves C5 to Th1. Its supraclavicular section consists of a superior, a medial and an inferior trunk (primary chords). These trunks form within or somewhat lateral to the gap between the anterior and medial scalene muscle (interscalene gap). Inferior to the clavicle the three plexus fascicles (medial, lateral and posterior or dorsal) are formed by interchange of axons between the different trunks and they are named according to their relationship to the axillary artery (secondary chords). Out of these fascicles the three main nerves of the upper extremity (median, ulnar and radial nerve) and the axillary, the musculocutaneous and several cutaneous nerves are formed.

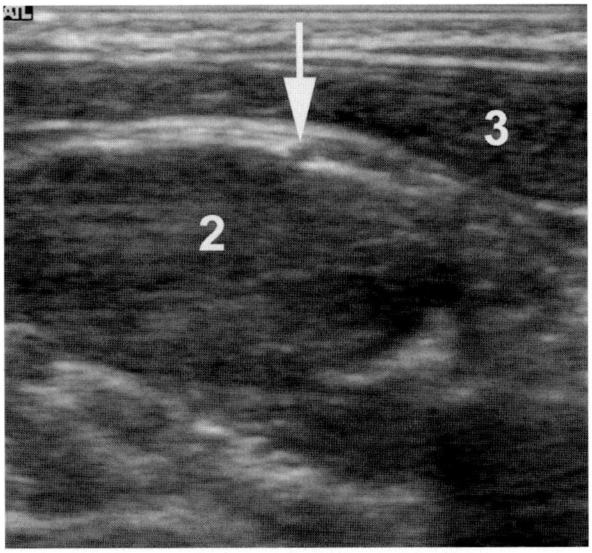

a

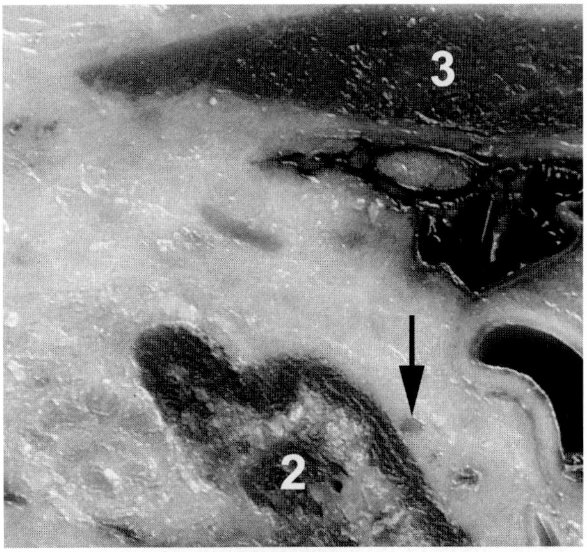

b

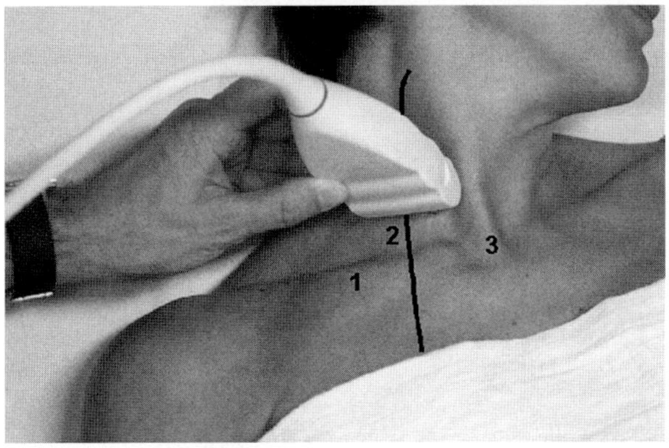

c

Fig. 2.4a–c. Transverse US scan (**a**) and the corresponding cryosection (**b**) showing the phrenic nerve (*arrow*) in its typical position directly ventral to the anterior scalene muscle (*2*) (depending on the scanning level) covered by the sternocleidomastoid muscle (*3*). **c** Scheme with the projection of the phrenic nerve onto the skin surface with the corresponding landmarks: clavicle (*1*), anterior scalene muscle (*2*), medial head of the sternocleidomastoid muscle (*3*)

The sonographic identification of the plexus trunks is best achieved in a transverse plane through the interscalene gap, with a slight cranial tilt to the transducer (Fig. 2.5). The three trunks present as hypoechoic nodules positioned on a virtual line from dorsocranial to ventrocaudal. They are embedded in loose connective and fatty soft tissue and must not be mixed up with small lymph nodes of the region on transverse sonograms. Orientation of the probe in a longitudinal plane along the course of the trunks reveals the typical fascicular pattern of peripheral nerves (Yang et al. 1998).

Two distinct nerves leave the plexus trunks at this level: the long thoracic nerve with fibers from the superior and medial trunks and the thoracodorsal nerve with fibers from the medial and inferior trunks. These two nerves are responsible for the lateral, superficial rump muscles (serratus anterior muscle and dorsal latissimus muscle) and run downwards almost perpendicular to each other. The thoracodorsal nerve is usually accompanied by a branch of the axillary artery (thoracodorsal artery) in its distal course. Due to only minimal difference in echotexture against the surrounding tissue a clear visualization of these nerves is only achieved in selected cases.

The plexus fascicles in proximity to the axillary artery can be visualized best with an abducted or elevated arm and with the transducer oriented along the course of the axillary artery. The posterior fascicle continues into the axillary and radial nerve, and the lateral fascicle together with axons of the medial fascicle (median loop) – after releasing the musculocutaneous nerve directly underneath the clavicle – into the median nerve. The medial fascicle forms the ulnar nerve and the nerves responsible for the sensibility of the medial arm.

2.3.2 Nerves of the Upper Arm

The *musculocutaneous nerve* originates from the lateral fascicle of the brachial plexus and from the

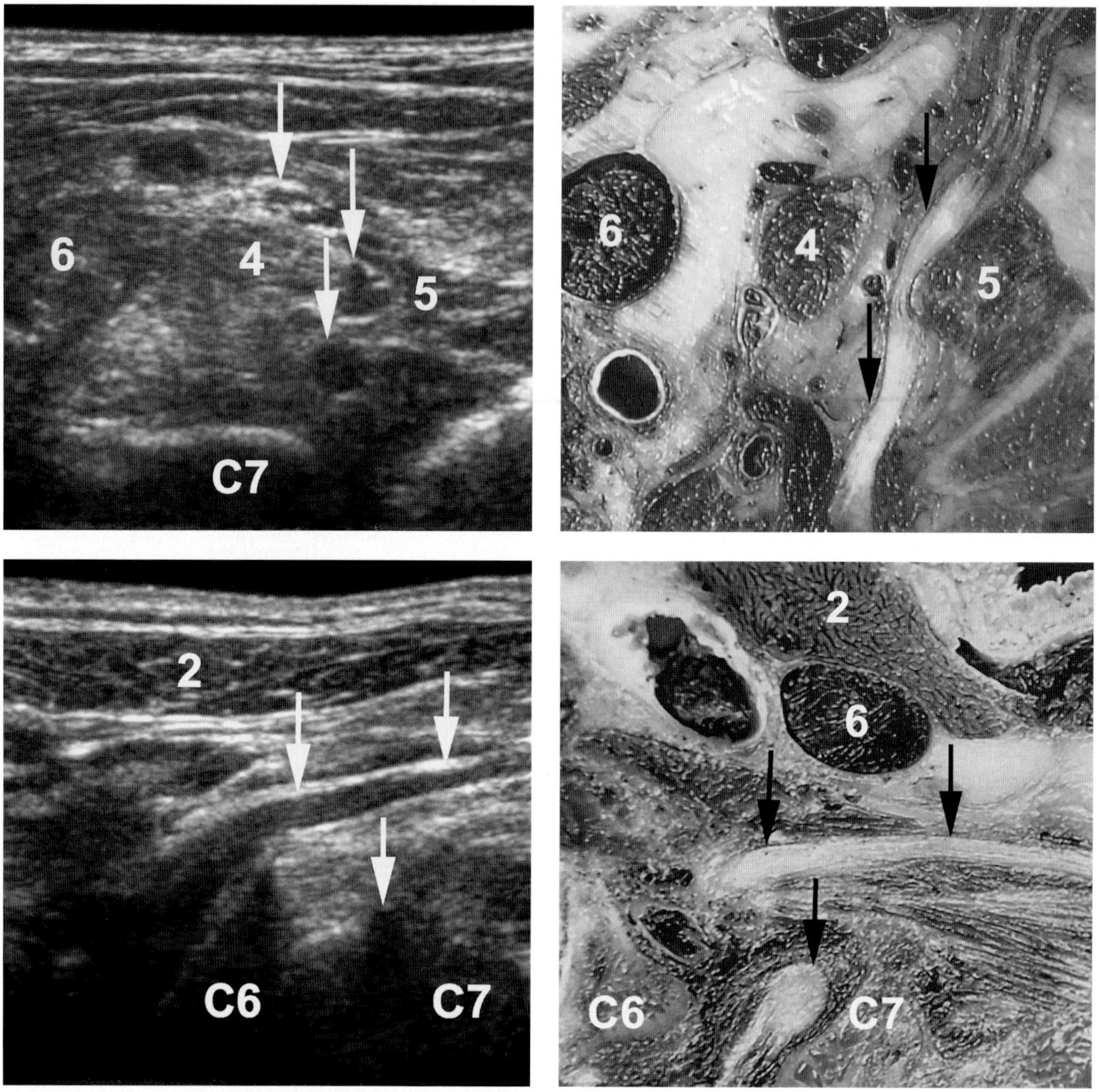

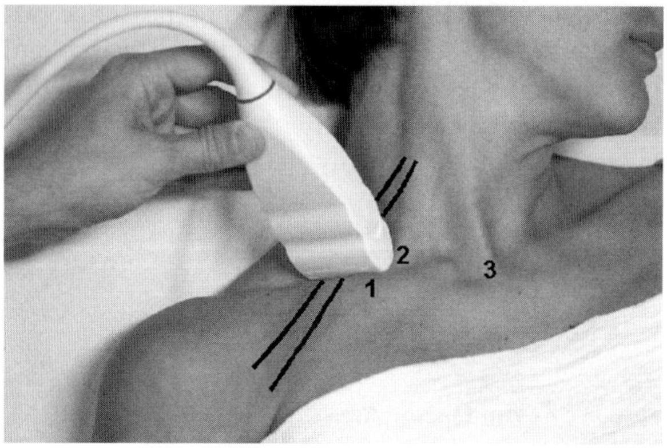

Fig. 2.5a–e. Transverse US scan (**a**) and the corresponding cryosection (**b**) showing the roots and trunks of the brachial plexus (*arrows*) between the anterior (*4*) and middle (*5*) scalene muscle in its typical topographic relationship to the internal jugular vein (*6*) (*C7* body of the seventh cervical vertebra). US scan (**c**) and corresponding cryosection (**d**) corresponding to the course of the roots and the proximal trunks of the brachial plexus (*arrows*) (*2* sternocleidomastoid muscle, *6* internal jugular vein, *C6 C7* bodies of the sixth and seventh vertebra). **e** Scheme with the projection of the trunks of the brachial plexus onto the skin surface with the corresponding landmarks: lateral (*2*) and medial (*3*) parts of the sternocleidomastoid muscle, clavicle (*1*)

roots C5 to C7. It runs at the medial side of the coracoid process and dorsally enters the coracobrachial muscle. Passing through the coracobrachial muscle the nerve reaches the fascial space between the brachial biceps and the brachial muscle. Usually covered by the muscle belly of the short head of the brachial biceps muscle it heads for the region of the radial epicondyle of the humerus (Fig. 2.6). In this region it comes closer to the surface exiting between the radial onset of the biceps muscle and the underlying brachial muscle, and continuing subcutaneously ends in the lateral cutaneous antebrachial nerve, which supplies the skin of the lateral forearm (sensory branches). The musculocutaneous nerve is a very small nerve identified most easily with sonography at its course medial to the coracoid process or between the brachial biceps and brachial muscle. From here it may be followed proximally and distally – depending on local contrast and sonographic resolution. It usually is well contrasted by the embedding muscles along a fair distance.

The *median nerve* is formed out of parts of the lateral and medial fascicle of the brachial plexus (median loop). It runs in the medial bicipital groove ventral to the brachial artery directly heading downward to the elbow, where it usually lies between the two heads of the pronator teres muscle (Lanz and Wachsmuth 1972) in 95%, between the ulnar head of the muscle and the ulna in 3% or even perforates the humeral head of the muscle in 2% of cases. The pronator teres muscle is the most proximal muscle supplied by the median nerve. Very seldom the perforation of parts of the pronator teres muscle by the median nerve may lead to a kind of entrapment syndrome, resulting in an impairment of the ventral forearm muscles. Being the largest nerve of the upper arm the median nerve may be easily identified with sonography along its course within the medial bicipital groove ventral to the brachial artery (Fig. 2.7).

The *ulnar nerve* as the main branch of the medial fascicle of the brachial plexus (roots C8 to Th1) also heads directly downward to the elbow within the medial bicipital groove, and reaches the "groove of the ulnar nerve" (sulcus nervi ulnaris) where it is bent around the lower margin of the medial epicondyle of the humerus. In the upper arm the nerve does not release any motor or sensory branches. Sonographic identification of the ulnar nerve is most easily achieved along its course within the medial bicipital groove posterior to the brachial artery, or as the sole structure within the groove of the ulnar nerve (Fig. 2.8).

The medial fascicle of the brachial plexus is responsible for two additional sensory nerves supplying the medial skin of the upper extremity: the medial brachial cutaneous nerve and the medial antebrachial cutaneous nerve – both originating from roots C8 and Th1 and both running downwards epifascially and subcutaneously. Sonographic identification of these nerves is only possible in selected cases with transducers of at least 15 MHz due to only minimal differences in echotexture between the nerves and their surroundings.

a

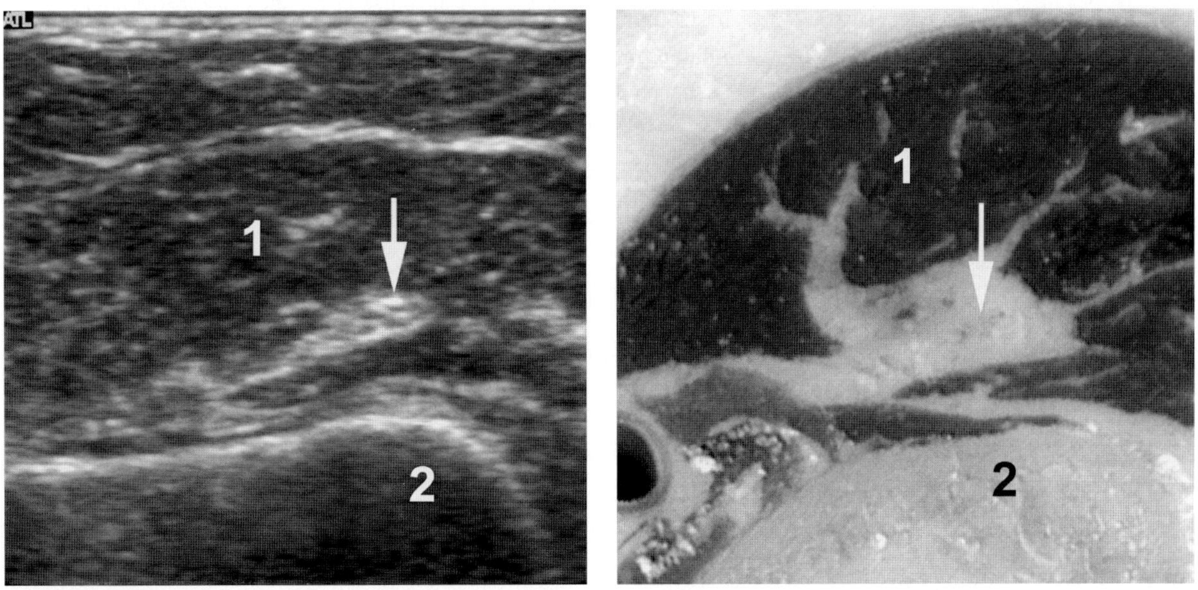

b

Fig. 2.6a, b. Transverse US scan (**a**) and the corresponding cryosection (**b**) showing the musculocutaneous nerve (*arrow*) lying within the brachial biceps muscle (*1*) ventral to the humerus (*2*)

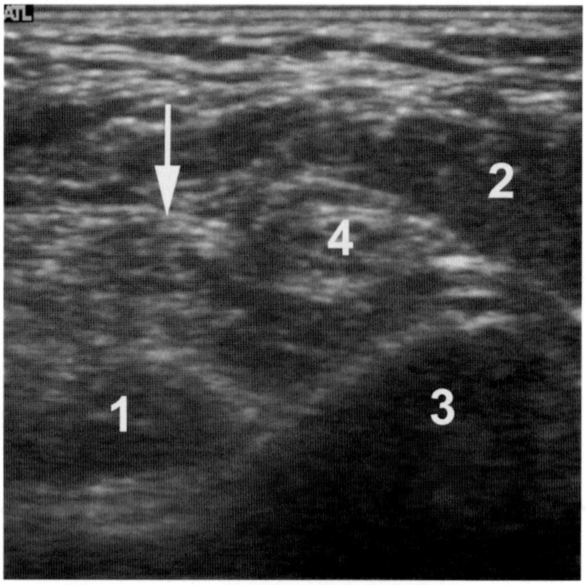

a

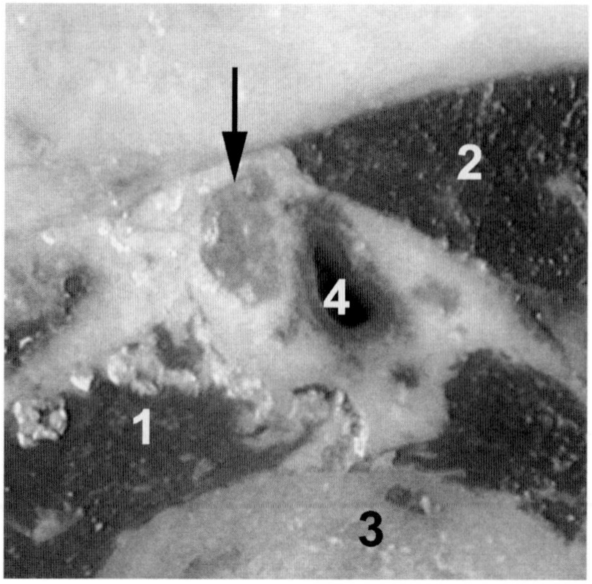

b

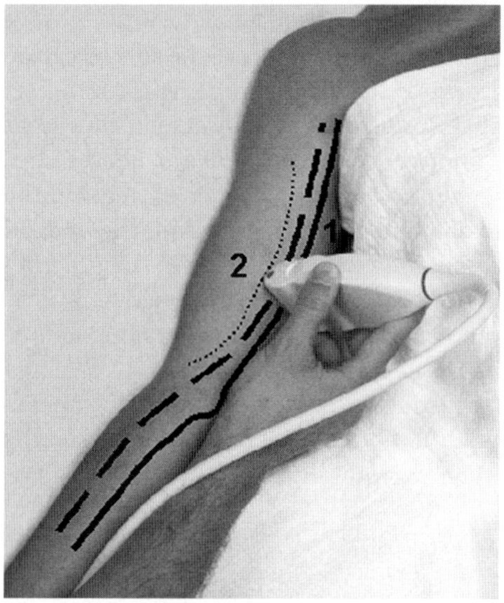

c

Fig. 2.7a–c. Transverse US scan (**a**) and the corresponding cryosection (**b**) showing the median nerve (*arrow*) next to the brachial artery (*4*) is between the triceps (*1*) and brachial biceps (*2*) muscles (*3* humerus). **c** Scheme with the projection of the typical course of the median (*broken line*) and the ulnar (*solid line*) nerves onto the skin surface (*2*, *dotted line* ventral brachial biceps muscle)

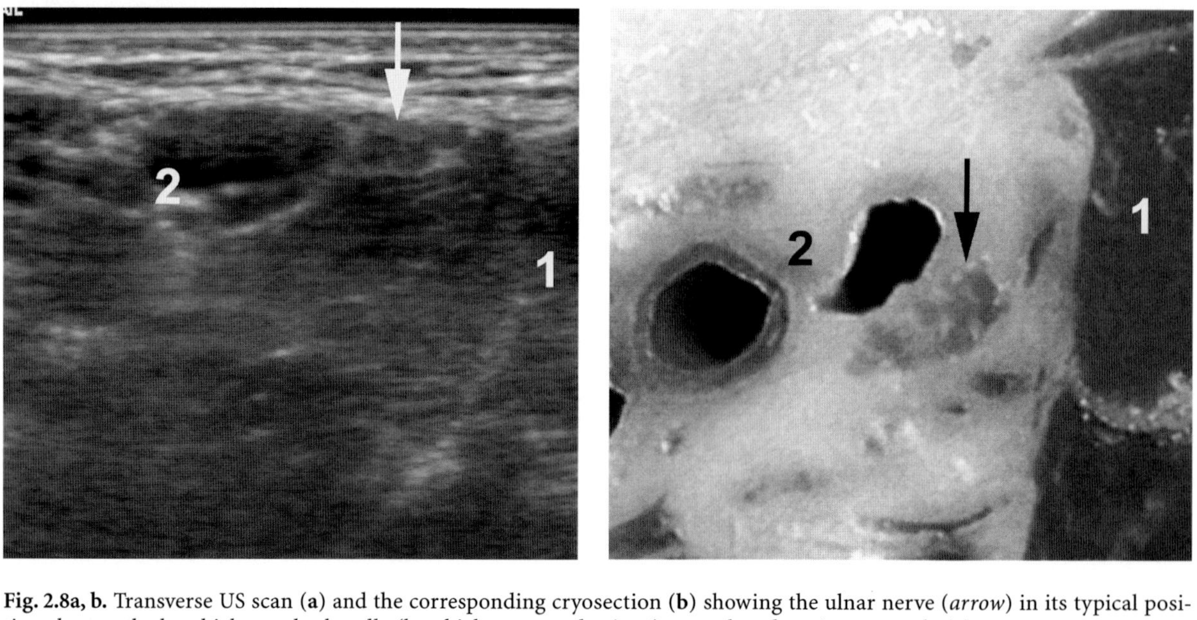

a b

Fig. 2.8a, b. Transverse US scan (**a**) and the corresponding cryosection (**b**) showing the ulnar nerve (*arrow*) in its typical position close to the brachial vascular bundle (brachial artery and vein, *2*) ventral to the triceps muscle (*1*)

The dorsal fascicle of the brachial plexus releases two nerves: the axillary nerve and the radial nerve being both mixed nerves (motor and sensory elements) supplying the shoulder and the complete dorsal aspect of the upper extremity.

The *axillary nerve* formed out of roots C5 and C6 leaves the dorsal fascicle at or slightly below the clavicle and runs dorsally along the inferior aspect of the articular capsule of the shoulder (humeroscapular joint) to bend around the surgical neck of the humerus (collum chirurgicum humeri). It exits the lateral axillary hiatus (foramen axillare laterale, defined laterally by the humerus, proximally by the minor teres muscle, distally by the minor teres muscle and medially by the long head of the triceps muscle) where motor branches take off for the teres muscles. The axillary nerve reaches the deltoid muscle posteriorly with several branches for the muscle and additionally provides sensory branches for the skin of the shoulder. A short way after its exit from the dorsal fascicle the axillary nerve is accompanied by the posterior circumflexing artery and veins of the humerus, which supply the deltoid muscle and the muscles at the border of the lateral axillary hiatus. The axillary nerve may be detected sonographically with elevation of the arm in the posterior axillary fold (lateral axillary hiatus). Here it is seen as a rounded, tubular structure entering the deltoid muscle accompanied by two vessels. From here it may be followed upward to its reunion with the radial nerve in the dorsal fascicle (Fig. 2.9).

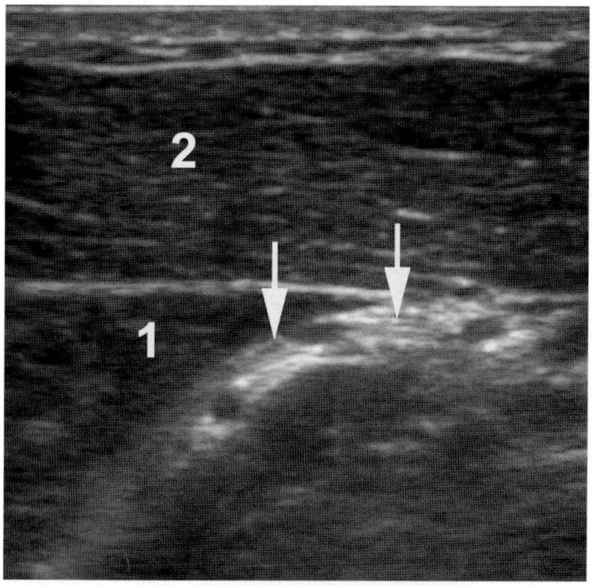

a

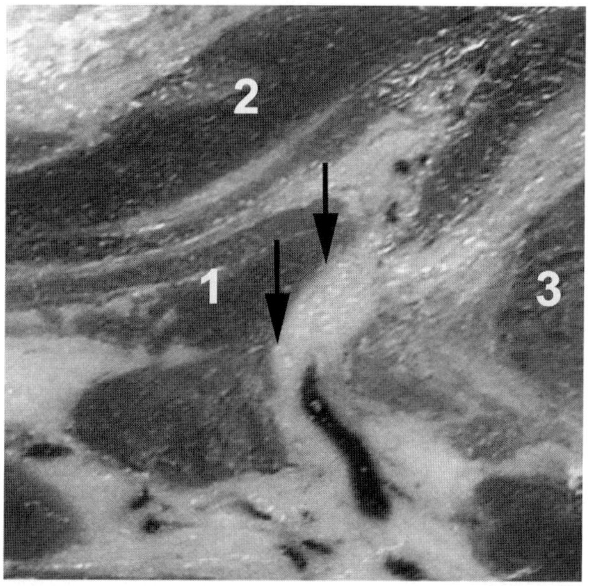

b

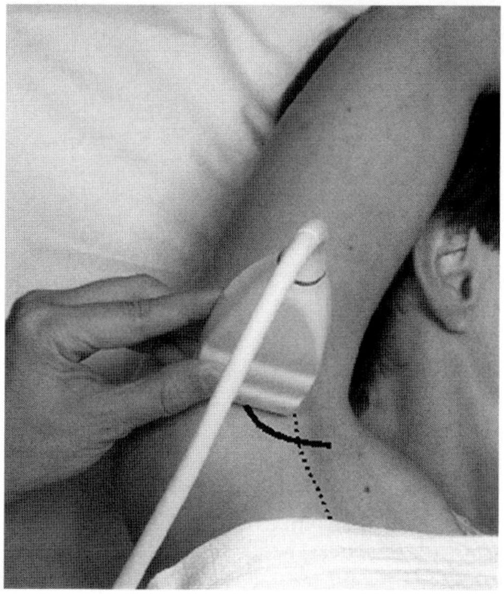
c

Fig. 2.9a–c. Transverse US scan (**a**) and the corresponding cryosection (**b**) showing the axillary nerve and accompanying vessels (*arrows*) ventrally covered by the lateral parts of the latissimus dorsi muscle (*1*) and the pectoral muscle (*2*) inferior to the glenoid part of the scapula (*3*). **c** Scheme with the projection of the course of the axillary nerve (*solid line*) onto the skin surface with the posterior axillary fold (*dotted line*) mainly formed by the underlying latissimus muscle

The *radial nerve* (roots of C5 to C8) supplies the extensor muscles of the whole upper extremity plus the dorsal skin. It pursues the course of the dorsal fascicle in relation to the axillary and brachial artery. Ventral to the tendinous origin of the dorsal latissimus muscle it bends to the posterior surface of the humerus continuing to the proximal end of the osseous "groove of the radial nerve" (sulcus nervi radialis). It is accompanied by the profound brachial artery with the corresponding vein. In its spiral course directly at the surface of the humerus between the proximal lateral and distal medial head of the brachial triceps muscle, it reaches the region of the lateral epicondyle where it finally lies at the flexor side of the elbow (cubita) between the brachial and brachioradial muscle. Along its whole course the radial nerve releases motor and sensory branches to the extensor muscles and dorsal skin. The nerve is most easily assessed with sonography in its course within the musculo-osseous channel formed by the bellies of the brachial triceps muscle and the humerus (Fig. 2.10) (Bodner et al. 1999, 2001). From this region it may be followed proximally and distally with adherence to the anatomic landmarks mentioned above (axillary/brachial artery, muscular interposition).

2.3.3 Nerves of the Forearm

In the forearm the *median nerve* after passing the pronator teres muscle enters the fascial space between the main flexor groups of the upper extremity. It runs downward to the wrist between the superficial and the profound finger flexors. In its course many muscular branches supply different ventral muscle groups of the forearm. Several ulnar flexors of the forearm, however, are omitted by this nerve and their supply is mentioned later in this chapter. One remarkable

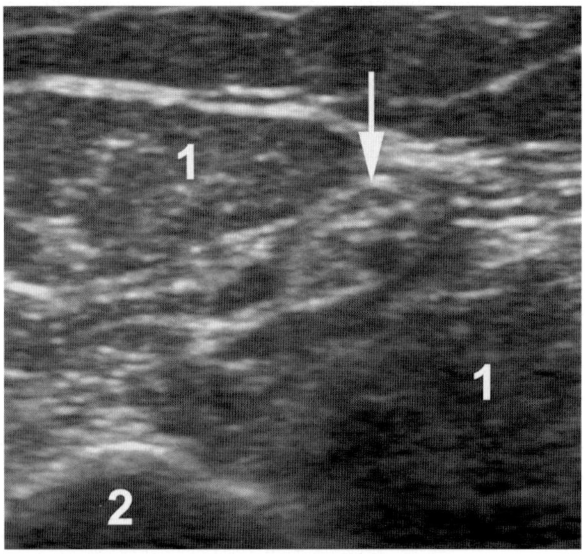

a

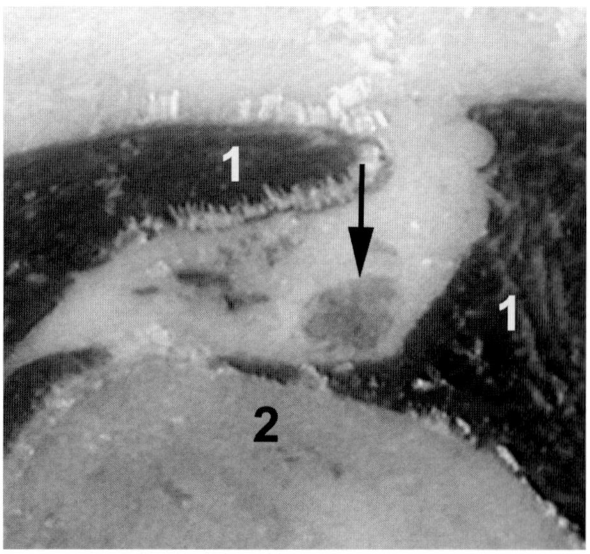

b

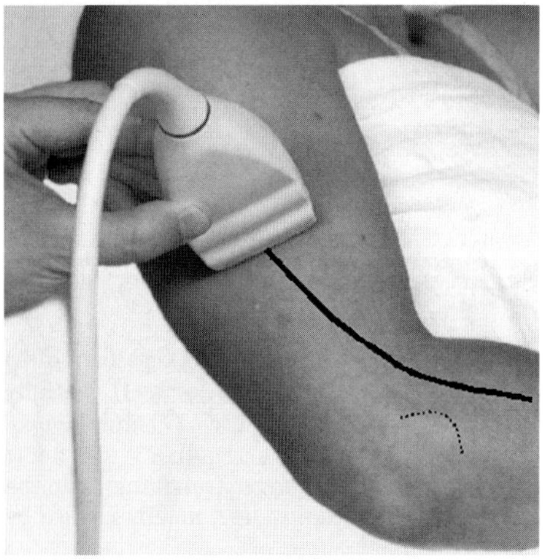

c

Fig. 2.10a–c. Transverse US scan (**a**) and the corresponding cryosection (**b**) showing the radial nerve (*arrow*) in its groove between the heads of the triceps muscle (*1*) running directly on the surface of the humerus (*2*). **c** Scheme with the skin projection of the course of the radial nerve (*solid line*) in the dorsal upper arm with the lateral epicondyle (*dotted line*) as a relevant landmark for positioning of scanhead branch of the median nerve is the anterior antebrachial interosseous nerve which is released in the cubita region and runs downward to the carpus lying directly on the interosseous membrane. This branch finally reaches the square pronator muscle, and along its course supplies the long flexor of the thumb and the radial parts of the deep finger flexors.

In the region of the wrist the median nerve lies directly under the tendon of the long palmar muscle, interposed between the flexor tendons and covered by a thin layer of the forearm fascia (Fig. 2.11). In this region the median nerve may already have split into two parts (common digital nerve trunks), in which case an interposed persistent median artery may coexist as an anatomical variant (GASSNER et al. 2002).

Sonographic identification of the median nerve is easiest at the wrist, as its distal course between the forearm flexors may sometimes be obscured by a variable amount of surrounding fatty tissue. In the cubita it is usually positioned medially to the deep lying brachial artery and veins. Due to its small caliber the anterior antebrachial interosseous nerve cannot always be visualized by sonography.

Passing the groove of the ulnar nerve the *ulnar nerve* usually lies between the two heads of the ulnar carpal flexor. Covered by this muscle it runs straight to the wrist. It supplies the ulnar carpal flexor and the three ulnar parts of the deep finger flexor muscle, which end in the deep flexor tendons of the three ulnar fingers. In the distal part of the forearm the ulnar nerve lies between the tendon of the ulnar carpal flexor muscle medially and the ulnar artery and veins laterally. The ulnar artery and the ulnar nerve both lie superficially to the thin layer of the forearm fascia only covered by loose subcutaneous fat and connective tissue. Sonographic visualization of the ulnar nerve is easiest before its entrance into the ulnar carpal flexor muscle at the elbow and in the distal third of the forearm in its typical position between the tendon of the ulnar carpal flexor muscle and the ulnar artery (Fig. 2.12). As it is embedded in inhomogeneous echogenic tissue in the wrist region and is smaller than the neighboring median nerve its identification at this site may sometimes be difficult.

On its course in the cubita and the forearm the *radial nerve* runs at the ventral side between the brachial and the brachioradial muscle. At the level of the radial head (caput radii) it bifurcates into its terminal branches: the superficial and the profound branch. The superficial branch of the radial nerve runs further distally at the medial border of the brachioradial muscle and medial to the long and short radial carpal extensor muscles. The proximal part of the superficial branch always stays ventral to the supinator muscle in the proximal forearm and is accompanied medially by the radial artery and veins along an individually variable distance. The distal section of this branch returns to the dorsal subcutaneous region of the extremity through the distal part of the brachioradial muscle and crosses the extensor retinaculum dorsally. The profound branch of the radial nerve enters the supinator

a 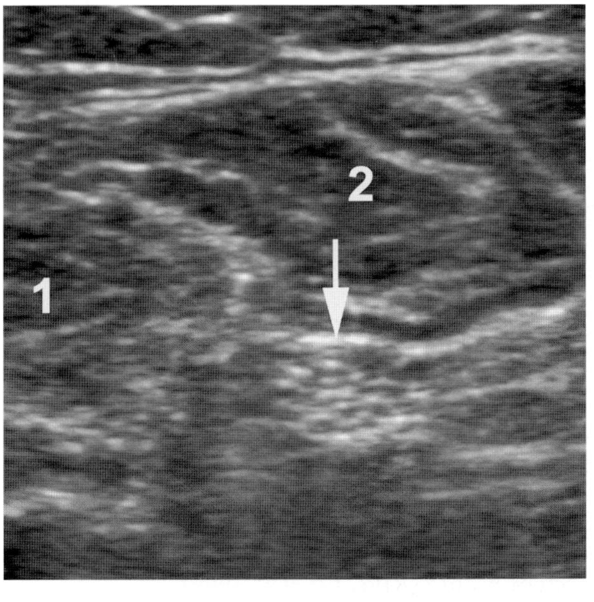

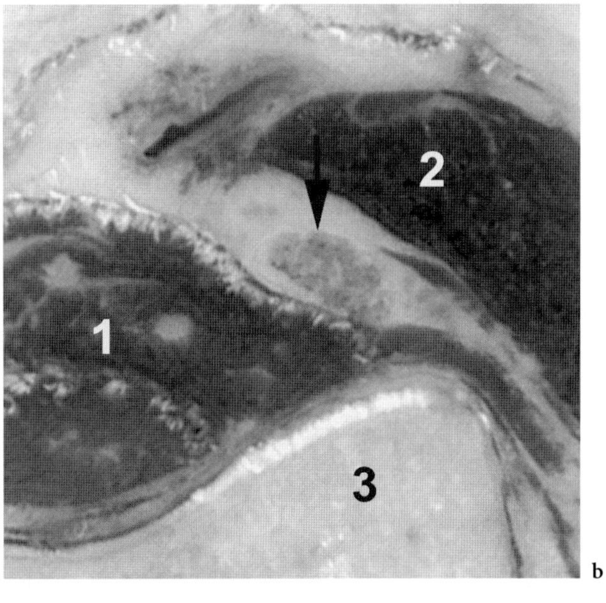 b

Fig. 2.11a, b. Transverse US scan (**a**) and the corresponding cryosection (**b**) showing the median nerve (*arrow*) lying between the distal brachial muscle (*1*) and the flexor of the radial carpus (*2*) muscle (*3* trochlea of the humerus)

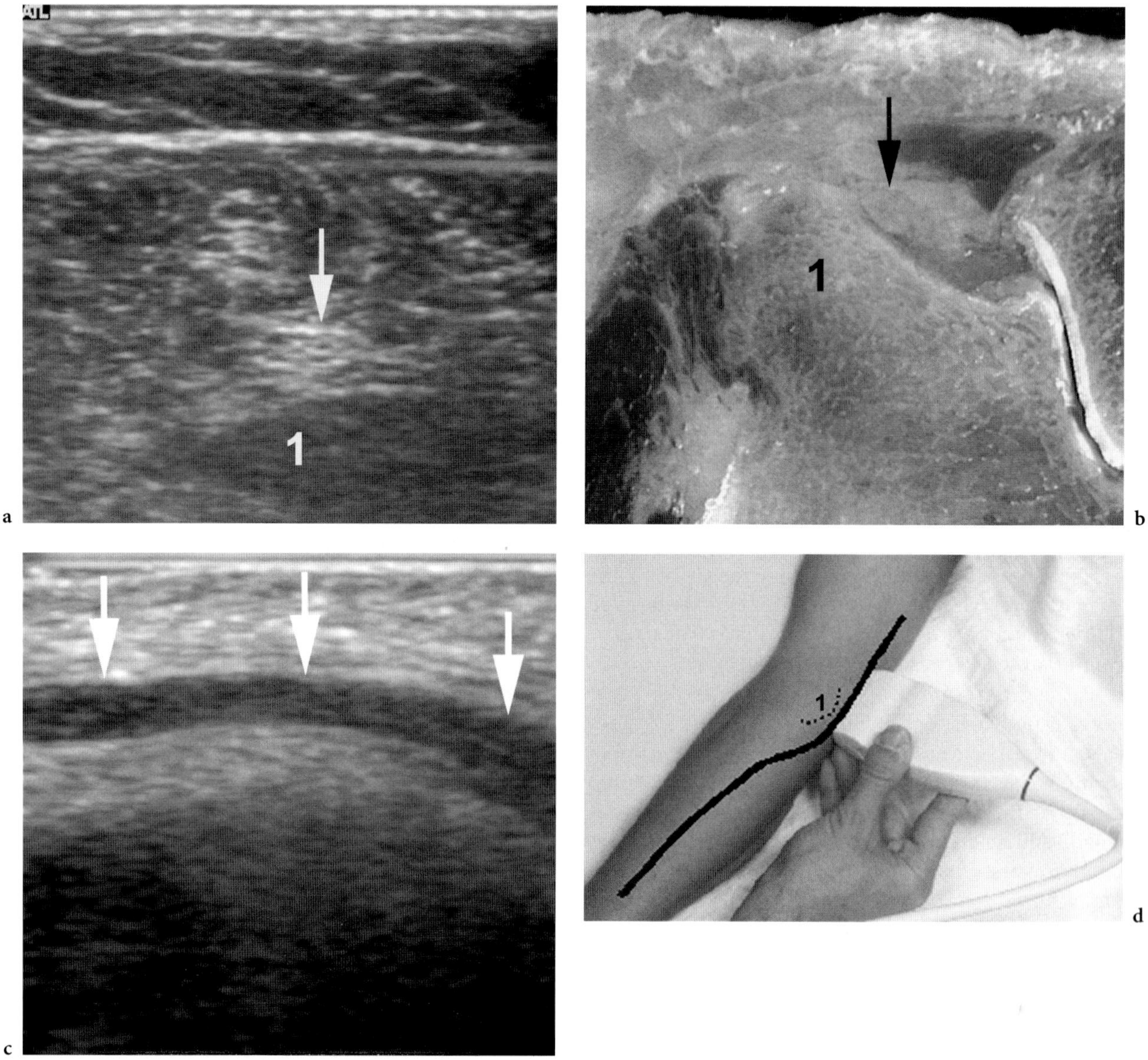

Fig. 2.12a–d. Transverse US scan (**a**) and the corresponding cryosection (**b**) showing the ulnar nerve (*arrow*) in its course within the “sulcus nervi ulnaris” formed by connective tissue and the distal humerus (*1*). **c** Longitudinal US scan of the ulnar nerve (*arrows*) within the “sulcus nervi ulnaris”. **d** Scheme with skin projection of the ulnar nerve (*solid line*) in the cubita relative to the ulnar epicondyle of the humerus (*dotted line*)

muscle at an individually variable distance from the radial nerve bifurcation passing through a small, tendinous arch (the arch of Frohse). If this arch is too small the profound branch of the radial nerve may be compressed – especially during hand extension and pronation which further reduces the width of the supinator arch (Thomas et al. 2000). On its course through the supinator muscle the profound branch releases several muscular branches and finally enters the space between the superficial and profound hand extensors. It ends as the posterior antebrachial interosseous nerve lying on the posterior surface of the interosseous membrane. Sonographic identification of the radial nerve and its branches in the forearm is easiest at their course between the brachial and brachioradial muscle where they show a high contrast difference compared with the surrounding muscular tissue. In most asymptomatic subjects the profound branch of the radial nerve shows a relative change in caliber at its entry into the supinator muscle through the arch of Frohse (Riffaud et al. 1999).

The superficial branch is best assessed medially to the brachioradial muscle. The terminal branches of the superficial radial nerve branch can only be visualized with the use of transducers with a frequency of at least 15 MHz. The profound branch of the radial nerve is easily visualized inside the supinator muscle due to the high sonographic contrast difference between the nerve and the surrounding muscle (Fig. 2.13). The posterior antebrachial interosseous nerve is only detectable with present sonographic equipment in rare cases due to its small size and insufficient contrast.

2.3.4 Nerves of the Hand

In some subjects the division of the *median nerve* begins in the region of the distal forearm, and at the latest in the region of the carpal tunnel. Usually the first common digital palmar nerve (for the thenar and the thumb) is the first branch leaving the nerve. The infrequently found median artery, which

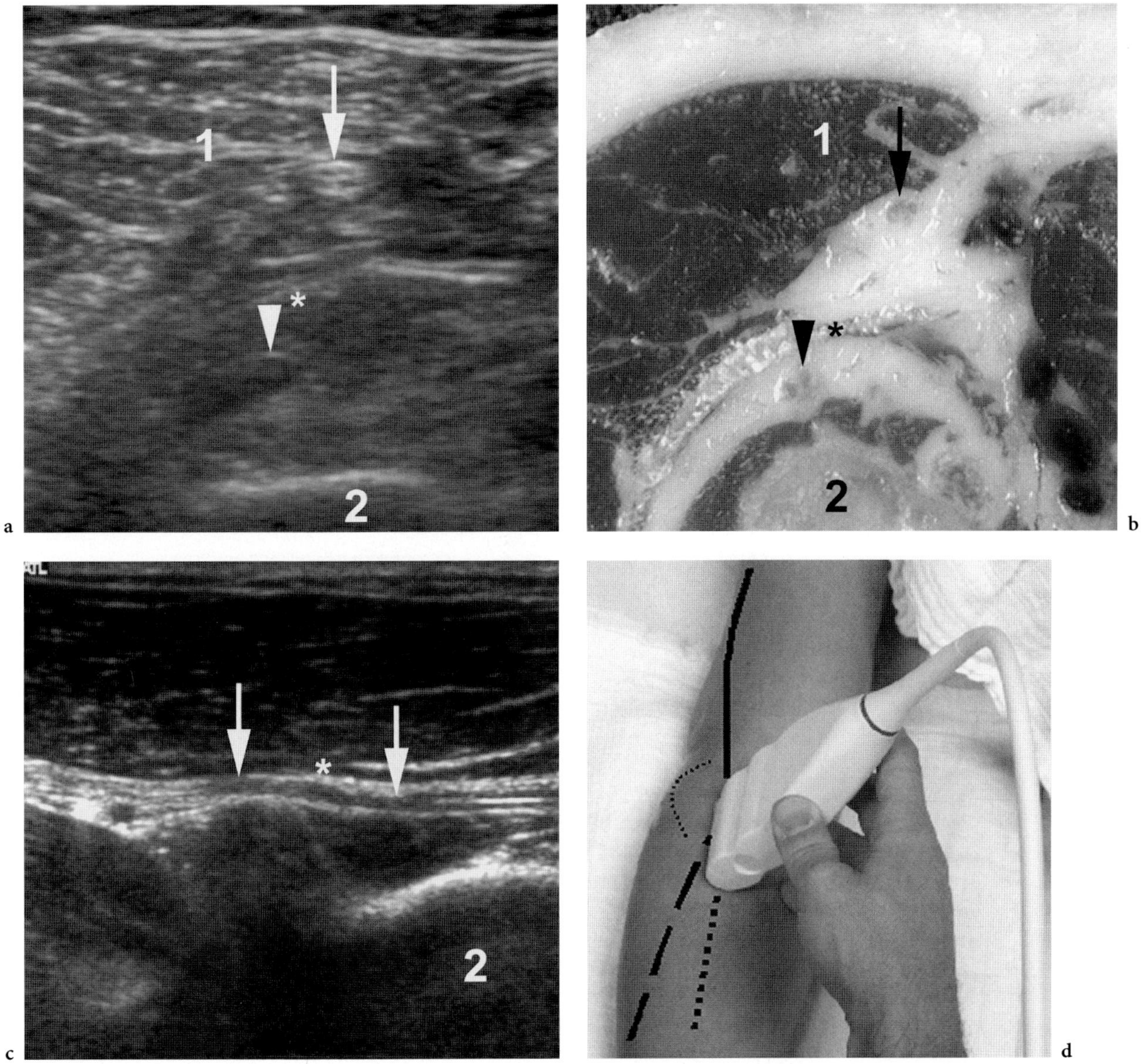

Fig. 2.13a–d. Transverse US scan (**a**) and the corresponding cryosection (**b**) showing the division of the radial nerve superficial branch (*arrow*) and profound branch (*arrowhead*). The profound branch is typically covered by the arch of Frohse (*asterisk*) and the superficial branch by the proximal parts of the brachioradial muscle (*1*) (*2* proximal radius). **c** Longitudinal US scan of the profound branch of the radial nerve (*arrows*) with the arch of Frohse (*asterisk*) (*2* radius). **d** Scheme with the skin projection of the course and division of the radial nerve in the cubita: radial nerve (*solid line*), superficial branch (*broken line*), profound branch (*thick dotted line*). Radial epicondyle of the humerus (*thin dotted line*) as landmark

is a variable branch of the proximal section of the ulnar artery and leads into the also variable superficial palmar arterial arch (Hafferl 1969; Lanz and Wachsmuth 1972; Platzer 1982), may be found inside the carpal tunnel interposed between the first common digital palmar nerve and the median nerve remnant. The bifurcation of the residual median nerve into the second (second finger and radial part of third finger motor and sensory supply) and third (ulnar third and radial fourth finger motor and sensory supply) common digital palmar nerve usually takes place inside or directly distal to the carpal tunnel. The median nerve and its terminal branches always appear more or less oval or flattened, with considerable individual variation in healthy subjects (Sarria et al. 2000; Duncan et al. 1999) (Fig. 2.14).

The terminal peripheral branches of the median nerve – the paired proper palmar finger nerves

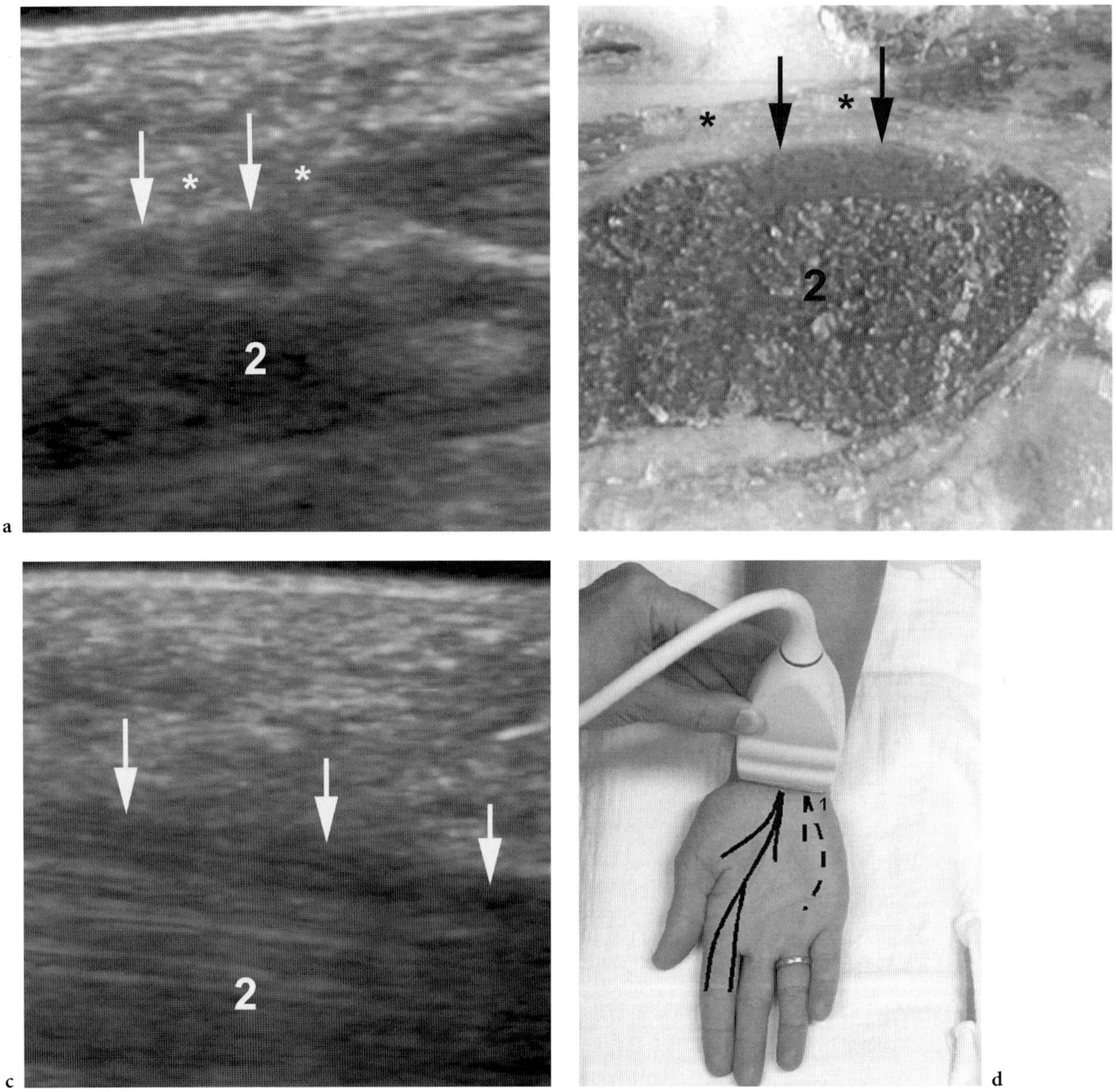

Fig. 2.14a–d. Transverse US scan (**a**) and the corresponding cryosection (**b**) showing the median nerve in the hand (*arrows*) together with the cross sections of the finger flexor tendons within the carpal tunnel (*2*) covered by the transverse ligament of the carpus (*asterisks*). **c** Longitudinal US scan of the distal median nerve (*arrows*) with the underlying finger flexor tendons (*2*). **d** Scheme with skin projection of representative branches of the median nerve (*solid lines*) and the ulnar nerve (*broken lines*) in the hand. Pisiform bone (*1*) as landmark

(palmar supply of the first to the third fingers and the radial palmar side of the fourth finger) – are sensible branches emerging of the common digital palmar nerves, which are directly positioned on the tendons or tendon sheaths of the long flexor muscles. They may only be visualized with transducers of at least 15 MHz. Each of them is accompanied by a proper palmar finger artery, usually lying more superficially (Fig. 2.15).

The *ulnar nerve* reaches the hand running superficially to the flexor retinaculum and is accompanied laterally by the ulnar artery. Here it bifurcates releasing the profound branch, which forms a neural arch supplying the muscles of the hypothenar, the interosseous muscles and finally even part of the thenar muscles, between the proximal parts of the small flexor and the abductor of the small finger. The residual ulnar nerve (fourth common digital palmar nerve) ends in

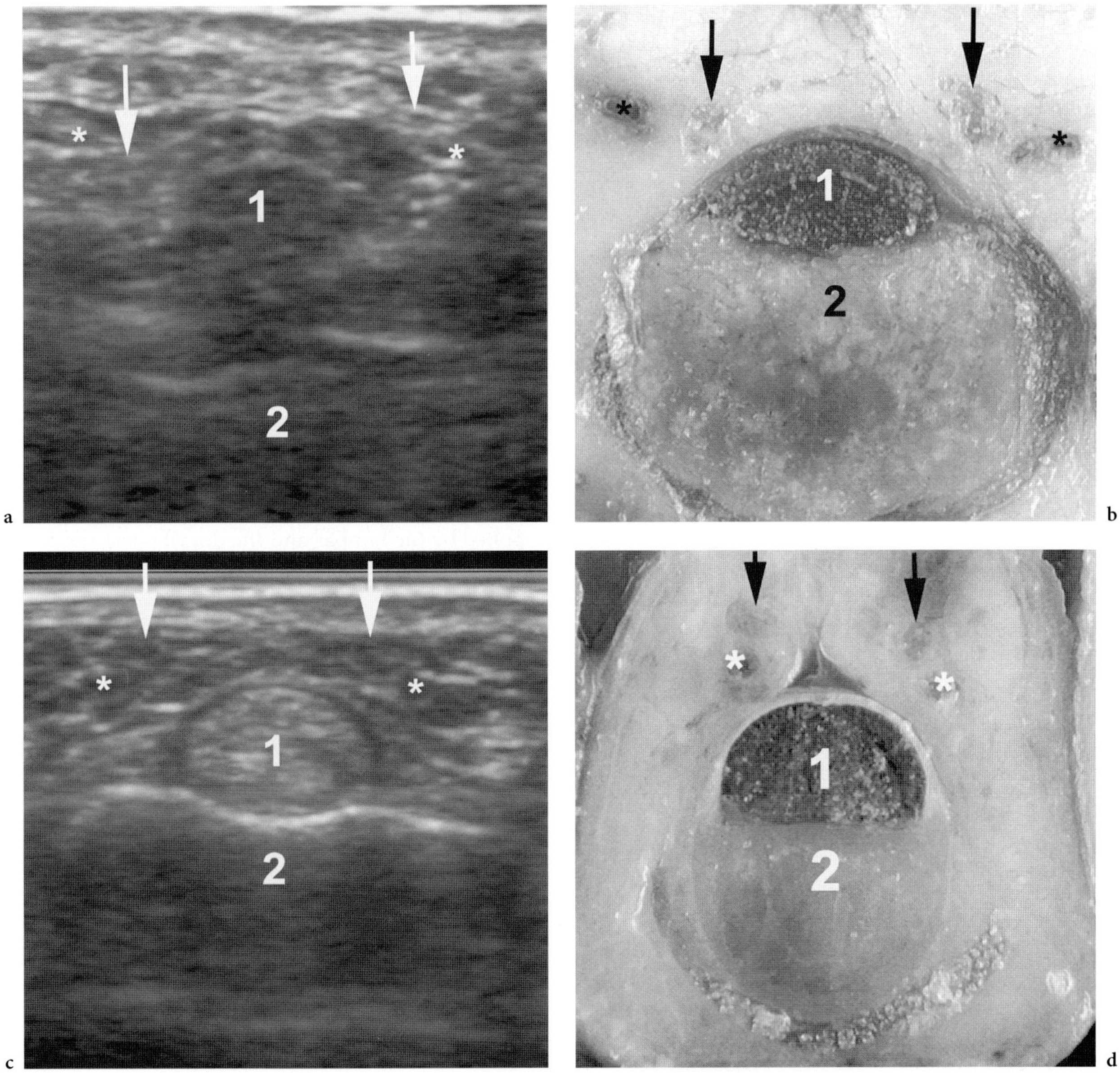

Fig. 2.15a–d. Transverse US scan (**a**) and the corresponding cryosection (**b**) showing the metacarpal section of the branches of the median nerve (proper digital nerves, *arrows*) together with the accompanying arteries (*asterisks*) (*1* flexor tendons, *2* underlying metacarpal bone). Transverse US scan (**c**) and the corresponding cryosection (**d**) showing the digital section of the branches of the median nerve (proper digital nerves, *arrows*) together with the closely accompanying arteries (*asterisks*) (*1* flexor tendons, *2* underlying digital bone)

the paired proper palmar finger nerves (supplying the radiopalmar aspect of the fourth and the palmar aspect of the fifth finger). Just like the terminal median nerve branches, the terminal ulnar branches are accompanied by the proper palmar finger arteries (the terminal arterial branches of the superficial palmar arch). A very small side-branch of the ulnar nerve – the dorsal branch of the ulnar nerve – which exits the ulnar nerve in the middle of the forearm, reaches the hand subcutaneously and dorsomedially to the styloid process of the ulna. It ends in the sensory proper finger nerves for the dorsal aspect of the fourth and fifth finger being accompanied by subcutaneous veins. The sonographic visualization of the terminal branches (proper palmar finger nerves) and their proximal nerve stems only succeeds with high-frequency transducers of at least 15 MHz (Fig. 2.16).

The *radial nerve* ends in three common dorsal finger nerves, having already formed in the region of the distal forearm. Each of these neural branches lies subcutaneously and crosses the extensor retinaculum superficially. The split in the proper dorsal finger nerves, which are again paired (for the dorsal thumb and the dorsoproximal parts of the second to the fourth fingers – the second and third dorsal fingers are usually supplied by the median nerve), takes place at variable locations. The terminal dorsal branches are accompanied by the barely visible terminal arterial branches of the dorsal carpal branch of the radial artery. Visualization of these flimsy branches of the radial nerve is achieved best in the region of the lateral extensor retinaculum. The branches are embedded in subcutaneous fat and connective tissue, which is why their presentation may be insufficient. The posterior antebrachial interosseous nerve and its terminal branches for the sensory supply of the dorsal carpal and digital joints may not be visualized by present state-of-the-art ultrasonography.

2.4 The Lower Extremity

Just like the proximal extremity the lower extremity forms paddle-like during the fetal period. It is supplied by the corresponding neural segments (metameric segmentation) of the rump wall. In later life this ontological specialization results in the distinct distribution of the sensible dermatomes in correlation with the supplying spinal roots. For the lower extremity these are the segments L1 to S3. The annular organization of the dermatomes on the rump wall is transferred to a somewhat longitudinal representation in the lower extremity just as it is in the upper extremity, but with some kind of inward rotation of the dermatomes. The recombination of the axons with formation of the peripheral nerves itself takes place at the level of the lumbar and sacral plexus, with the ventral parts of the lower extremity supplied by the lumbar and the dorsal parts and the pelvic floor by the sacral plexus.

a
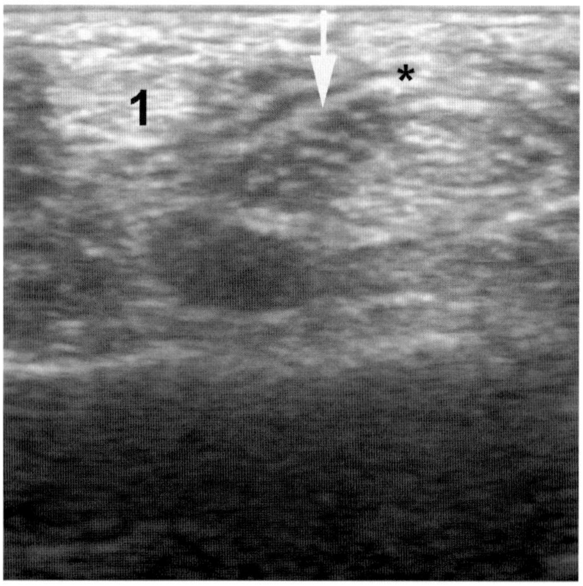

b
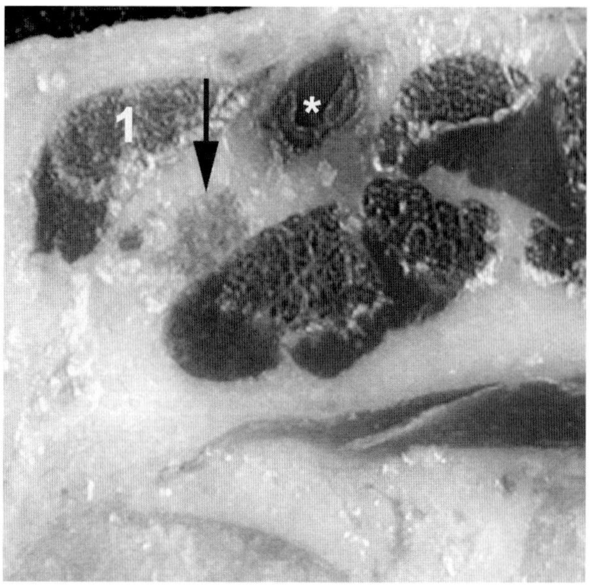

Fig. 2.16a, b. Transverse US scan (**a**) and the corresponding cryosection (**b**) showing the ulnar nerve (*arrow*) in its carpal section accompanied closely by the ulnar artery (*asterisk*) next to the tendon of the ulnar flexor of the carpus (*1*)

2.4.1 Nerves of the Groin and the Thigh

The most cranial nerve descending from the lumbar plexus is the sensory *lateral femoral cutaneous nerve*. It forms out of the ventral branches of the spinal nerves of segments L2 and L3. It runs downward on the iliac muscle to the medial side of the anterior iliac spine and uses the very lateral part of the muscle's lacuna to get to the ventrolateral subcutaneous space. It can be identified with sonography in the muscle's lacuna, where it enters the subcutaneous space between the sartorial and tensor fasciae latae muscle. Because of its small size its sonographic visualization may be very difficult.

One of the largest peripheral nerves of the human body is the *femoral nerve*. It contains the fascicles for the musculature, and is the sole innervater of the knee extensors and is responsible for the sensibility of almost the whole ventral and medial aspect of the lower extremity. The femoral nerve is usually formed out of the ventral branches of the spinal nerves of segments L1 to L4. The recombination of the neural fascicles of the femoral nerve takes place within the psoas muscle, where it is split into a superficial and a profound section. The proximal part of the nerve leaves the psoas muscle at its lateral border, running downward to the inguinal region in the retroperitoneum inside a groove formed by the psoas muscle medially and by the iliac muscle laterally. It leaves the muscle's lacuna as the most medial structure separated from the adjacent femoral artery only by the iliopectineal arch (Fig. 2.17). The latter is a thin tendinous structure, which is part of the inguinal ligament complex, and connects the inguinal ligament and the body of the iliac bone.

After a variable distance the nerve spreads into its several terminal branches: ventral and medial cutaneous nerve branches and motor branches for the supplied muscles. The main direction of the course of the femoral nerve and its branches is always parallel to the sartorial muscle beneath. The final branch of the femoral nerve, the saphenous nerve lies adjacent to the superficial femoral artery and perforates the vastoadductorial membrane in its distal third of the thigh together with the descendent knee artery, a branch of the superficial femoral artery. The saphenous nerve supplies the knee and the medial aspect of the lower leg with sensory fibers and runs subcutaneously to the region of the superficial pes anserinus. The femoral nerve is best assessed with sonography in its groin section. Here it can be found next to the pulsating femoral artery with an oval or triangular cross-sectional appearance.

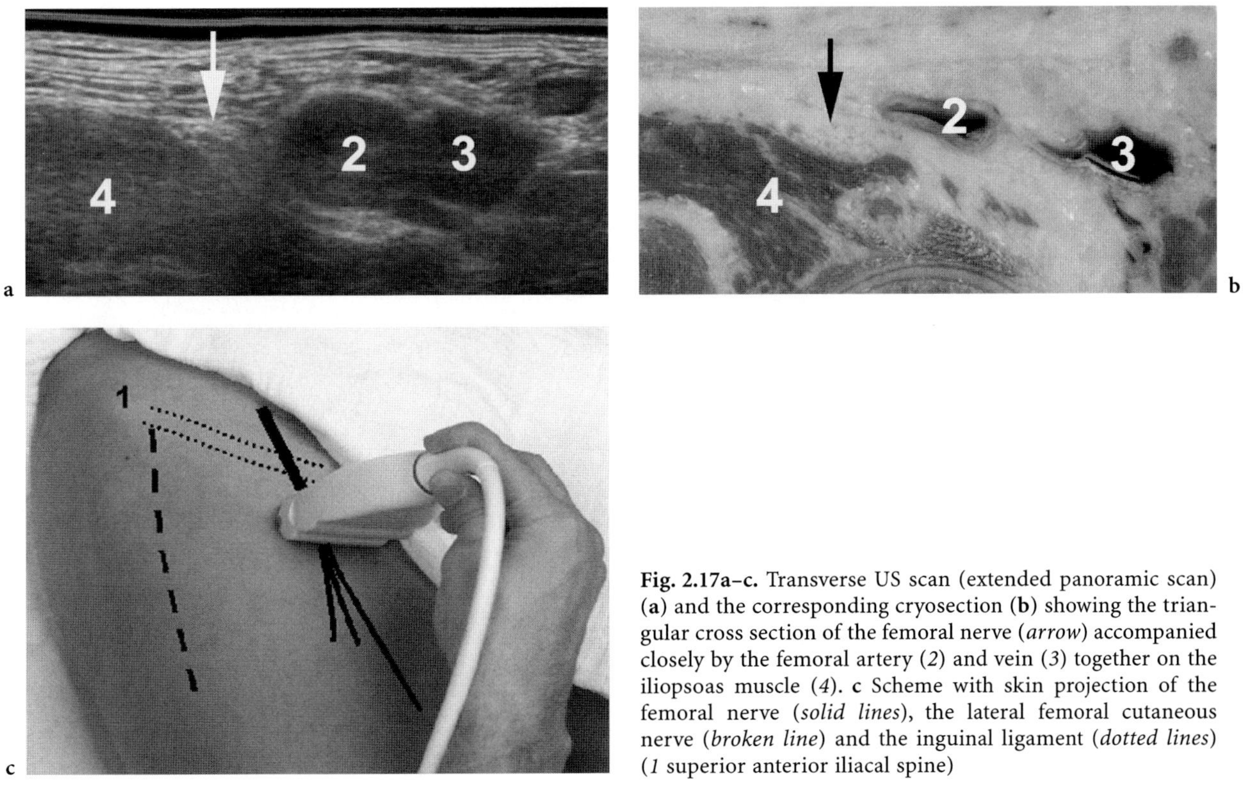

Fig. 2.17a–c. Transverse US scan (extended panoramic scan) (**a**) and the corresponding cryosection (**b**) showing the triangular cross section of the femoral nerve (*arrow*) accompanied closely by the femoral artery (*2*) and vein (*3*) together on the iliopsoas muscle (*4*). **c** Scheme with skin projection of the femoral nerve (*solid lines*), the lateral femoral cutaneous nerve (*broken line*) and the inguinal ligament (*dotted lines*) (*1* superior anterior iliacal spine)

The section of the femoral nerve in its pelvic course up to 10 cm proximal to the inguinal ligament may also be visualized by sonography after sufficient evacuation of air in the hypogastric bowel. The proximal thigh section of the nerve may sometimes be difficult to assess due to early branching as well as to low contrast differences between the nerve and surrounding soft tissues. The saphenous nerve may only be visualized in favorable conditions in its subcutaneous course at the medial aspect of the knee.

The deep muscle-supplying branches of the femoral nerve cannot be visualized with present sonographic equipment (Gruber et al. 2003).

The largest peripheral nerve of the human body is the *sciatic nerve* (Fig. 2.18). In fact it consists of two large nerves combined by a common epineural sheath: the laterally positioned common fibular nerve and the medially positioned tibial nerve. The sciatic nerve forms out of the branches of the lumbar and the sacral plexus of segments L4 to S3, whereby

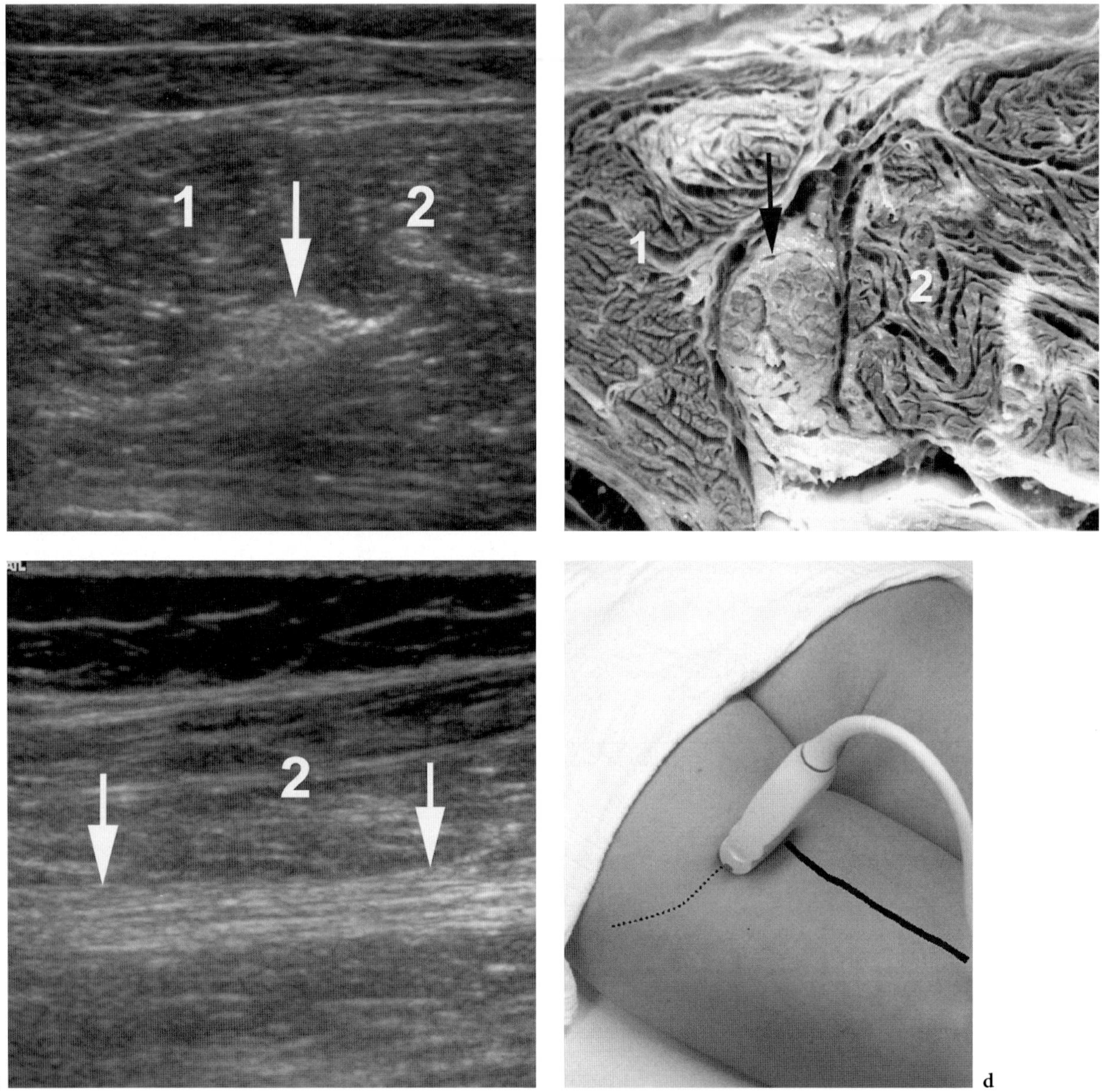

a b c d

Fig. 2.18a–d. Transverse US scan (**a**) and the corresponding cryosection (**b**) showing the sciatic nerve (*arrow*) interposed between the femoral biceps (*1*) and the semitendinous and semimembranous muscles (*2*), respectively. **c** Longitudinal US scan of the sciatic nerve (*arrows*) with the overlying semitendinous and semimembranous muscles, respectively (*2*). **d** Scheme and skin projection of the sciatic nerve (*solid line*). Inferior gluteal fold (*dotted line*) as landmark the common fibular nerve elements derive from the branches of the segments L4 to S2, and the tibial nerve elements from the branches of L4 to S3 after recombination of nerve fibers in the retroperitoneal and subperitoneal lumbosacral plexus. The sciatic nerve exits the subperitoneal space through the major sciatic foramen, which is formed by the major incisura of the sciatic bone and by the sacrospinous ligament, coursing underneath the piriform muscle (infrapiriform compartment of the major sciatic foramen). Here it is accompanied medially by the pudendal and inferior gluteal vessels and the corresponding nerves, altogether surrounded by a considerable amount of loose connective tissue and fat. In the subgluteal space (only covered by the maximus gluteal muscle) it takes a slightly lateral convex course crossing the underlying small deep gluteal muscles (gemellus muscles and internal obturator muscle) and the quadratic femoral muscle (connecting the sciatic tuber and the intertrochanteric crest of the femur). It traverses laterally to the sciatic tuber and is crossed by the gluteal vessels. In this region the nerve becomes covered by proximal parts of the sciatic-crural muscles (mainly by the long head of the femoral biceps muscle), while it lies on top of the minimus adductor muscle and further distally the magnus adductor muscle. In this region the sciatic nerve is accompanied by arterial and venous branches of the profound femoral artery (perforating vessels) which supply the sciatic-crural muscles (Graif et al. 1991).

In the more distal parts of the dorsal thigh the sciatic nerve divides into its intrinsic neural sections at a very individually variable height. These sections (the lateral common fibular nerve and the medial tibial nerve) are interposed between the two heads of the femoral biceps muscle, whereby the *common fibular nerve* follows the tendon of the femoral biceps muscle medially and further down dorsomedially to the tendon attachment at the head of the fibula.

After releasing the sensory sural nerve dorsally the *tibial nerve* is accompanied medially by the popliteal vessels in its course through the tendinous adductorial hiatus. In this section the tibial nerve as well as the common fibular becomes almost subcutaneous covered only by the thin popliteal and crural fascia. In the most distal thigh, or better in the region of the dorsal knee, the nerve is interposed between the two heads of the gastrocnemius muscle together with the directly underlying popliteal vein and even more deeply positioned artery. The sonographic identification of the sciatic nerve and the common fibular and tibial nerve is most easily achieved at the distal third of the dorsal thigh (Fig. 2.19). After its identification

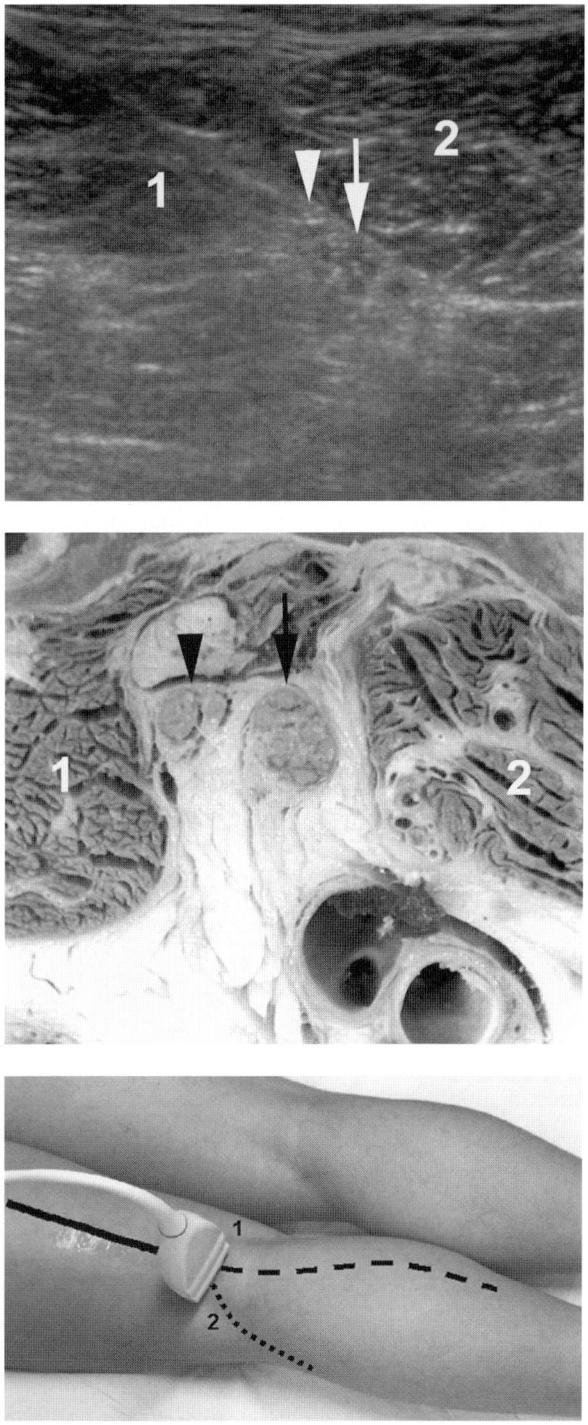

a b c

Fig. 2.19a–c. Transverse US scan (**a**) and the corresponding cryosection (**b**) showing the common fibular (*arrowhead*) and the tibial nerve (*arrow*) next to the distal parts of the femoral biceps (*1*) and the semitendinous and semimembranous muscles (*2*), respectively. **c** Scheme and skin projection of the sciatic nerve (*solid line*) and its division into the common fibular nerve (*dotted line*) and the tibial nerve (*broken line*) with the tendons of the semimembranous and semitendinous muscle (*1*) and femoral biceps muscle (*2*) as landmarks in this region the sciatic nerve may be followed proximally with ease. In the gluteal region its presentation becomes worse because of the thick overlying bulk of muscle.

A very small and thin but important branch of the lumbar plexus is the *pudendal nerve*. It is formed out of the ventral branches of segments S2 to S4 and supplies the external genitals as well as the constrictor muscles of the urinary and intestinal tract and several muscles of the pelvic floor. It forms in the subperitoneal space in the sacral plexus, exits the pelvic space together with the sciatic nerve ventromedially to it accompanied by the pudendal artery and vein, bends around the sacrospinous ligament to get to the medial surface of the sciatic tuber directly inferior to the anal levator muscle running within a fibro-osseous channel: the pudendal channel or channel of Alcock (Gruber et al. 2001; Kovacs et al. 2001). A clear visualization of the complete course of the pudendal nerve by sonography is not feasible at present. However identification of the nerve succeeds in about 50% of subjects in the deep gluteal region. Reliable topographic relationships to the pudendal artery and bony and ligamentous landmarks, however, may be identified by sonography, which is important for guidance of a pudendal block (Gruber et al. 2001; Kovacs et al. 2001). The latter is discussed in more detail in Chapter 6.

2.4.2 Nerves of the Lower Leg

Three nerves are responsible for the sensory and motor supply of the lower leg: the mere sensory saphenous nerve (terminal branch of the femoral nerve) for the medial aspect, the motor and sensory tibial nerve for the dorsal aspect, and the motor and sensory common fibular nerve with both its terminal branches (superficial and profound fibular nerve) for the ventrolateral aspect.

The saphenous nerve runs subcutaneously downward to the inner ankle usually accompanied dorsomedially by the saphena magna vein. It cannot always be visualized by sonography because of its small size and insufficient contrast against its surroundings.

The *fibular nerve* positioned medially and further distally positioned dorsomedially to the tendon of the femoral biceps muscle bends around the dorsal and dorsolateral neck of the fibula to enter the fibular muscles. In this bend it divides into its terminal branches: the profound and the superficial fibular nerve. The more dorsally and caudally positioned profound fibular nerve enters the space between the dorsally lying long and the ventrally lying short fibular muscle accompanied by the anterior tibial vessels medially. It supplies the two muscles and the overlying skin. The more ventrally, cranially and medially positioned superficial fibular nerve enters the space between the short fibular muscle and the fibular bone to run to the ventral side of the shank between the fibular muscles and long digital extensor muscle or their tendons. Crossing the tendons of the ventral extensor musculature the superficial fibular nerve becomes subcutaneous and splits into its terminal sensory skin branches. The common fibular nerve is easily visualized in the popliteal region and in its course around the fibular neck before it enters the fibular muscles (Fig. 2.20).

The sonographic visualization of the course of both terminal branches within the fibular muscles is only possible with transducers of at least 12 MHz. The superficial fibular nerve in the ventral shank, however, cannot always be visualized by sonography.

The *tibial nerve* enters the space between the two heads of the gastrocnemius muscle in the thigh to run downward in the dorsal shank. In the proximal fourth of the lower leg, crossing the underlying oblique popliteal muscle, it perforates the proximal soleus muscle to enter the space between the superficial and profound foot flexor muscles. Usually before perforating the soleus muscle it releases multiple muscular and cutaneous branches for the dorsal shank. The subcutaneous main branch of the dorsal shank – the sural nerve – also runs further distally almost centrally, usually lateral to the saphena parva vein and heads for the posterior region of the outer ankle. The tibial nerve becomes more and more oriented medially in the distal fourth of its course together with the accompanying posterior tibial vessels and aims for the posterior medial malleolar region (Fig. 2.21). Here the nerve is usually the most posterior structure escorted ventrally by the vessels, interposed between the loose superficial and the tense profound stratum of the retinaculum of the flexor muscles. Sonographic visualization of the tibial nerve is easiest in the distal shank, but with the posterior tibial vessels as landmarks there is no problem in identification of the nerve in any section of its course.

2.4.3 Nerves of the Foot

The nerves of the foot are the terminal branches of the sciatic or better the tibial and fibular nerve,

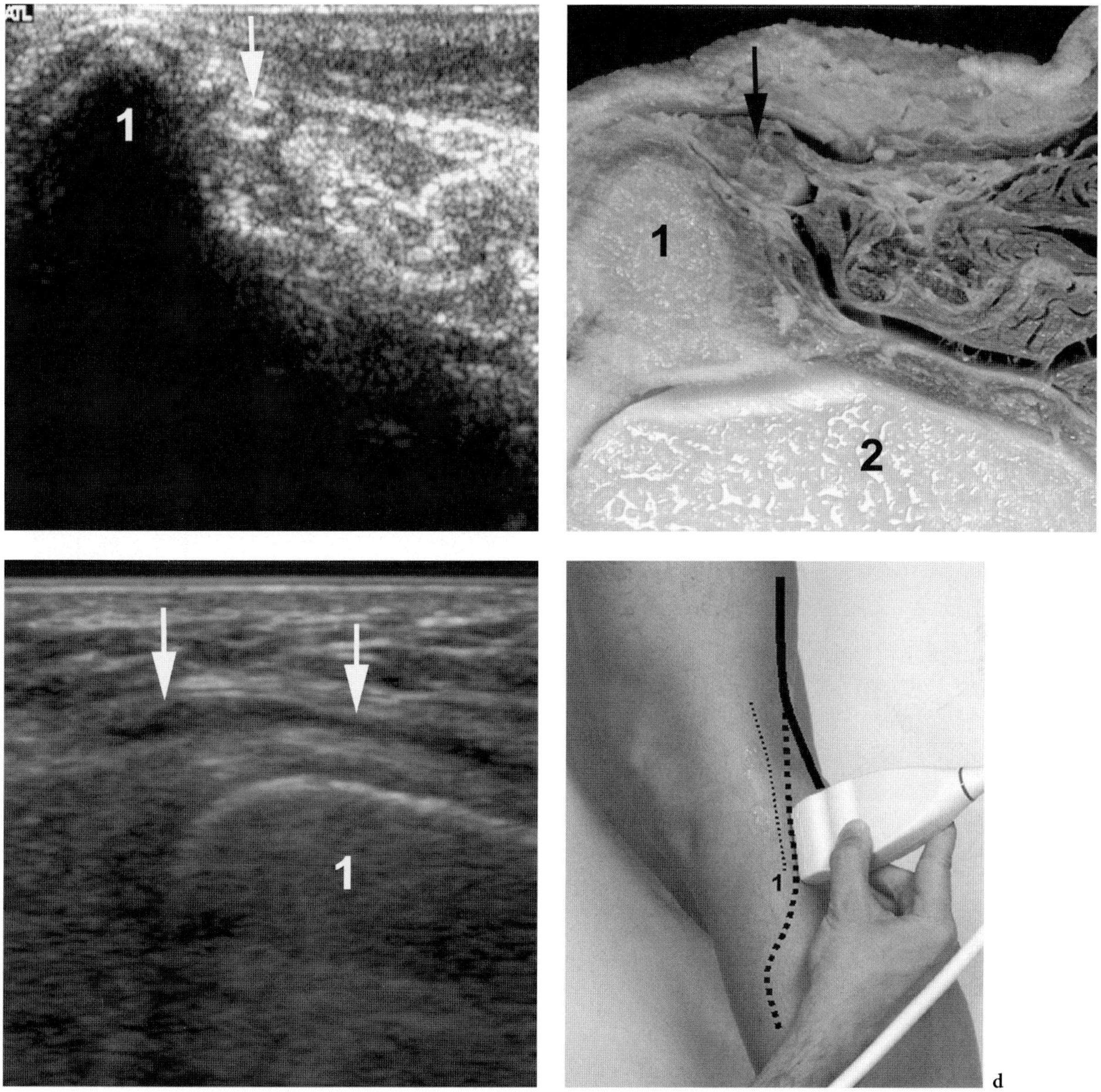

Fig. 2.20a–d. Transverse US scan (**a**) and the corresponding cryosection (**b**) showing the proximal part of the common fibular nerve (*arrow*) in the lower leg in its course around the neck of the fibula (*1*) (*2* tibia). **c** Longitudinal US scan corresponding to the course of the common fibular nerve (*arrows*) at the neck of the fibula (*1*). **d** Scheme with skin projection of the course of the common fibular nerve (*thick dotted line*) in the lateral lower leg. Tendon of the femoral biceps muscle (*thin dotted line*), sciatic or tibial nerve (*solid line*), fibular head (*1*) as landmarks

whereas the terminal endings of the saphenous nerve as end-branch of the femoral nerve reach the metatarsophalangeal joint of the hallux at the medial foot border.

The terminal branches of the superficial fibular nerve reach the dorsum of the foot subcutaneously, usually accompanying the tendons of the long digital extensors of the second and third toe. These very tiny nerves can only seldom be identified by sonography.

The main sensory and motor supply to the foot is provided by the tibial nerve with both its terminal branches: the medial and the lateral plantar nerve. These two branches usually form in the region of the medial malleolus. The medial plantar nerve runs plantomedially directly on the tendons and sheaths of the long flexor of the toes accompanied medially by the medial plantar vessels. The nerve branches into common and proper plantar toe nerves sup-

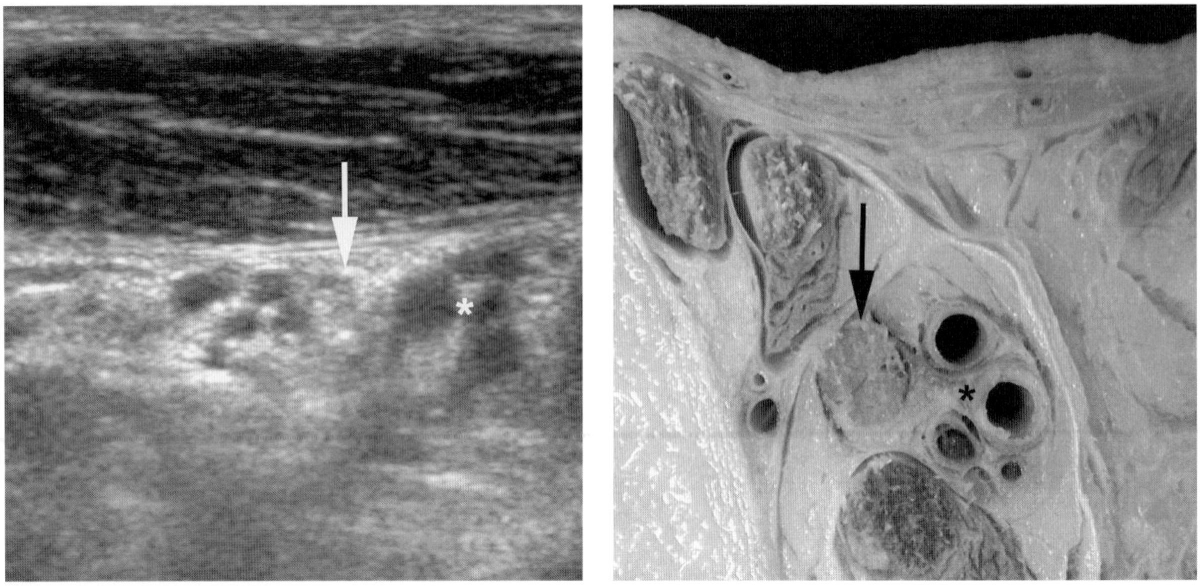

a b

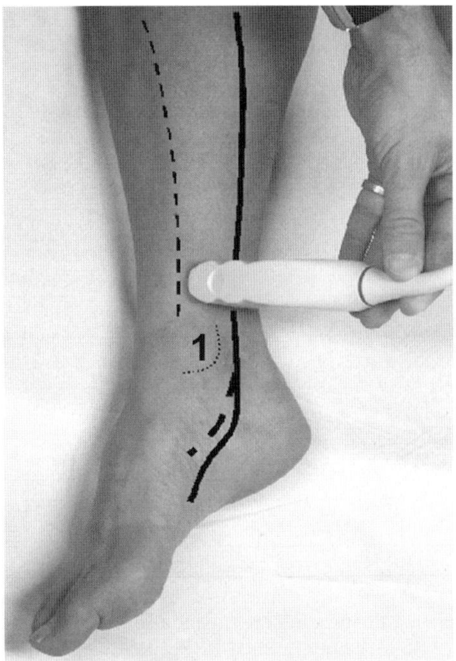

c

Fig. 2.21a–c. Transverse US scan (**a**) and the corresponding cryosection (**b**) showing the distal tibial nerve (*arrow*) accompanied by the posterior tibial vascular bundle (*asterisk*). **c** Scheme and skin projections of the distal tibial nerve (*solid line*) and its terminal plantar medial (*thick broken line*) and lateral (*solid line*) branches (the medial and lateral plantar nerves). Edge of the tibia (*thin broken line*) and medial malleolus (*dotted line, 1*) as landmarks

plying sensation to the skin of the first to the medial surface of the fourth toe. The medial and the lateral plantar nerve are covered by the tight plantar fascia until it is penetrated by the common plantar finger nerves in its distal third. The subcutis of the planta is a very structured space with lobulated fatty tissue and tense connective tissue fibers, connecting the plantar fascia to the plantar skin. That is why the sonographic visualization of the terminal branches of the plantar toe nerves is very difficult and not always achieved clearly.

The lateral plantar nerve usually continues the course of the tibial nerve together with the now more laterally positioned main plantar vessels. It usually splits into three terminal branches for the supply of the lateral and intertarsal plantar intrinsic muscles, with the supply of the skin of the fibular aspect of the fourth and plantar aspect of the fifth toe, after branching into common and proper plantar toe nerves. The discussion above for the branches of the medial plantar nerve equally applies to the sonographic visualization of these subcutaneous branches.

2.5 The Trunk

In the trunk the primordial metameric organization of the human body stays unaltered as far as peripheral nerves are concerned. The primary segmentation of the body as expressed in the segmental organization of the vertebral column and the musculature therefore applies logically to the peripheral nerves. The usual spinal nerve exiting the intervertebral foramen splits into two main branches: the ventral root and the dorsal root. The ventral roots are mainly responsible for any motor and sensory supply of structures ventral to and the dorsal roots dorsal to the respective intervertebral foramen. The thoracic nerves may be subdivided into a superior "intercostal" group (segments Th1 to Th6) and an inferior "subcostal" group (segments Th7 to Th12). These nerves are functionally mixed nerves (motor and sensory elements) and supply more or less the corresponding metameric rump wall segments (muscles and overlying skin) with anterior and lateral cutaneous branches.

The thoracic nerves of the superior group – the intercostal nerves – are positioned beneath the corresponding rib together with the cranial segmental intercostal vessels in a space defined by the external and internal intercostal muscles. The thoracic nerves of the inferior group show a segmental pattern similar to that of the intercostal nerves innervating the less-segmented lateral and ventral abdominal musculature and the corresponding overlying skin, also accompanied by corresponding segmental vessels. The most inferior of these nerves is *the* subcostal nerve (Th12) which ends in the region of the iliac crest. The nerves supplying the inguinal region of the trunk (iliohypogastric, ilioinguinal and genitofemoral nerve) show an almost "segmental" course in the rump wall, but are the most cranial branches of the lumbar plexus and are not accompanied by segmental vessels. The most cranial nerves of the superior group (intercostal nerves 1 to 3) are somehow incompletely integrated in the formation of the brachial plexus so that they release accessory sensory branches for the supply of the inner proximal upper extremity (intercostobrachial nerves). The sonographic visualization of these segmental nerves can be performed easily for the intercostal nerves despite their smallness as they are accompanied by clearly identifiable vessels (Fig. 2.22).

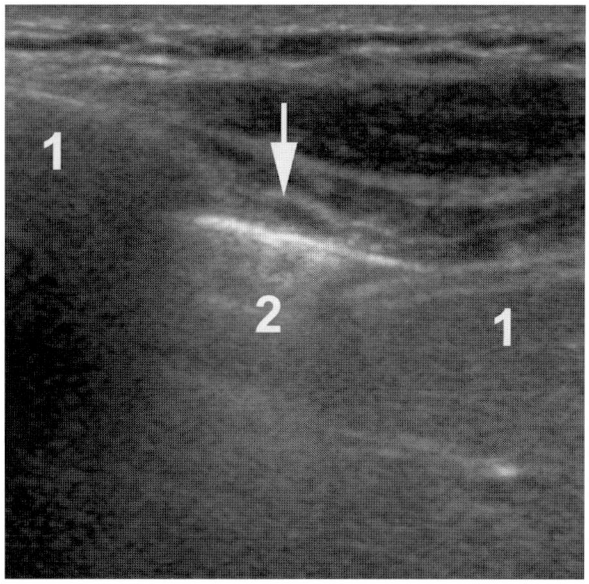

Fig. 2.22. Transverse US scan of the chest wall showing echogenic rib bones (*1*) with acoustic shadows covering the also echogenic lung (*2*) and the cross section of an intercostal nerve (*arrow*) inferior to its corresponding rib

The thoracic nerves of the inferior group and the "inguinal region trunk nerves" of the lumbar plexus (iliohypogastric, ilioinguinal and genitofemoral nerve) are usually only visible in pathological conditions with enlargement of the nerve, such as for example neuroma – the normal nerves are generally too small to be reliably assessed with sonography.

The dorsal root usually ends in a mixed segmental peripheral nerve releasing the posterior cutaneous branches – in the inferior dorsal region forming the superior and medial clunium nerves – and supplying the autochthon musculature with very fine terminal branches. The sonographic visualization of these nerves is also only achieved in the case of pathological alterations.

References

Bodner G, Huber B, Schwabegger A, et al (1999) Sonographic detection of radial nerve entrapment within a humerus fracture. J Ultrasound Med 18:703–706

Bodner G, Buchberger W, Schocke M, et al (2001) Radial nerve palsy associated with humeral shaft fracture: evaluation with US – initial experience. Radiology 219:811–816

Bodner G, Harpf C, Gardetto A, et al (2002) Ultrasonography of the accessory nerve. Normal and pathological findings in cadavers and patients with iatrogenic accessory nerve palsy. J Ultrasound Med 21:1159–1163

Duncan I, Sullivan P, Lomas F (1999) Sonography in the diagnosis of carpal tunnel syndrome. AJR Am J Roentgenol 173:681–684

Gassner E, Schocke M, Peer S, et al (2002) Persistent median artery in the carpal tunnel – color Doppler ultrasonographic findings. J Ultrasound Med 21:455–461

Graif M, Seton A, Nerubai J, et al (1991) Sciatic nerve: sonographic evaluation and anatomic-pathologic considerations. Radiology 181:405–408

Gruber H, Kovacs P, Piegger J, et al (2001) New, simple, ultrasound-guided infiltration of the pudendal nerve: topographic basics. Dis Colon Rectum 44:1376–1380

Gruber H, Peer S, Kovacs P, et al (2002) The ultrasound appearance of the femoral nerve and cases of iatrogenic impairment. J Ultrasound Med (in press)

Hafferl A (1969) Lehrbuch der Topographischen Anatomie, 3rd edn. Springer, Berlin Heidelberg New York

Kahle W (1991) Nervensystem und Sinnesorgane, 6th edn. Thieme, Stuttgart

Kovacs P, Gruber H, Piegger J, et al (2001) New, simple, ultrasound-guided infiltration of the pudendal nerve: ultrasonographic technique. Dis Colon Rectum 44: 1381–1385

Platzer W (1982) Atlas der topographischen Anatomie. Thieme, Stuttgart

Riffaud L, Morandi X, Godey B, et al (1999) Anatomic basis for the compression and neurolysis of the deep branch of the radial nerve in the radial tunnel. Surg Radiol Anat 21:229–233

Sarria L, Cabada T, Cozcolluela R, et al (2000) Carpal tunnel syndrome: usefulness of sonography. Eur Radiol 10:1920–1925

Silvestri E, Martinoli C, Derchi LE, et al (1995) Echotexture of peripheral nerves: correlation between US and histologic findings and criteria to differentiate tendons. Radiology 197:291–296

Thomas SJ, Yakin DE, Parry BR, et al (2000) The anatomical relationship between the posterior interosseous nerve and the supinator muscle. J Hand Surg [Am] 25:936–941

Von Lanz T, Wachsmuth W (1972) Praktische Anatomie, 4th edn. Springer, Berlin Heidelberg New York

Yang WT, Chui PT, Metreweli C (1998) Anatomy of the normal brachial plexus revealed by sonography and the role of sonographic guidance in anesthesia of the brachial plexus. AJR Am J Roentgenol 171:1631–1636

3 Nerve Compression Syndromes

S. Peer, S. Kiechl, G. Bodner

CONTENTS

3.1 Introduction 37
3.2 Ulnar Nerve Compression
S. Kiechl, S. Peer 38
3.2.1 Cubital Tunnel Syndrome 38
3.2.2 Guyon's Canal 44
3.3 Radial Nerve Compression 46
G. Bodner, S. Peer
3.3.1 Epidemiology and Clinical Presentation 46
3.4 Median Nerve Compression
S. Kiechl, S. Peer 48
3.4.1 Carpal Tunnel Syndrome 48
3.5 Peroneal Nerve Compression 54
S. Peer
3.5.1 Peroneal Tunnel Syndrome 54
3.6 Tibial Nerve Compression
S. Kiechl, S. Peer 55
3.6.1 Tarsal Tunnel Syndrome 55
References 57

3.1 Introduction

Generally speaking neuropathy caused by extrinsic compression may occur anywhere in the body and affect a variety of peripheral nerves. Special anatomic conditions, however, may result in an increased risk for the development of so-called entrapment neuropathies at certain locations. These conditions are various:

- Nerves may travel through narrow passageways together with tendons and vessels. Osteofibrous tunnels in the upper or lower limb, for example, are spaces superficially confined by tight fibrotic retinacula and at the bottom either by bone or musculotendinous structures. The retinacula, which are anchored on bony ridges or osseous prominences on either side of the tunnel prevent dislocation of the structures contained inside. Nerves traveling inside such tunnels may be affected by chronic external wear and tear often of uncertain origin, or by the presence of abnormal tissue inside the tunnel such as an ulnar artery aneurysm inside Guyon's canal for example.
- A nerve may also be compromised by an abnormally tight ligament or an anatomic muscle or vessel variant running across the nerve in an oblique course.
- At the forefoot, compression of the interdigital nerve against the transverse intermetatarsal ligament, associated with forefoot deformities or certain clothing habits, may lead to the development of Morton's metatarsalgia.
- Nerve compression may also occur secondary to trauma or surgery at certain sites, such as the posttraumatic tarsal tunnel syndrome, with development of neuropathy in a previously asymptomatic individual due to narrowing of the tarsal tunnel caused by malaligned fractures or callus formation.

No matter which underlying mechanism results in a compression syndrome, the reaction of a nerve to external compression has some common features. Chronic irritation of a nerve due to stretching or persistent compression is thought to interfere with the local intraneural microvasculature (Stewart 1993). Ischemia due to compression of the vasa nervorum and venous congestion results in epineural and endoneural edema. As the disease progresses to a more chronic state, fibrotic reactions in the nerve sheath result in further compromise to the fascicles.

S. Peer, MD
Professor, Department of Radiology, Section for Diagnostic and Interventional Sonography, University Hospital Innsbruck, Anichstrasse 35, 6020 Innsbruck, Austria
G. Bodner, MD
Professor, Department of Radiology, Section for Diagnostic and Interventional Sonography, University Hospital Innsbruck, Anichstrasse 35, 6020 Innsbruck, Austria
S. Kiechl, MD
Professor, Department of Neurology, Section for Electrodiagnosis (EMG/NLG), University Hospital Innsbruck, Anichstrasse 35, 6020 Innsbruck, Austria

Sonographic findings in patients with entrapment neuropathies reflect these pathophysiological reactions. Changes in echotexture and in shape and alignment of nerves may be detected. The nerve commonly shows an abrupt change in diameter, with flattening at the site of direct compression. This sonographic sign was first described for the detection of median nerve compression in the carpal tunnel by Buchberger and coworkers (Buchberger et al. 1991) and is now also considered to be a reliable measure for entrapment neuropathy in other locations (Chiou et al. 1998; Martinoli et al. 1996, 2000; Sarria et al. 2000). Proximal to the level of nerve entrapment localized enlargement of the nerve with swelling of fascicles is an expression of vasocongestion and edema (Martinoli et al. 2002; Nakamichi and Tachibana 2000; Peer et al. 2002). An increase in intraneural and perineural flow signals in color Doppler or power Doppler images is commonly seen and represents the hypervascular state seen in nonspecific, reactive inflammation (Martinoli et al. 2000). Changes in echotexture accompany a general change in nerve diameter with loss of fascicular discrimination at the site of maximum compression and flattening of the nerve, and swelling of individual fascicles or often coalescence of fascicles to a single large hypoechoic cord at the level of edema and vasocongestion.

In comparison with MRI, which is the only competing imaging modality for the work-up of nerve compression syndromes, sonography is low cost and generally available. At the same time sonography is nondiscomforting, quickly performed and easily adjusted to a patient's complaints in static as well as dynamic examinations. The latter are an important adjunct to the standard evaluation of peripheral nerve diseases, and especially valuable for the diagnosis of functional disorders such as the snapping triceps syndrome with ulnar nerve dislocation (Jacobson et al. 2001). This functional evaluation is beyond the abilities of MRI. A huge advantage of sonography in comparison with MRI is its ability to image longer nerve segments in a single study and its superior resolution. In contrast to these benefits, the quality of the information provided by sonography is user-dependent and the time to achieve a sufficient level of expertise in examination technique and interpretation of results is essentially longer than for MRI.

The next sections discuss the typical clinical and sonographic features of the most common compression syndromes in more detail.

3.2 Ulnar Nerve Compression

S. Kiechl, S. Peer

Ulnar nerve entrapment occurs at two distinct sites, at the elbow where the nerve courses around the medial humeral epicondyle (within or associated with the so-called cubital tunnel), and at the wrist (in Guyon's canal). The cubital tunnel is the most frequent site of ulnar nerve compression and, in relation to entrapment neuropathies of other nerves, second in frequency only to median nerve compression in the carpal tunnel. In contrast, ulnar nerve entrapment in Guyon's canal is rare (Campbell 2000).

3.2.1 Cubital Tunnel Syndrome

The cubital tunnel is an osteofibrous tunnel at the medial side of the elbow. Its roof is formed by a fibrous band called the cubital tunnel retinaculum (also called the Osborne fascia), which traverses from the medial epicondyle to the tip of the olecranon (see also Chapter 2). In this region the ulnar nerve in its course from the medial aspect of the upper arm to the palmar aspect of the forearm bends around the medial epicondyle in direct contact with the bone. Then the nerve runs between the ulnar and humeral head of the flexor carpi ulnaris muscle. The two muscle bellies are connected by an extension of the cubital tunnel retinaculum, the so-called arcuate ligament (Mazurek and Shin 2001). A certain amount of motion with stretching of the nerve and a decrease in the ulnar tunnel diameter is an anatomical feature of this site, which occurs in the normal, asymptomatic individual (Bozentka 1998). Certain additional conditions lead to decompensation with development of neuropathy (Bozentka 1998).

3.2.1.1 Epidemiology and Clinical Presentation

Ulnar nerve compression at the elbow is the second most common mononeuropathy of the upper extremities. As the initial clinical feature, patients typically note numbness in the fifth and medial half of the fourth fingers sometimes spreading to the medial hand (Fig. 3.1). Typically sensory disturbances do not extend much beyond the wrist. Pain and tenderness occur at the medial epicondyle and radiate along the ulnar forearm to the hand. Complaints may be provoked or enhanced by trigger situations such as rest-

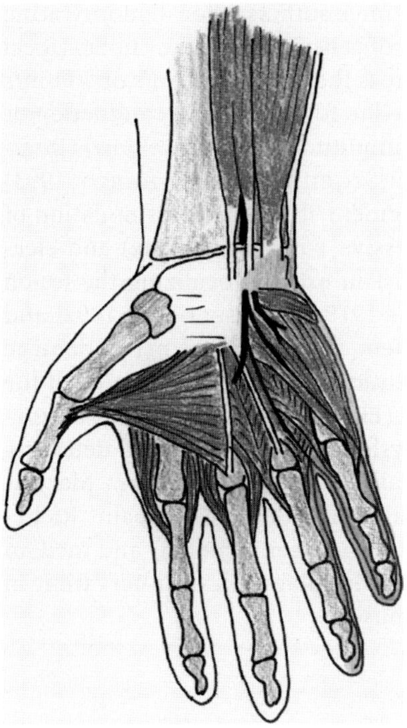

Fig. 3.1. Anatomy of the ulnar nerve (*dark gray* motor innervation, *light gray* sensory innervation)

ing of the elbow on a hard surface, applying external pressure to the groove, maximal flexion of the elbow or repetitive flexion and extension movements.

In the common case of progressive nerve damage, weakness of ulnar-innervated hand muscles occurs and causes an abnormal posture of the hand ("ulnar clawing") and significant disability in the performance and fine control of finger movements. Abduction of the little finger due to paresis of the fourth interosseous muscle is recognized as Wartenberg's sign (Mumenthaler et al. 1998). Forearm flexors (flexor carpi ulnaris and digitorum profundus muscles) are less-prominently involved or exceptionally even spared. Muscle wasting is best visible at the first interosseous space and hypothenar eminence. In some patients, motor deficits develop insidiously without sensory symptoms.

3.2.1.2 Etiology

On passing through the ulnar groove at the elbow the nerve is susceptible to compression injury (Miller 1991). The precise mechanisms of nerve damage and the nature of the compressive pathology are highly heterogeneous:

1. External compression is the most common cause and derives from repeated or sustained leaning on the elbow. It may cause substantial (cumulative) nerve injury particularly in the cases of a predisposing shallow condylar groove, subluxated nerve or sustained pressure in coma or anesthetized patients (Miller and Camp 1979).
2. Real entrapment occurs in the *ulnar sulcus* if the nerve is constricted by scar tissue, in the *cubital tunnel* ("cubital tunnel syndrome") (Campbell et al. 1991; Miller and Hummel 1980) where the ulnar nerve passes under the aponeurotic origin of the flexor carpi ulnaris muscle (1–3 cm distal to the epicondyle) or in the *flexor pronator aponeurosis* (more than 4 cm distal to the epicondyle).
3. Tardy ulnar nerve palsy typically develops years after fracture or luxation of the elbow based on bone exostosis or cubitus varus or valgus abnormalities. Other causative bone abnormalities are advanced arthrosis, osteoarthritis or hyperostosis in Paget's disease, to name just a few.
4. Recurrent prominent luxation of the ulnar nerve over the medial condyle can directly damage the nerve or predispose it to repetitive trauma.
5. Soft tissue masses in the condylar groove or cubital tunnel such as organized hematoma, scarring, accessory muscles (anconeus epitrochlearis muscle) or intraneural ganglia are further potential sources of ulnar nerve compression.

3.2.1.3 Diagnosis

The diagnosis of ulnar neuropathy is – in most cases – reliably established by an experienced clinician after reviewing the patient's history (emphasis put on trigger situations) and performing a thorough neurological examination. A sensitive and highly characteristic clinical test is Froment's maneuver (Fig. 3.2). When attempting to pinch a piece of paper between the thumb and index finger, the patient primarily utilizes the median-innervated long flexor of the thumb as a compensation for the ulnar hand weakness, and a typical flexed thumb posture emerges.

Other diagnoses mimicking ulnar neuropathy such as lower trunk or medial cord brachial plexus palsy, combined C8 and Th1 radiculopathy or distal ulnar nerve entrapment can be differentiated based on the pattern of sensory and motor deficits. Diagnostic work-up of patients with ulnar compression at or adjacent to the elbow should include a palpatory examination of the ulnar nerve at the ulnar groove for an abnormal thickening, tenderness, decreased

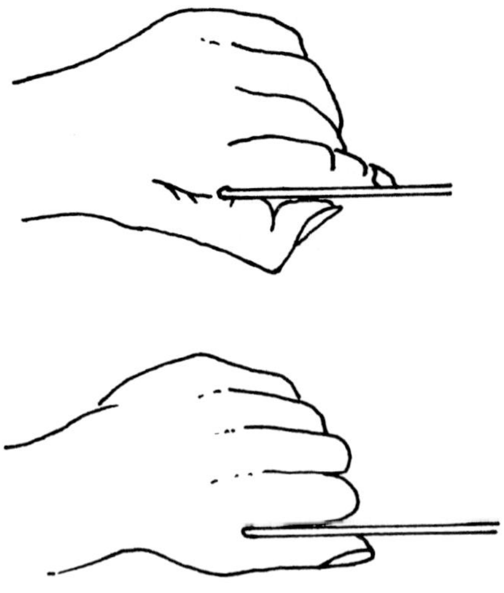
a
b

Fig. 3.2. Froment's maneuver. *a* In the case of ulnar nerve palsy a typical flexed thumb posture emerges when the patient attempts to pinch a piece of paper between the thumb and index finger. *b* Maneuver in a normal subject

mobility or luxability. Subsequently, provocation tests (maximal elbow flexion for the cubital tunnel syndrome and assessment of Tinel's sign), radiography of the elbow and high-resolution sonography of the nerve and neighboring tissues have to be performed.

Electrodiagnostic studies play a central role in evaluating suspected ulnar nerve lesions. Standard nerve conduction studies performed in a flexed elbow position are sometimes sufficient for demonstrating segmental slowing of sensory and motor fibers (focal demyelination) across the elbow (<45 m/s or >11 m/s difference compared to forearm nerve conduction or >20% drop in the amplitude across the elbow) (LIVESON and MA 1992; STOEHR and BLUTHARDT 1993) (Fig. 3.3). Short segment stimulation (stimulation of the nerve in successive 1-cm increments) and electromyography assist in exactly localizing the lesion (MILLER and CAMP 1979; CAMPBELL et al. 1992) and estimating the extent and acuity of nerve damage relevant to therapeutic decisions and planning of the surgical approach (Fig. 8.14). In addition, the experienced electrophysiologist is capable of detecting innervation anomalies such as the forearm Martin-Gruber anastomosis (Fig. 8.15) or the palm Riche-Cannieu anastomosis between the ulnar and median nerves, and of defining the origin of innervation in the various hand muscles.

3.2.1.4 Therapy

Careful exploration for relevant trigger events and behaviors causing external nerve compression are crucial to a successful therapy. In such cases strict avoidance strategies are often sufficient for a reversal of symptoms and prevention of progressive nerve damage (DELLON et al. 1993). In the absence of external traumata conservative therapy for ulnar

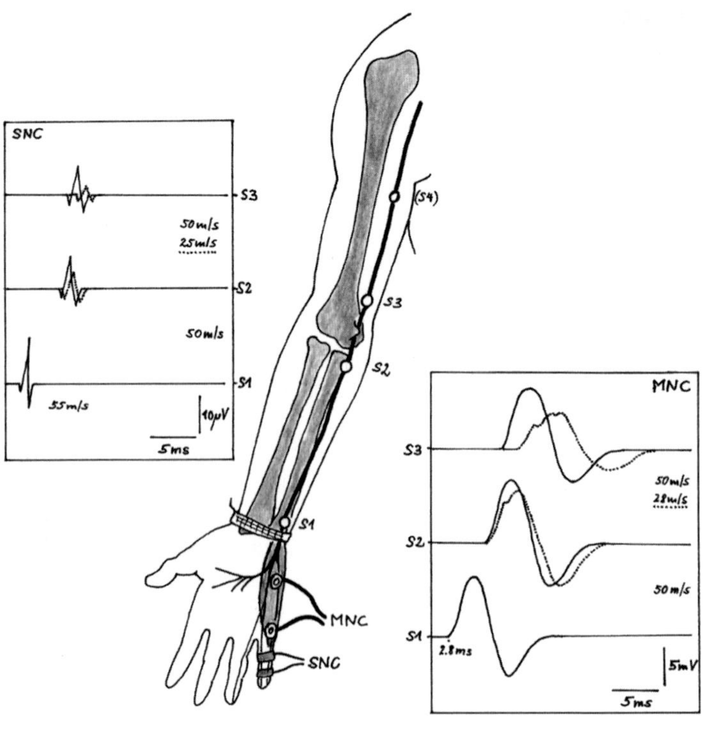

Fig. 3.3. Ulnar nerve. Motor nerve conduction (*MNC*) and antidromic sensory nerve conduction (*SNC*) studies. Routinely, stimulation is performed at the wrist (*S1*), and below (*S2*) and above the elbow (*S3*). Motor potentials are recorded from the abductor digiti minimi muscle (*disk electrodes*) and sensory potentials from the fifth finger (*ring electrodes*). The recordings presented are from a normal subject (*full line*) and a patient with ulnar neuropathy at the elbow (*dotted line*)

nerve compression is limited. Steroid injection and oral antiinflammatory drugs are not useful.

Surgical treatment of cubital tunnel syndrome consists either of complete decompression of the nerve (releasing the nerve from compressive adhesions and bands), or of decompression with transposition of the nerve under the flexor muscle (ARLE and ZAGER 2000). A surgical procedure (release of the nerve at the ulnar groove or cubital tunnel or submuscular transposition of the nerve) (CAMPBELL et al. 1988) is reserved for patients with significant sensorimotor deficits or a severe pain syndrome. Results are generally satisfactory unless substantial damage has already been done prior to intervention.

3.2.1.5 *Sonography*

From a technical point of view sonography of the cubital tunnel is best performed with a high-resolution linear scanhead of 12 to 15 MHz. For example, on the ATL HDI5000 (ATL-Philips, Bothell, Wash., USA) – which is our standard equipment – we prefer to use the small size 15 MHz intraoperative transducer. Because of its small build this transducer allows easy access to the somewhat restricted space at the medial epicondyle. A standoff pad may also be used for improvement of image quality. Standard documentation of findings is in transverse and longitudinal planes at the medial aspect of the upper arm, medial epicondyle and at the forearm just distal to the cubital tunnel.

The best sonographic access to the ulnar nerve is gained with the patient lying supine on the examination table, with the arm to be examined close to the sonographer. We normally use an additional small pillow to position the fully stretched arm in about 45 degrees of abduction with forced supination (Fig. 3.4). This maneuver results in a stable position, which is easily held by the patient for longer times and allows access to the ulnar nerve along its complete course at the upper arm and forearm. Forced supination and external rotation of the outstretched arm positions the nerve in an almost straight course from above the elbow to the proximal forearm, which facilitates the acquisition of longitudinal sonograms inside the cubital tunnel. The latter is of considerable importance if panoramic images are taken, as the sweep of the scanhead along the nerve is much more easily accomplished with the nerve in an elongated position (Fig. 3.5).

Tension on the nerve is minimal in this position, as the outstretched arm limits tractional forces (BOZENTKA 1998), which is why we recommend this position for measurements of nerve diameters. With elbow flexion the nerve gets flattened even in healthy individuals, which must not be mistaken for compression (OKAMOTO et al. 2000). After documentation of the nerve's shape and echotexture in this basic position, functional sonograms are acquired with passive flexion and/or rotation of the elbow. With these maneuvers we aim to detect of reduced longitudinal nerve motion or subluxation as well as changing nerve diameter in certain positions of the elbow.

We usually start the examination with identification of the ulnar nerve in a transverse plane at the inner side of the upper arm, where it courses in a superficial position alongside the dorsal margin of the biceps muscle. From here we follow the nerve down to the ulnar sulcus and onward to the proximal forearm. During this first sweep we record any changes in nerve diameter, with standard measurements acquired about 3 cm above and below, as well

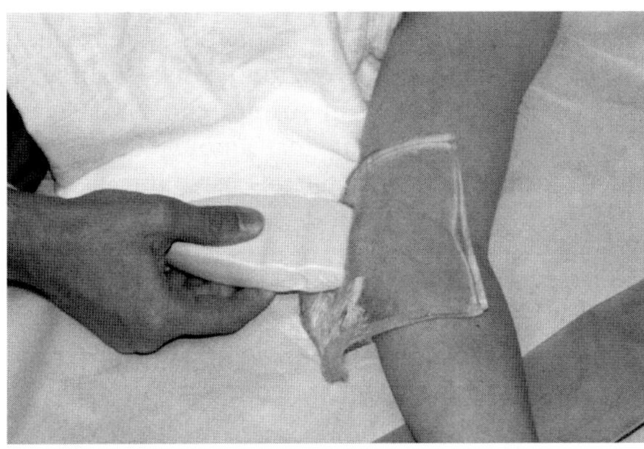

Fig. 3.4. Position of transducer for identification of the ulnar nerve at the level of the upper arm. With positioning of the transducer posterior to the medial epicondyle, the superficially coursing nerve is easily identified

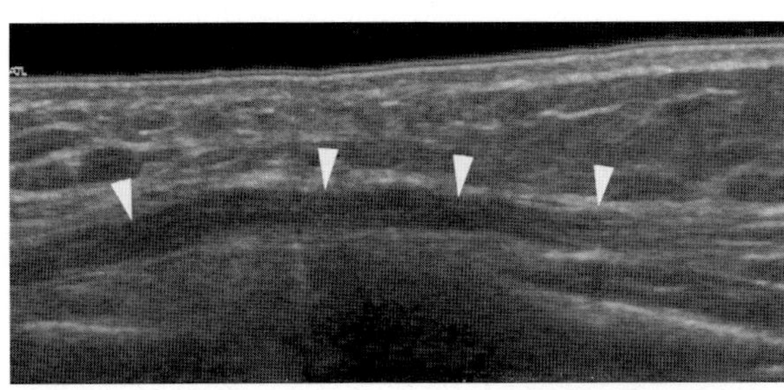

Fig. 3.5. Longitudinal panoramic sonogram in a patient with cubital tunnel syndrome. The ulnar nerve (*arrowheads*) shows mildly edematous, hypoechoic fascicles along its course inside the sulcus, with a smooth transition to a more normal appearing echotexture at the level of the upper arm (at the right hand margin of image)

as inside the cubital tunnel. While the nerve has a more oval shape at the level of the upper arm and forearm, it typically appears to be round inside the cubital tunnel. In a study by Chiou et al. on ten healthy volunteers, short and long axis diameters of the ulnar nerve as well as cross-section areas were measured at the level of the epicondyle and 5 cm above and below the elbow (Chiou et al. 1998). Their measurements are presented in Table 3.1 and show an increase in cross-section area at the level of the epicondyle where the nerve is more rounded in shape.

Table 3.1. Ulnar nerve diameter and cross-sectional areas in normal subjects (Chiou et al. 1998)

	Short axis (cm)	Long axis (cm)	Cross-sectional area (cm^2)
Upper arm	0.189	0.3	0.057
Epicondyle	0.182	0.374	0.068
Forearm	0.208	0.297	0.062

The sonographer has to be aware of this typical increase in ulnar nerve size inside the cubital tunnel and not mistake it for cubital tunnel disease. Indeed, we believe this increase in size to represent a reaction of the nerve to a normal amount of traction and stretching inside the narrow osteofibrous canal, without any implication of disease. Changes in nerve diameter have traditionally been used for the diagnosis of carpal tunnel disease (Buchberger et al. 1991; Lee et al. 1999; Martinoli et al. 2000), and the same has been advocated for the cubital tunnel. In contrast to healthy asymptomatic subjects, patients with cubital tunnel syndrome show an enlarged ulnar nerve at the level of the epicondyle, while measurements at the upper arm and forearm do not differ significantly (Chiou et al. 1998).

The normal ulnar nerve shows the characteristic findings of peripheral nerves on transverse planes, which is a hyperechoic epineurium and perineurium with a number of individually discernible fascicles (Fig. 3.6). This pattern is always observed at the upper arm and forearm, while at the epicondyle the nerve may appear more hypoechoic, with some enlargement of single fascicles. The latter may be due to some amount of anisotropy because of a more curvilinear course of the nerve in this region (Martinoli et al. 2000). Together with the slight increase in nerve diameter inside the cubital tunnel, this may as well reflect a "normal amount" of localized edema, with gradual transition towards a symptomatic state. Our experience has led us to favor the second explanation, but this has not been confirmed in clinically controlled trials. As a general rule, we always observe a distinct hyperechoic superficial epineurium in normal nerves, no matter how thick the nerve or its fascicles are.

In symptomatic patients we observe diminished fascicular discrimination and an indistinct outer surface due to epineural edema with infiltration of surrounding soft tissues (Fig. 3.7a).

While the described features of the ulnar nerve are more easily seen in the transverse plane, subsequently acquired longitudinal planes or panoramic views are better suited for evaluation of abrupt changes in nerve diameter at the level of compression (Fig. 3.8).

Color Doppler and/or power Doppler scans are acquired in nerves with B-mode findings suggestive for neuropathy. Particularly in the longitudinal plane an increase in epineural and perineural vessels may be detected representing a hypervascular inflammatory state. We also try to obtain Doppler flow spectra from the ulnar collateral artery, which is considered the main arterial source for the ulnar nerve (Balogh et al. 1997; Prevel et al. 1993). Our preliminary experience indicates a change from a normal monophasic

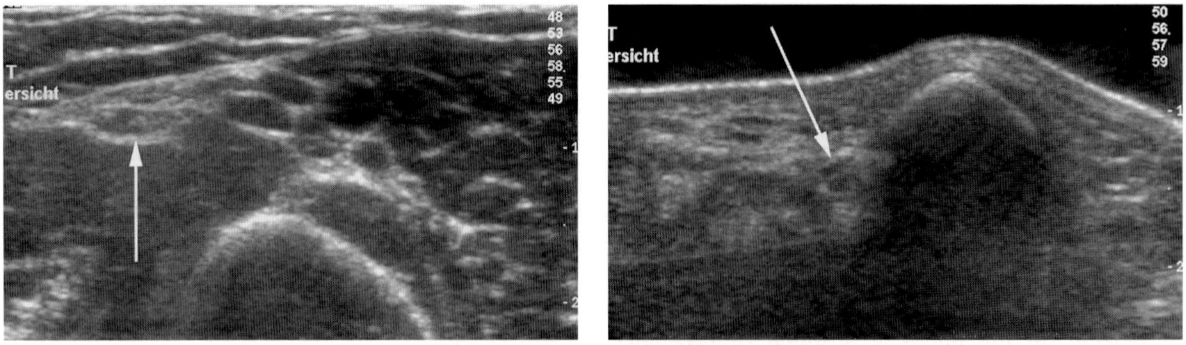

Fig. 3.6. Transverse sonograms through normal ulnar nerve (*arrows*) at the level of the upper arm (*left*) and cubital tunnel (*right*) showing typical appearance with distinct epineurium and a variable number of individually discernible fascicles

a 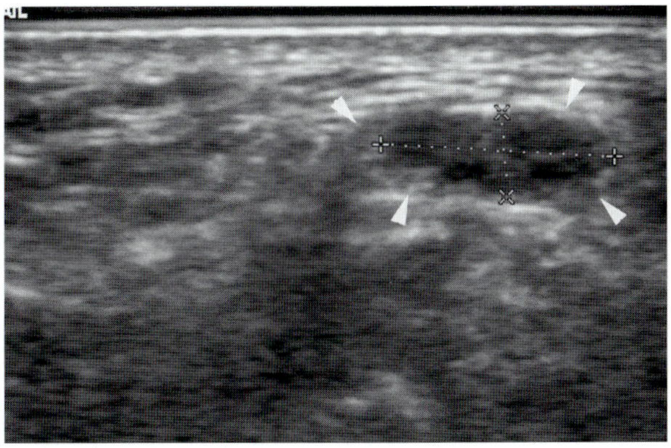

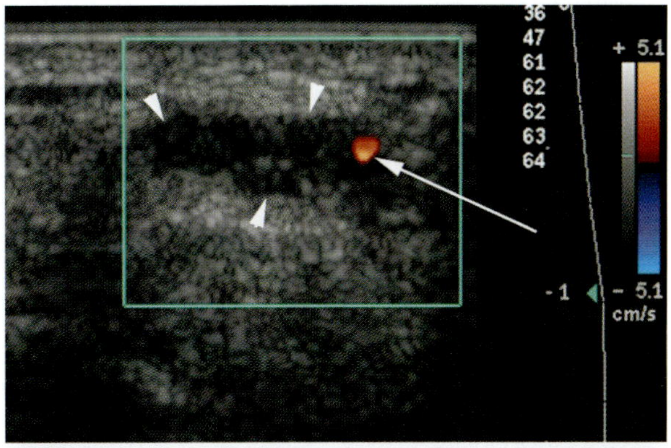

b

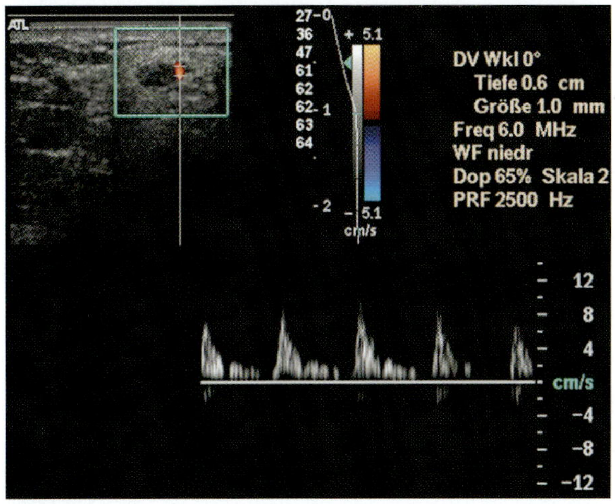

c

Fig. 3.7a–c. Transverse sonogram (**a**), color Doppler sonogram (**b**) and spectral wave analysis in a patient with cubital tunnel disease. **a** Enlargement of the nerve with loss of fascicular discrimination and surrounding hypoechoic edema (*arrowheads*) is seen. **b** With color Doppler sonography an enlarged perineural vessel (*arrow*) is detected inside the nerve (*arrowheads*). **c** With spectral wave analysis this vessel shows a biphasic spectrum with positive diastolic flow

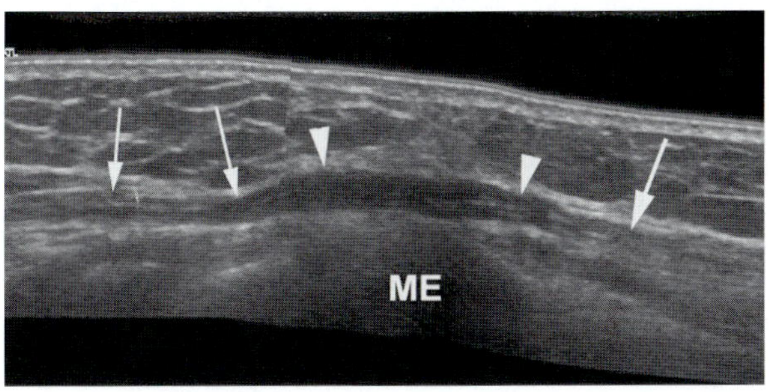

Fig. 3.8. Longitudinal panoramic sonogram through ulnar nerve at the elbow in a patient with cubital tunnel disease. Marked swelling of the nerve on its course through the cubital tunnel is seen (*arrowheads*) with normal caliber and echotexture proximally and distally (*arrows*) (*ME* medial epicondyle)

or triphasic high-resistance peripheral flow spectrum to a biphasic spectrum with continuous positive diastolic flow in symptomatic patients, which may reflect the hyperemia in neuropathy (Fig. 3.7b, c).

There are essentially four different sites of potential ulnar nerve compression in the region of the elbow. From proximal to distal they are: the medial intermuscular septum, the retroepicondylar groove, the humeroulnar arcade and the point of exit of the nerve from the flexor carpi ulnaris (Campbell 2000). Of these anatomic locations the ulnar groove is the site most frequently responsible for entrapment, while compression at the other sites is rare. Pathological conditions such as arthrotic bone spurs in the condylar groove, ganglia, heterotopic ossifications or loose bodies, or an accessory anconeus epitrochlearis muscle (Fig. 3.9) may promote development of entrapment neuropathy (O'Driscoll et al. 1992; Puig et al. 1999).

In contrast to the carpal tunnel retinaculum, the normal cubital tunnel retinaculum is only infrequently visualized with sonography. In cases of cubital tunnel syndrome, however, a thickened retinaculum may occasionally be detected. In the case of compression, the ulnar nerve presents with abrupt narrowing at the site of compression and marked swelling with loss of fascicular texture proximal to this level (Fig. 3.10a). Marked edema in the epineurium and surrounding soft tissues are additional characteristic findings (Fig. 3.10b).

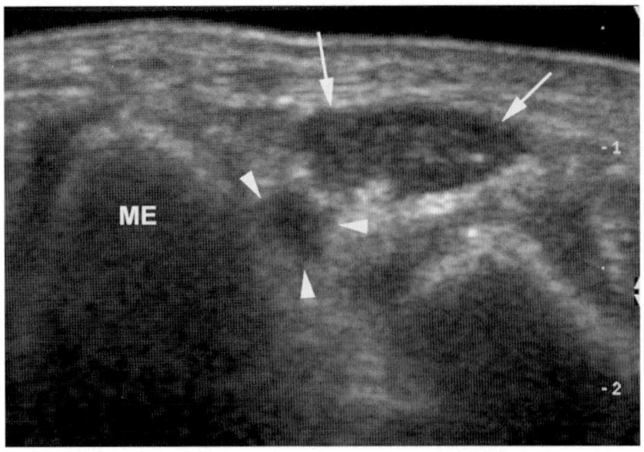

Fig. 3.9. Transverse sonogram at medial side of the elbow in a patient with a palpable mass and associated evidence of ulnar nerve compression. A large accessory muscle belly (*arrows*) overlying the ulnar nerve is demonstrated consistent with anconeus epitrochlearis muscle. Note loss of fascicular discrimination in the ulnar nerve with epineural edema (*arrowheads*) (*ME* medial epicondyle)

a

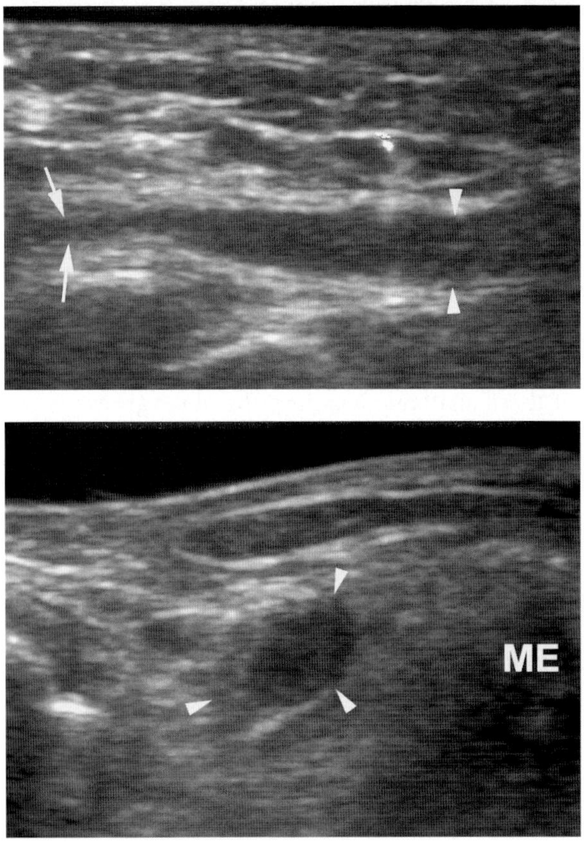

b

Fig. 3.10a, b. Longitudinal (**a**) and transverse (**b**) sonograms in a patient with cubital tunnel disease. Marked swelling of the ulnar nerve above the level of compression (**a** *arrowheads*) with return to normal size distal to the medial epicondyle (**a** *arrows*). Loss of fascicular discrimination and perineural edema is seen on the transverse scan (**b** *arrowheads*) (*ME* medial epicondyle)

Hypervascularization of the nerve and changes in Doppler spectra of recurrent ulnar artery and/or ulnar collateral artery may further be detected.

The typical features of cubital tunnel syndrome are:

- Abrupt narrowing of the ulnar nerve at site of compression
- Swelling of the nerve above level of compression
- Loss of fascicular texture
- Indistinct outer surface of the nerve
- Edema in surrounding soft tissues
- Hypervascularization

A special condition that may be present in asymptomatic individuals but also account for ulnar neuropathy at the elbow is ulnar nerve dislocation. This represents an abnormal movement of the ulnar nerve out of the cubital tunnel and anterior to the medial epicondyle during flexion of the elbow (Childress 1975), which is caused by absence of the cubital tunnel retinaculum. Neuropathy is induced by abnormal friction and tear to the nerve during recurrent dislocation. Ulnar nerve dislocation shares a clinical feature – a transient snapping sensation during flexion of the elbow – with snapping triceps syndrome, which represents medial dislocation of the medial head of the triceps muscle. Both syndromes may exist side by side or in an isolated form. Because of the overlap in clinical findings they are not easily distinguished during physical examination (Spinner and Goldner 1998). However, differentiation of the two entities is necessary as the approach for surgical treatment will differ. Dynamic sonography is helpful in this regard, as it allows direct visualization of ulnar nerve and/or triceps muscle dislocation during active flexion and extension of the elbow (Jacobson et al. 2001; Okamoto et al. 2000). However, the diagnosis of ulnar nerve dislocation may be missed if excessive transducer pressure is applied, which can prevent the nerve from dislocating. Sonography typically shows abnormal movement of the nerve and/or muscle at the level of the medial epicondyle (Fig. 3.11). In addition, the characteristic snap may be felt with the transducer. In symptomatic individuals an enlarged cross section of the nerve and edema are signs of neuropathy, just as in the traditional cubital tunnel syndrome (Jacobson et al. 2001).

3.2.2 Guyon's Canal

Proximal to the wrist the ulnar nerve runs superficially to the flexor retinaculum and lies under the tendon of the flexor carpi ulnaris. Then it turns

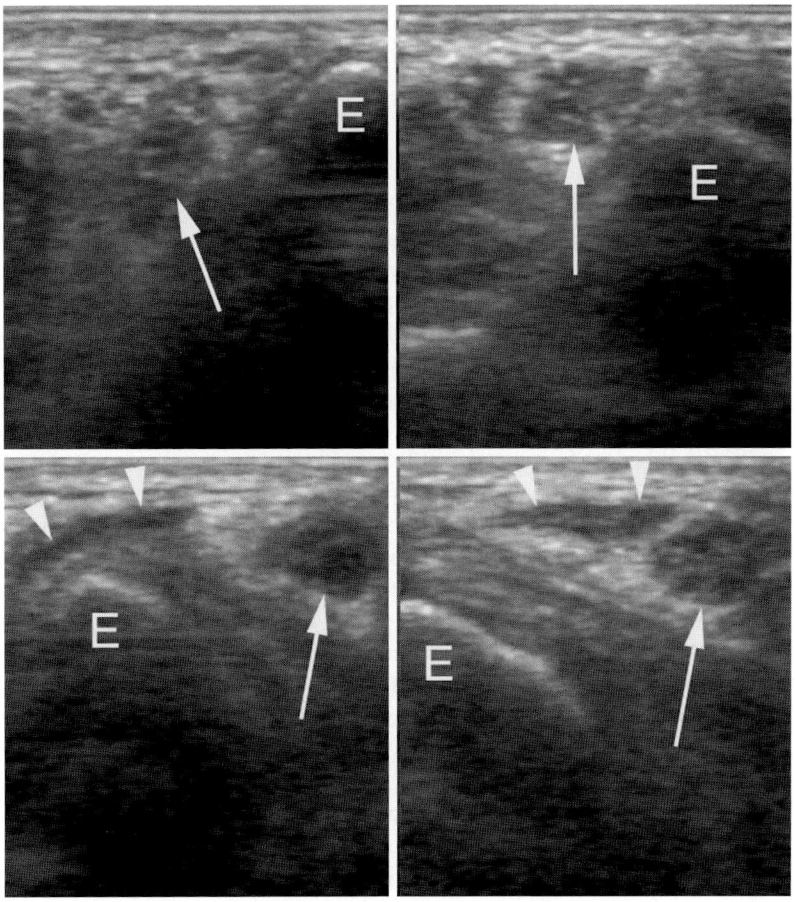

Fig. 3.11. Series of transverse sonograms acquired during flexion of the elbow (*left to right* extension to maximum flexion). The ulnar nerve (*arrow*) dislocates ventrally to the epicondyle during elbow flexion and is followed by the medial head of the triceps muscle (*arrowheads*) later in the movement (*E* epicondyle)

radial to the pisiform bone entering a fibrous tunnel called Guyon's canal. The roof of this canal consists of the palmar carpal ligament and the palmaris brevis muscle, the floor is formed mostly by the flexor retinaculum with contributions from the flexor digitorum profundus, the pisohamate and pisometacarpal ligaments and the opponens digiti minimi. It is bordered by the pisiform and the hook of the hamate (Mazurek and Shin 2001). On its course through the canal, the ulnar nerve is accompanied by the ulnar artery and vein. In the distal portion of the tunnel the nerve bifurcates into a deep motor branch and a superficial sensory branch. Compared with cubital tunnel syndrome, entrapment of the ulnar nerve inside Guyon's canal is rare.

3.2.2.1 Clinical Considerations

The ulnar nerve may be compressed anywhere along its course through Guyon's canal resulting in sensory, motor or sensorimotor symptoms. According to the level of compression, three distinct neurological syndromes are discerned. More proximal compression at the entrance of the nerve into the canal results in weakness of intrinsic hand muscles innervated by the ulnar nerve (all interossei, lumbricalis II and IV, hypothenar muscles) plus a sensory deficit in the hypothenar and ulnar half of the ring finger, both on the palmar surface only. Compression along the deep branch results in mere motor deficits, whereas compression in the distal canal results in sensory deficits only.

There are a variety of reasons for ulnar neuropathy at the level of Guyon's canal including, among others: reduction in the canal's diameter by space-occupying lesions such as ganglia (Shea and McClain 1969), lipoma (Bui-Mansfield et al. 2002), or pseudoaneurysms (Lorea and Schuind 2000); posttraumatic nerve irritation, for example by hook of the hamate fractures or Galeazzi fracture-dislocation (Pecina et al. 2001); and occupationally related external compression, vascular disturbances and hypertrophy of the flexor carpi ulnaris muscle.

A trial of conservative treatment is usually instituted in patients with neuropathy, which will take up to 6 months to work. If no improvement is achieved within this time the lesion should be treated surgically with decompression of the nerve.

3.2.2.2 *Sonography*

From a technical standpoint (sonographic equipment) what has been said for sonography of the ulnar nerve at the elbow is equally true for examination of Guyon's canal. With the patient lying supine or sitting, the hand is positioned on a pillow with the palm facing up, and a standoff pad is always used. After identification of the nerve at the distal forearm in a transverse plane, it is followed to the canal, where it is easily visualized and consists of a tiny ovoid structure with a hyperechoic epineurium and only two or three small fascicles. The latter will only be discriminated if a high-frequency transducer is used, otherwise the nerve will only appear as a thin rounded or ovoid structure. With high-resolution equipment the bifurcation of the nerve and its branches may also be visualized and followed for a certain distance. While the sensory branch tends to follow the ulnar artery, the motor branch runs more deeply.

As already mentioned above, ulnar neuropathy at Guyon's canal is rare and in many cases due to additional pathologies, such as tiny ulnar artery aneurysms, ganglia related to the pisotriquetral joint or malaligned fractures. These space-occupying lesions are easily assessed with sonography. In all of these situations the nerve in addition shows the characteristic findings for peripheral nerve compression, which are mentioned above: swelling, edema, etc. (Fig. 3.12).

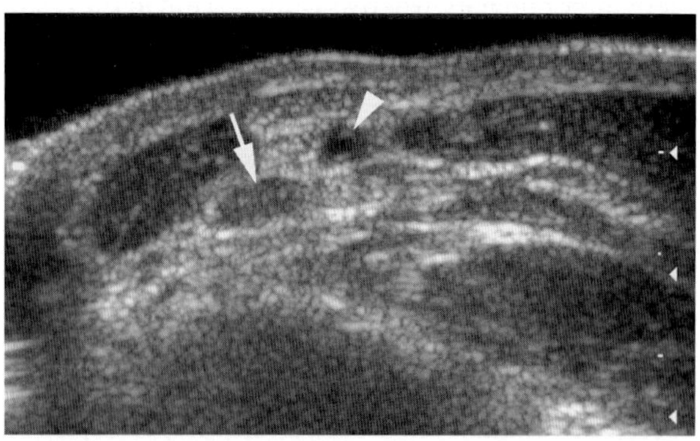

Fig. 3.12. Transverse sonogram in patient with numbness and paresthesias in the fifth finger. Swelling of the ulnar nerve (*arrow*) with loss of fascicular discrimination is shown on its course through Guyon's canal (*arrowhead* ulnar artery)

3.3 Radial Nerve Compression

G. Bodner, S. Peer

The syndrome of radial nerve compression mainly centers around a possible pathology along the course of the nerve inside the so-called radial tunnel, which was first described as an infrequent cause of persistent tennis elbow (Roles and Maudsley 1972). This syndrome is known as supinator syndrome, "radial tunnel syndrome" or "posterior interosseous nerve paralysis". This type of nerve palsy is often misdiagnosed as lateral epicondylitis. It has to be mentioned that the radial tunnel syndrome is heavily disputed in the literature (Kalb et al. 1999; Rosenbaum 1999). Today there is some evidence that misdiagnosis of radial nerve compression may have occurred in several cases, and even postsurgical improvement of a patient's symptoms is not considered evidence of the true existence of radial tunnel disease by some authors (Rosenbaum 1999). High-resolution sonography may prove helpful in this regard with direct demonstration of radial nerve compression and subsequent structural changes inside the nerve bundle (Bodner2002).

Other extrinsic compression syndromes of the radial nerve may occur due to external forces or coexisting pathology such as ganglia at the elbow or musculoskeletal tumors.

3.3.1 Epidemiology and Clinical Presentation

3.3.1.1 *Etiology*

A frequent external radial nerve compression syndrome among chronic drinkers is caused by the abnormal position of the upper limb, when the arm is stretched across a hard support (Sturzenegger and Rutz 1991). This syndrome is commonly referred to as "Saturday night nerve palsy". Other causes for nerve compressions may be ganglia at the elbow (Ogino et al. 1991) or an anomalous triceps muscle (Wilhelm 1985), which can impinge on the nerve or strain the nerve during arm motion or muscle contraction. Other rare cases for radial nerve palsy are tumors, lymph node metastases and persistent pressure from crutches (Phalen et al. 1971).

The radial tunnel is not a bony or osteofibrous tunnel in its true sense. It is defined as the potential space created by structures surrounding the radial nerve and its posterior interosseous branch as they travel through the proximal forearm from the humeroradial joint past the proximal edge of the supinator muscle. Along approximately 5 cm various anatomical structures may lead to radial nerve compression: fibrous bands, a fan of branches from the radial artery, edges of the extensor carpi radialis and supinator muscles. The last of these may sometimes be of a tendinous nature The proximal edge of the supinator muscle, known as the arcade of Frohse, is tendinous in about half the population (Spinner 1968). At the "radial tunnel" two distinct and probably completely different nerve compression syndromes exist. The first is the so-called "radial tunnel syndrome", which appears to be a mere painful syndrome at the proximal forearm. The second syndrome with definite muscular weakness is called "posterior interosseous nerve syndrome".

3.3.1.2 Clinical Considerations

The clinical work-up of a patient with radial nerve palsy includes a detailed physical and neurological examination. As a general guideline sensory and motor radial deficiency relates to a proximal (axillary) compression. Motor radial deficiency, sparing the triceps muscle, appears in compression syndromes at the spiral groove. Weakness of finger extension, sparing the extensor carpi radialis supports the presence of a compression syndrome of the deep branch of the radial nerve.

Electroneurographic examination is currently the method of choice to indicate the level of nerve compression and to assess functional nerve recovery. In most cases of a radial nerve palsy, conduction studies show activity and therefore integrity of the nerve. Follow-up EMG can assess the amount of recovery. Nerve conduction tests, however, are unable to differentiate the cause of nerve compression, for example if the nerve is dissected in traumatic lesions, impinged or severely encased by callus. In these cases no or only minimal neurological activity can be measured. It is, however, important to diagnose the cause of the nerve compression at an early stage, as irreversible degeneration of the motor end plate of the muscle may occur after 6 to 12 months. According to the literature, a nerve without signs of recovery has to undergo surgical inspection. The lack of information from electroneurographic testing regarding integrity of the nerve calls for a noninvasive method such as sonography to accurately visualize the nerve itself.

The radial tunnel syndrome is characterized by pain and tenderness in the region of the radial tunnel, with an increase in pain during certain maneuvers, such as resisted extension of the middle finger or resisted supination with extension of the elbow. These maneuvers contract the extensor carpi radialis and/or supinator muscle with possible impingement of the radial nerve. Patients with radial tunnel syndrome differ clinically from patients with true compression neuropathies in so far as they do not show any prominent focal tenderness, any neurological deficit or pathological findings during electrodiagnostic testing (Rosenbaum 1999).

The posterior interosseous nerve syndrome or "true neurogenic radial tunnel syndrome" (Rosenbaum 1999) manifests with muscle weakness typically sparing the extensor carpi radialis (no wrist drop!), but during wrist extension the hand may deviate radially because of weakness of the extensor carpi ulnaris. There is impairment of finger extension at the metacarpophalangeal joints, as well as reduced function of the abductor pollicis longus, and extensor pollicis longus and brevis muscle. This clinical syndrome may be caused by a variety of structures compressing the nerve along the radial tunnel and compression at the arcade of Frohse is most common.

3.3.1.3 Sonography

Using a 5–12 MHz broad-band linear array the radial nerve is easily detected in a transverse scan at the lateral aspect of the mid-humerus, and may afterwards be followed upward or downward from this level. In addition color Doppler sonography allows visualization of the accompanying deep brachial artery, which may serve as a guideline for identification of the nerve. It consists of four to eight hypoechoic tubular structures (fascicle groups) surrounded by an echoic rim. The nerves normal transverse diameter ranges from 4.0 to 4.2 mm and the normal anteroposterior diameter ranges from 2.3 to 3.5 mm. The nerve changes its form from a more rounded shape at the proximal part to oval at the central part and rounded again at the distal part of the humerus. At the level of the lateral condyle between the brachioradialis and brachialis muscle, the nerve splits into two branches, the deep and superficial branches, which may also be assessed with sonography (Bodner et al. 2002).

The impingement of the deep branch of the radial nerve at the level of the supinator muscle can be detected with sonography. In our own case series of four patients with a supinator syndrome, sonography allowed clear visualization of an edematous nerve with a caliber change proximal to the supinator muscle in all cases. The echotexture of the affected nerve was hypoechoic and rich vascularity was seen at the superficial epineurium. Intraoperative nerve inspection confirmed the sonographic findings (Fig. 3.13) (BODNER et al. 2002).

3.3.1.4
Therapy

In cases with proven radial nerve compression inside the radial tunnel surgical decompression is advocated (RITTS et al. 1987). While the normal patient work-up implies clinical and electrodiagnostic follow-up examinations for at least 6 weeks and surgery if no improvement of deficits is obtained under conservative management, this rationale may change with the introduction of sonography. If an underlying anatomical and surgically treatable cause for radial nerve paralysis is detected early surgery may be advocated based on sonographic findings.

3.4
Median Nerve Compression

S. KIECHL, S. PEER

Compression neuropathy of the median nerve is the most common of all entrapment neuropathies and is practically only found at the carpal tunnel. At this site the median nerve travels through a narrow passage together with the flexor tendons and is therefore subject to entrapment if any coexisting condition results in a further decrease of the space underneath the flexor retinaculum. These secondary neuropathies caused by ganglia of the wrist, tendonitis of the flexor tendons, etc. are rare and so is compression of the median nerve in another location along its course from the shoulder to the wrist. The main disease entity we focus on in this paragraph, therefore, is the so-called idiopathic carpal tunnel syndrome (CTS).

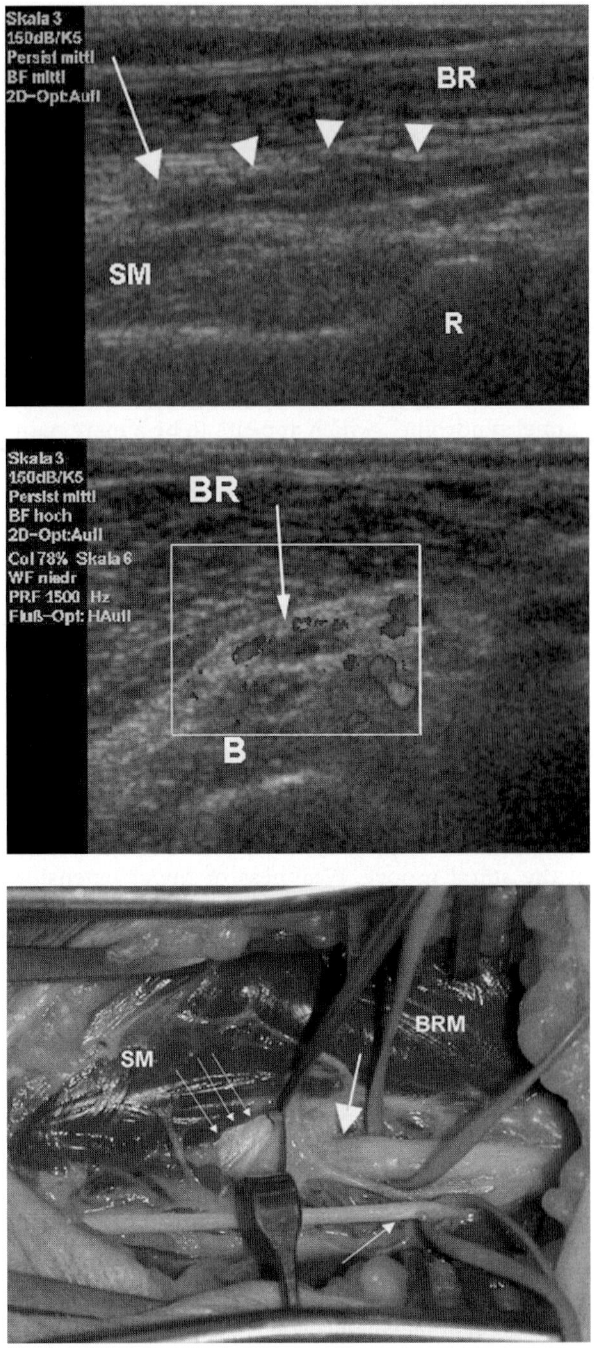

Fig. 3.13a–c. Longitudinal sonogram (**a**) in a patient with clinical evidence of supinator syndrome shows a hypoechoic tubular structure (*arrowheads*) with a reduction in nerve diameter (*arrow*) at the entry into the supinator muscle (*SM*) (*BR* brachioradialis muscle, *R* radial head). Transverse sonogram (**b**) shows a hypoechoic structure corresponding to the deep radial nerve branch which is surrounded by multiple vessels. Intraoperative nerve inspection (**c**) shows an edematous deep branch of the radial nerve (*arrow*) at the level of the arcade of Frohse (*arrows*) (*small arrow* normal superficial branch of radial nerve, *SM* supinator muscle, *BR* brachioradialis muscle)

3.4.1
Carpal Tunnel Syndrome

3.4.1.1
Epidemiology and Clinical Presentation

CTS is the most common entrapment syndrome of the upper extremities with an estimated incidence in the general community of 125 per 100,000 per year (STEVENS et al. 1988). Typically, the dominant hand is affected first. The clinical hallmark and usual presenting feature of CTS is a pain syndrome called brachialgia paresthetica nocturna (MUMENTHALER et al. 1998). Patients are awakened from sleep in the early morning hours with pain radiating from the wrist proximally into the forearm and arm, and report numbness and tingling in the hand, stiffness of the fingers, and characteristic swelling sensations. All complaints rapidly resolve after repeated hand movements such as shaking. Episodes of pain in the night may be exacerbated by prolonged strenuous manual work. With more severe nerve compression the patient experiences permanent paresthesias or sensory loss over the palmar thumb and digits innervated by the median nerve (Fig. 3.14), and in advanced disease weakness and wasting of part of the thenar muscles (Fig. 3.14). Significant vasomotor disturbances are comparatively rare.

3.4.1.2 Etiology

CTS arises from compression of the median nerve in the canal formed by the transverse carpal ligament and carpal bones. Under pathological circumstances tissue pressure in the carpal tunnel reaches 30 mmHg, i.e. four times the normal level (SZABO and CHIDGEY 1989). Chronic or recurrent compression of the median nerve causes focal demyelination and eventually axon degeneration as the pathological counterpart to the emerging clinical deficits. Temporary ischemia due to compression of the vasa nervorum accounts for the reversible pain manifesting during the night. Factors contributing to the development of CTS are numerous and often coexist in individuals: (1) congenital smallness of the tunnel or anatomical peculiarities (persistent arteria mediana, abnormal course or insertion of finger flexor and palmaris muscles); (2) susceptibility of the nerve to pressure (diabetic or other neuropathies, etc); (3) systemic and endocrine disorders (pregnancy, hypothyroidism, acromegaly, amyloidosis, etc), and (4) reduced space in the carpal tunnel due to space-occupying lesions (osteophytes, exostosis, ganglia, hematoma, tenosynovitis, articular deformities in rheumatoid arthritis, etc) (ROSENBAUM and OCHOA 1993; STEVENS et al. 1992). The application of high-resolution ultrasound has expanded our knowledge of the diversity of the pathological conditions underlying CTS.

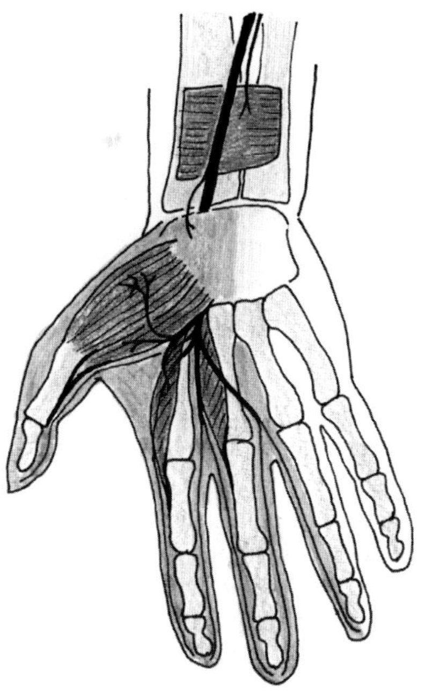

Fig. 3.14. Anatomy of the median nerve (*dark gray* motor innervation, *light gray* sensory innervation)

3.4.1.3 Diagnosis

In most instances, the diagnosis of CTS is reliably settled by an experienced clinician based on a review of the patient's history and complaints, and a careful neurological examination. Clinical assessment should include Phalen's maneuver (emergence of paresthesias in the median territory elicited by maximal passive wrist flexion for one or more minutes (KUSCHNER et al. 1992; PHALEN 1966) and testing for Tinel's sign (paresthesias provoked by tapping with the finger over the carpal tunnel).

Electrodiagnostic testing is recommended when median nerve compression causes significant discomfort or sustained sensorimotor deficits. Standard nerve conduction studies usually allow the detection of distal conduction abnormalities (prolonged distal motor latency, i.e. >4.0 to 4.8 ms, and reduced distal sensory nerve conduction, i.e. <45 to 55 m/s) as indicators of nerve entrapment (STEVENS 1987; LIVESON and MA 1992) (Fig. 3.15). The sensitivity of the evaluation can be improved to near 100% by more sophisticated techniques such as short-segment studies (KIMURA 1979) (Fig. 3.16), palmar stimulations (STEVENS 1987) and costimulation of the ulnar nerve for a comparison of median versus ulnar distal motor latencies (FELSENTHAL 1977) (Fig. 3.15). The latter technique creates an ideal internal control for methodological problems.

An electrophysiological work-up is particularly useful to assess the damage to the median nerve (demyelination versus axon loss) relevant to therapeutic decisions, to rule out differential diagnoses

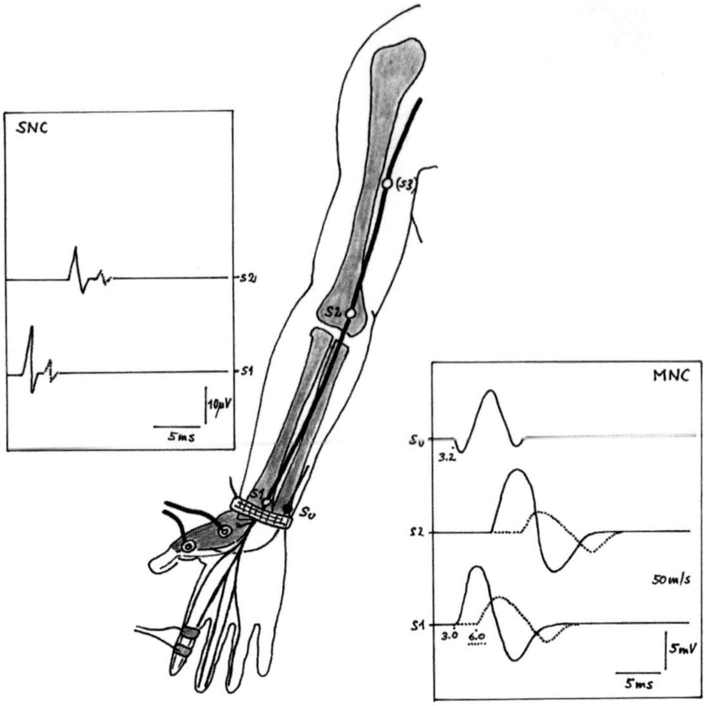

Fig. 3.15. Median nerve. Motor nerve conduction (*MNC*) and antidromic sensory nerve conduction (*SNC*) studies. Routinely, stimulation is performed at the wrist (*S1*) and elbow (*S2*), and over the ulnar nerve at the wrist (S_U, see text). Motor potentials are recorded from the abductor pollicis brevis muscle (*disk electrodes*) and sensory potentials from the index finger (*ring electrodes*). The recordings presented are from a normal subject (*full line*) and a patient with CTS (*dotted line*)

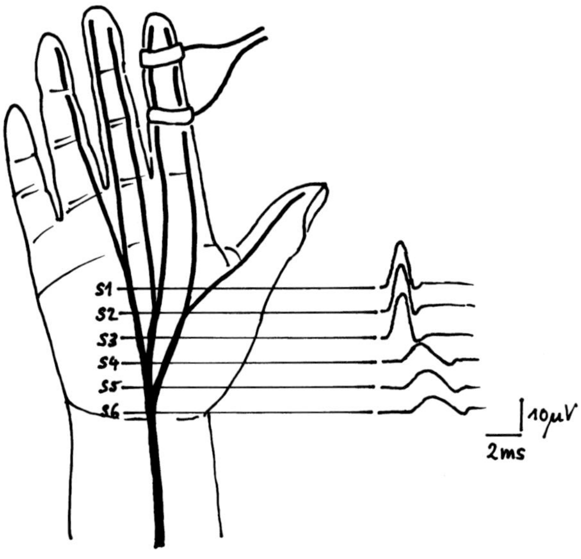

Fig. 3.16. Carpal tunnel studies: short segment stimulation

or coexistent disease, and to confirm the presence of CTS in the event of atypical complaints, pure motor deficits and prominent neuropathy.

3.4.1.4 Sonography

The value of sonography for the detection of median nerve entrapment inside the carpal tunnel has been recognized since 1991 when the first systematic approach to the sonographic diagnosis of CTS was reported based on data derived at our institution (Buchberger et al. 1991). Since then several reports in the literature have focused on the value of different sonographic criteria for CTS diagnosis (Duncan et al. 1999; Lee et al. 1999; Nakamichi and Tachibana 2000; Sarria et al. 2000; Dilley et al. 2001; Jamadar et al. 2001). All of these studies focused mainly on two sonographic techniques: measurement of median nerve diameter or cross-sectional area at distinct locations along the carpal tunnel and structural analysis of the median nerve and flexor retinaculum. If these reports are compared, one of the reliable findings for the diagnosis of CTS found by different authors is enlargement of the median nerve at the proximal level of the carpal tunnel (Fig. 3.17).

As discussed in other parts of this book, this enlargement of a nerve seems to be a common pathophysiological pathway to peripheral nerve damage and relates to vascular congestion and edema. While there is now general agreement that enlargement of the median nerve is a sign of CTS, there is some disagreement as to the amount of enlargement considered to be pathological. In the study by Buchberger et al. a cross-sectional area of the median nerve of 10 mm^2 measured in the proximal or middle carpal tunnel coincided with CTS (Buchberger et al. 1991, 1992). This was confirmed in recent study by Nakamichi and Tachibana (Nakamichi and Tachibana 2000), while in an EMG controlled study by Lee et al.

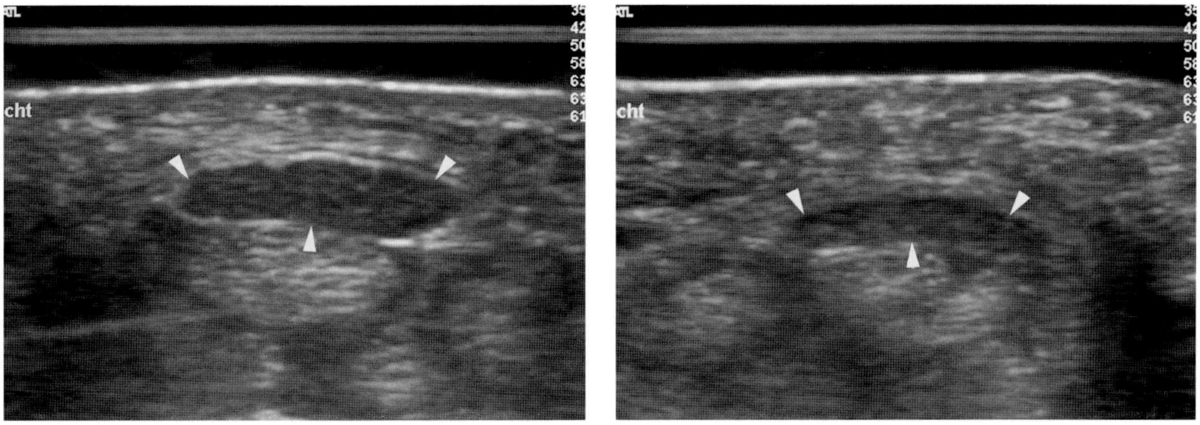

a b

Fig. 3.17a, b. Transverse sonograms through the median nerve in a patient with CTS acquired at the proximal (**a**) and distal (**b**) carpal tunnel. Marked swelling of the median nerve (*arrowheads*) is noted in the proximal carpal tunnel with loss of fascicular discrimination, whereas the nerve is somewhat flattened in the distal carpal tunnel

a cut-off value of 15 mm^2 was considered to be pathological (Lee et al. 1999). A further sonographic sign for CTS, which relates to median nerve enlargement and has been confirmed by various studies, is palmar bowing and thickening of the flexor retinaculum (Fig. 3.18). A reliable documentation of this finding, however, will only be achieved with the application of high-frequency sonographic transducers, which allow exact discrimination of the retinaculum.

In addition to median nerve enlargement, a distal flattening ratio above 3 has been defined as a cut-off value above which CTS has to be suspected (Buchberger et al. 1991, 1992). Patients with CTS included in their study had a mean distal flattening ratio of 4.6, whereas normal healthy subjects had a ratio of only 3.2. While the value of sonographic measurement of median nerve enlargement for CTS diagnosis was confirmed by other authors, the increased median nerve flattening ratio at the hook of the hamate was not confirmed in later studies to be suggestive of CTS (Nakamichi and Tachibana 2000; Sarria et al. 2000). Nevertheless, several reports agree on the finding of median nerve flattening in the distal carpal tunnel, or abrupt contour changes seen in patients with CTS (Lee et al. 1999; Nakamichi and Tachibana 2000). Based on our own experience with sonography in a large series of CTS patients, we are cautious with the interpretation of median nerve caliber changes. A considerable amount of distal median nerve flattening occurs in healthy asymptomatic volunteers. In addition the nerve often gets more hyperechoic in the flattened regions because of reduced fascicular discrimination (Fig. 3.19). From a technical point of view this median nerve flattening is best demonstrated with longitudinal panoramic sonograms (Fig. 3.19).

Similar results are known from the MRI literature, where the value of median nerve flattening in CTS diagnosis is disputed (Kleindienst et al. 1998;

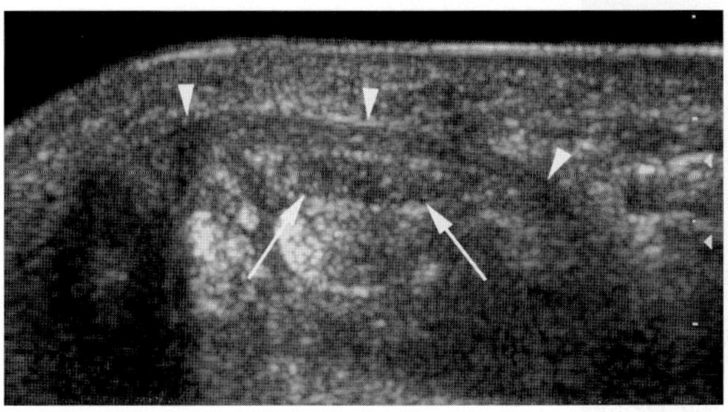

Fig. 3.18. Transverse sonogram through the carpal tunnel in a patient with CTS. Note the thickening and palmar bowing of the flexor retinaculum (*arrowheads*) and median nerve (*arrows*) with somewhat reduced fascicular discrimination

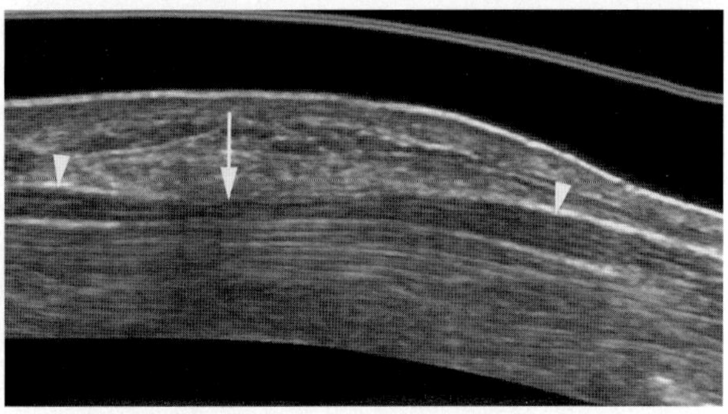

Fig. 3.19. Longitudinal panoramic sonogram through median nerve in a patient with clinical evidence of idiopathic CTS. A marked flattening of the median nerve (*arrowheads*) is noted inside the carpal tunnel (*arrow*) with normal caliber proximal (*right*) and distal (*left*) to the carpal tunnel

MONAGLE et al. 1999). Nevertheless an abrupt caliber change of the enlarged median nerve (a notch sign) at the entrance of the carpal tunnel showed a good correlation with EMG results in the study by Lee et al. (LEE et al. 1999) (Fig. 3.20).

The second important sonographic technique for CTS diagnosis, which we consider even more reliable, is the evaluation of changes in median nerve echotexture. Several studies have shown a loss of fascicular discrimination in the enlarged median nerve (LEE et al. 1999; NAKAMICHI and TACHIBANA 2000) together with marginal effacement from edema and longitudinal irregularities.

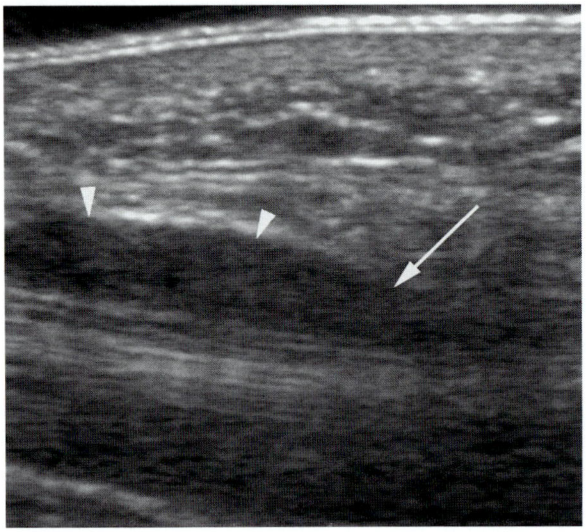

Fig. 3.20. Longitudinal sonogram through the median nerve (*arrowheads*) in a patient with CTS reveals abrupt narrowing (*arrow*) of the median nerve at its entrance into the carpal tunnel

With the advent of high-frequency transducers and newer sonographic software the identification of nerve vasculature has also become feasible, and according to our preliminary experience an increase in internal vascularization may be detected in median nerves of patients with neuropathy caused by median nerve compression (Fig. 3.21).

In summary, the sonographic diagnosis of CTS may be achieved based on the following signs (in order of reliability):

- Enlargement of the median nerve at the proximal carpal tunnel with an increased cross-sectional area above 12 mm^2.
- Changes in median nerve echotexture consistent with edema, i.e. loss of fascicular discrimination with more or less homogeneous hypoechoic appearance, and indistinct outer margins.
- Abrupt caliber change (notch sign) at the proximal margin of the flexor retinaculum.
- Demonstration of increased vascularization inside a nerve with color Doppler sonography (needs to be further defined in larger controlled trials).

Depending on the diagnostic possibilities available at a given institution the work-up of a patient with CTS may vary. Conventionally after obtaining a patient's history and physical examination, an electrodiagnostic study is ordered for evaluation of the median nerve. However, in agreement with Lee et al. (LEE et al. 1999), we propose a different algorithm, which favors the performance of a sonographic examination early in the work-up (Fig. 3.22).

Sonography is able to reliably diagnose idiopathic CTS in a high percentage of patients and to rule out secondary CTS due to abnormalities inside the carpal

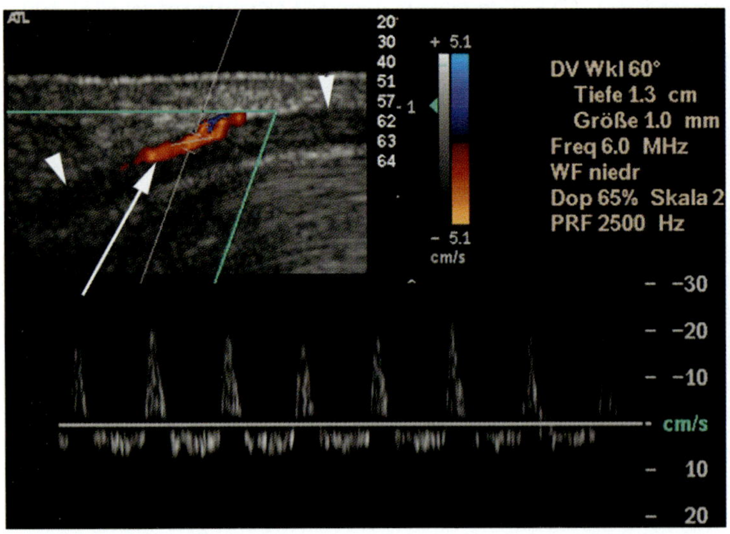

Fig. 3.21. Longitudinal color Doppler sonogram and spectral wave analysis in a patient with CTS. A large caliber vessel (*arrow*) is demonstrated inside the median nerve (*arrowheads*). Spectral wave analysis shows a relatively high velocity arterial waveform with a maximum flow velocity of approximately 20 cm/s

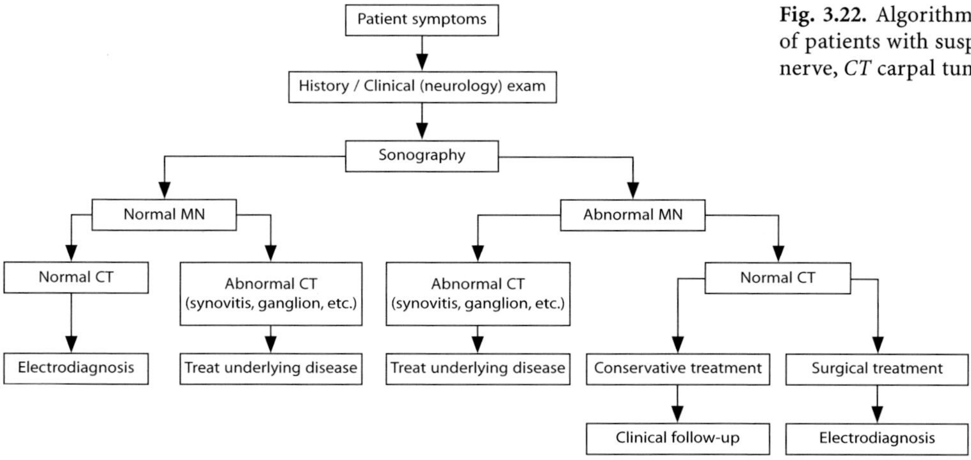

Fig. 3.22. Algorithm for diagnostic workup of patients with suspected CTS (*MN* median nerve, *CT* carpal tunnel)

tunnel such as flexor tendon synovitis, tumors or ganglia. According to this algorithm two distinct situations may result after taking a patient's history and carrying out a neurology examination: (1) clear signs and symptoms of CTS, and (2) indistinct findings. In the first situation sonography should be performed to rule out secondary CTS and to define the severity of the disease. Either conservative management or surgery may be instituted based on the sonographic findings. In the case of surgery for idiopathic CTS an electrodiagnostic study should be performed as this may be the best way to check for functional recovery during follow-up examinations, besides clinical improvement. In the second situation again sonography may be the first diagnostic study to be carried out. In patients with a normal sonogram or inconclusive sonographic findings an electrodiagnostic study should be done to exclude an intrinsic pathology of the median nerve or focal disease elsewhere along its course from the cervical roots to the hand.

A persistent median artery (PMA) with various combinations of median nerve shape is a special condition known at the carpal tunnel which merits further discussion. The median artery provides blood supply to the forearm and the hand during embryonic development. As the radial and ulnar arteries develop, the median artery atrophies to a small vessel accompanying the median nerve in the forearm. When extending into the carpal tunnel, a PMA may join the superficial volar arch, may supply the radial digits with an absent arch, or may end as a thrombosed thread. An enlarged, thrombosed, or calcified PMA and a PMA aneurysm in the carpal tunnel were considered causes of CTS (Eversmann 1988). In addition a vascular anomaly inside the carpal tunnel may be of importance in the case of carpal tunnel release, as an inadvertent transection of the vessel may result in severe bleeding. Furthermore, surgical transection of the median artery is not feasible without previous knowledge concerning the contribution of the vessel to the supply of the hand. According to the literature a PMA is found in 26% of asymptomatic volunteers and normally accompanied by variations in median nerve branching (high division or bifid median nerve) (Gassner et al. 2002) (Fig. 3.23). In a small series of patients with clinical evidence of CTS, this anomaly was detected sonographically at our department and postoperative patient outcome after carpal tunnel release was excellent (Gassner et al. 2002).

From a technical point of view, what has been said for imaging of the ulnar nerve in Section 3.2.1.5 equally applies to sonography of the median nerve as far as technical equipment is concerned. The use of a high-frequency transducer of at least 12 MHz and a stand off pad is highly recommended to achieve good results. Access to the median nerve at the wrist is easily achieved and identification of the nerve

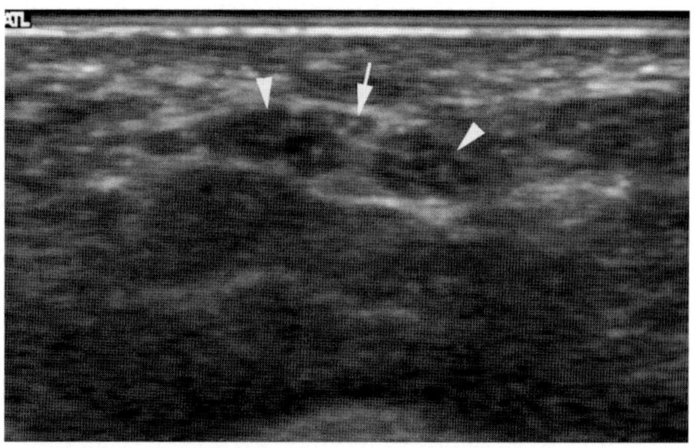

Fig. 3.23. Transverse sonogram through median nerve just proximal to the carpal tunnel. A bifid median nerve is shown (*arrowheads*) with an obliterated, not perfused median artery (*arrow*)

and flexor retinaculum hardly a problem except in postoperative patients. In the latter, identification of an incompletely cleaved retinaculum should always be attempted in subjects with persistent symptoms despite surgery. Other possibilities for inadequate postsurgical improvement of patients range from hematomas and infections over scar formation with renewed compression to direct nerve damage with partial or complete median nerve transection.

3.4.1.5 Therapy

The mainstays of treatment are the avoidance of wrist overuse, withdrawal of provoking factors, placement of neutral wrist splints during sleep, local corticosteroid injections adjacent to the carpal tunnel (Green 1984), and – if nonsurgical interventions fail or neurological deficits emerge – surgical sectioning of the volar carpal ligament. Pain and paresthesias bring most patients to medical attention before irreversible axonal loss has developed. Accordingly, overall prognosis of CTS is good to excellent in up to 80 to 90% of patients given adequate management (Campbell 1998).

3.5 Peroneal Nerve Compression

S. Peer

Depending on the site of nerve involvement (common peroneal nerve, superficial peroneal nerve, etc.) various syndromes of peroneal nerve compression may be discerned. As most of these subtypes are rare and experience with sonographic diagnosis is lacking, we only comment on common peroneal nerve compression at the level of the fibular neck.

3.5.1 Peroneal Tunnel Syndrome

The peroneal nerve leaves the sciatic nerve in the proximal portion of the popliteal fossa. However, a high division of the peroneal nerve at the thigh is known to exist in a number of patients. While the slightly larger tibial nerve continues in a more or less straight course, the peroneal nerve takes an oblique direction encircling the fibular head. It passes between the superficial head of the peroneus longus muscle and the bony surface of the fibular neck. While this region lacks features typically described for other osteofibrous tunnels, it is sometimes referred to as the peroneal tunnel (Pecina et al. 2001). Shortly after its course around the fibular neck the nerve divides into a superficial and a deep branch.

3.5.1.1 Clinical Considerations

The most common causes of compression neuropathy of the peroneal nerve are external, such as a tight short leg plaster cast, a malaligned fibular head fracture, or ganglia of the proximal tibiofibular joint. Although relatively rare, an idiopathic entrapment syndrome of the common peroneal nerve is known, which typically occurs in the restricted space between the bone and the fascia of the peroneus longus muscle. In many instances these lesions may be related to functional anatomic changes: inversion and plantar flexion of the foot tenses the peroneus longus muscle and squeezes the nerve towards the fibular neck. Repetitive actions with inversion and pronation (long distance running, operating machines with pedals) or habitual overuse (sleeping position, sitting with crossed legs) are therefore known to predispose the nerve to development of neuropathy (Kopell and Thompson 1960; Kumak 1987; LeGeyt and Ambrose 1998; Sidey 1969).

The peroneal nerve contains motor branches for the peroneus longus and brevis muscle (superficial branch) and the extensors and dorsiflexors of the foot and toes (deep branch). In addition the nerve contains sensory fibers for the anterolateral skin of the leg and the dorsal part of the great to the fourth toe (superficial branch). The deep branch has only minimal sensory function supplying the dorsal skin between the great and second toe. Common peroneal nerve compression consequently results in burning pain in the sensory regions mentioned above and motor weakness and atrophy with a gradual transition to a dropping foot in complete peroneal paralysis. Palpation or pressure over the peroneal tunnel typically increases a patient's pain (Pecina et al. 2001).

3.5.1.2 Sonography

With state of the art linear array transducers the common peroneal nerve may be followed along its course around the fibular neck. Despite the direct access to the nerve in this region, we prefer to identify it in the popliteal region using the biceps femoris tendon, which parallels the nerve over a long distance, as a characteristic landmark. From there on it is best followed in a transverse sonographic plane around the fibular neck to its bifurcation. While the superficial branch may often be visualized along its complete course at the lateral aspect of the leg, the deep branch is only infrequently identified diving deep between the tibialis anterior and extensor digitorum muscle.

The normal common peroneal nerve is a small round or ovoid structure with a mostly hyperechoic signal and only few and tiny hypoechoic fascicles. The approximation in signal between the mostly hyperechoic nerve and fatty tissue or the hyperechoic signal of atrophic muscle accounts for the problems encountered with sonography of the peroneal nerve in obese patients or patients with muscle atrophy caused by long-standing common peroneal nerve paralysis. In patients with peroneal nerve compression enlargement of the nerve with swelling of single fascicles is in most cases readily identified (Fig. 3.24).

The detection of coexisting abnormalities with external compression is straightforward, as ganglia, tumors, bony ridges, etc. are easily visualized with sonography (Fig. 3.25).

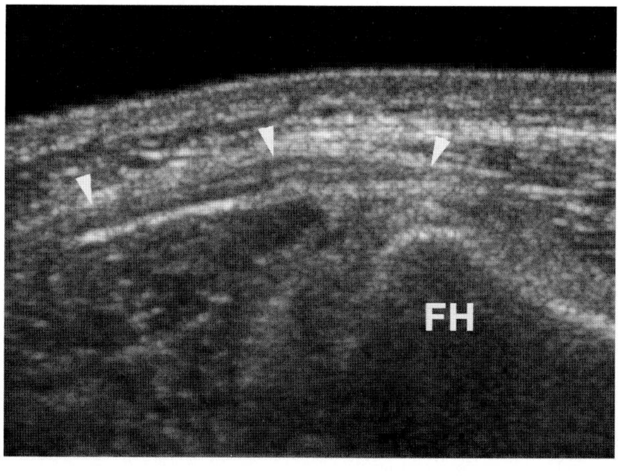

Fig. 3.24. Longitudinal sonogram through common peroneal nerve (*arrowheads*) proximal to the fibular head (*FH*) in a patient with muscle weakness at forefoot extension and hypesthesia at the dorsal part of the great toe. A short segment of enlargement of the nerve is seen proximal to its course around the fibular head consistent with nerve edema due to peroneal nerve compression

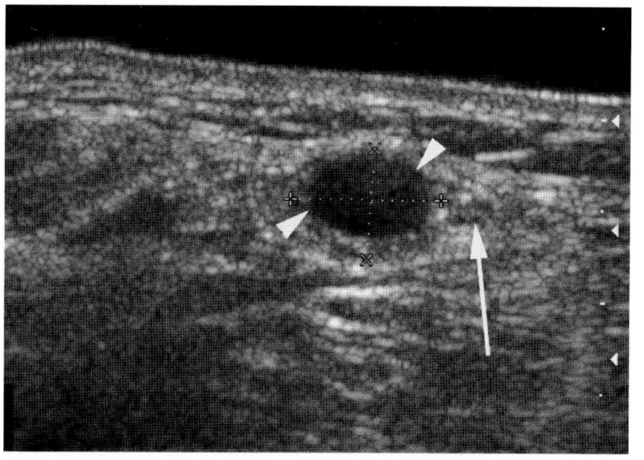

Fig. 3.25. Transverse sonogram through common peroneal nerve (*arrow*) at the level of the fibular head in a patient with fibular nerve palsy reveals nerve compression by a small intraneural ganglion (*arrowheads*)

3.6 Tibial Nerve Compression

S. Kiechl, S. Peer

From the sciatic nerve bifurcation the tibial nerve continues in a rather straight course down to the medial ankle accompanied by the tibial artery and vein. On its passage around the medial malleolus the nerve enters a fibro-osseous canal, referred to as the tarsal tunnel. On its passage through this canal, the nerve may be compressed resulting in tarsal tunnel syndrome (TTS), a recognized clinical entity first described in 1960 by Kopell and Thompson (Kopell and Thompson 1960).

3.6.1 Tarsal Tunnel Syndrome

The tarsal tunnel is a fibro-osseous canal consisting of a bony sulcus on the medial side of the calcaneus, the posterior talar process and the medial malleolus. According to Pecina the width of the bony sulcus at the bottom of the tarsal tunnel can vary, and patients with a small sulcus width are considered more prone to development of TTS (Pecina et al. 2001). The roof of the canal consists of the flexor retinaculum, which covers the tendons of the tibialis posterior, flexor digitorum and flexor hallucis longus muscles. The tibial artery and veins run together with these three tendons, and the tibial nerve and the tarsal tunnel may in fact be considered the hilum of the planta pedis, as it houses virtually all of its neurovascular supply. Before entering the tarsal tunnel the tibial nerve sends a small sensory branch towards the heel and at the upper margin of the retinaculum, or after a short distance in the canal, divides into its terminal branches, the medial and lateral plantar nerves.

3.6.1.1 Epidemiology and Clinical Presentation

TTS (Keck 1962; Mumenthaler et al. 1998) is clearly less frequent than the aforementioned entrapment syndromes of the upper extremities. The disorder is insidious in onset and mostly unilateral. Patients complain of a burning pain at the plantar side of the foot which sometimes radiates to the calf and typically increases while walking (DeLisa and Saeed 1983). The pain is often accompanied by paresthesias and foot numbness in the distribution of one or all of the terminal sensory branches. Sensory manifestations may worsen by foot eversion. Paresis of the small foot muscles with development of "claw digits" and abnormal posture of the foot is rare.

3.6.1.2 Etiology

The tibial nerve descends behind the medial malleolus and passes under the flexor retinaculum ("laciniate ligament") to the plantar side of the foot, where it divides into the calcaneal, medial and lateral plantar branches. In the tarsal tunnel, roofed by the flexor retinaculum, the nerve is prone to compression injury (Goodgold et al. 1965; Oh and Meyer 1999). In a majority of patients TTS is idiopathic with no clear precipitating factors detectable. The second most common cause is entrapment due to scare tissue or articular deformities originating from previous trauma (distortion or fracture of the ankle). Further sources of compression are an accessory flexor digitorum longus muscle and space-occupying lesions within the tunnel such as lipoma, varicose veins, ganglia, nontraumatic exostosis or neoplasm.

3.6.1.3 Diagnosis

If fully expressed (characteristic sensory and motor deficits), the TTS can easily be diagnosed on clinical grounds only. In cases of a pure pain syndrome, however, a correct diagnosis may be much more demanding and sometimes requires ancillary, e.g. radiological, testing. In such patients a positive compression test (provocation of typical complaints by manual pressure applied for 30 s to the tarsal tunnel) may be helpful. Standard electrodiagnostic testing consists of the measurement of distal motor latencies to the abductor hallucis and/or abductor digiti minimi muscles and electromyographic exploration of the muscles of the sole. Unilateral prolongation of the motor latency (>7 ms to the abductor digiti minimi muscle) and/or emergence of severe chronic or acute damage on electromyography strongly supports the diagnosis (Goodgold et al. 1965) (Fig. 3.26). However, normal results are not contradictive of the presence of TTS (sensitivity 50 to 80%) (Liveson and Ma 1992). Interpretability of electrodiagnostic

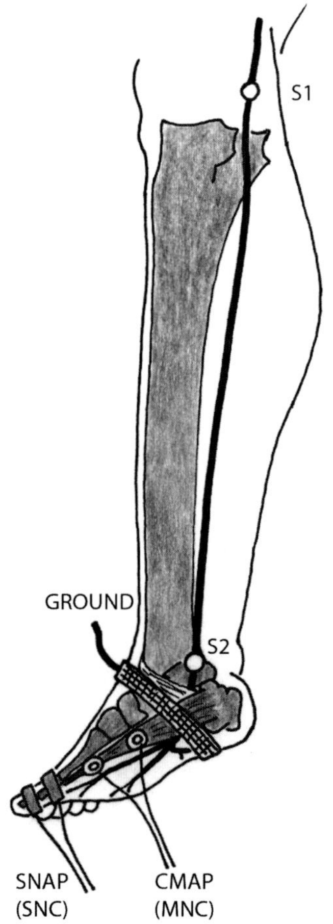

Fig. 3.26. Tibial nerve. Motor nerve conduction (*MNC*) and antidromic sensory nerve conduction (*SNC*) studies. Routinely, stimulation is performed at the ankle (*S1*) and in the popliteal fossa (*S2*). Motor potentials (*CMAP*) are recorded from the abductor hallucis muscle (*disk electrodes*) and sensory potentials (*SNAP*) from the big toe (*ring electrodes*)

testing may be difficult in the event of coexisting neuropathy or severe damage of the nerve root S1. The procedure with the highest diagnostic sensitivity is an anesthetic nerve block.

Finally, an orthopedic examination is mandatory to distinguish TTS from numerous differential diagnoses such as stress fractures, bursitis, inflammatory arthritis or plantar fasciitis. It has to be born in mind that some of these conditions may affect tibial nerve function in terms of a (noncompressive) local irritation.

3.6.1.4
Therapy

Potential sources of external compression such as ill-fitting shoes should be eliminated. Local corticosteroid injections are sometimes helpful. If TTS produces substantial discomfort or sensorimotor deficits and conservative treatment options fail operative release of the flexor retinaculum is the therapy of choice. Outcome after surgery is favorable in about three-quarters of patients (MONDELLI et al. 1998). A minority of patients develop chronic pain syndromes with features of reflex sympathetic dystrophy.

3.6.1.5
Sonography

Technical considerations for sonography of the tibial nerve at the tarsal tunnel are similar to what has been said for peroneal tunnel evaluation. A high resolution 12–15 MHz transducer is certainly recommended for this region. Identification of the distal tibial nerve is easily achieved in a transverse scan plane just above the medial malleolus if the transducer is positioned in the groove between the Achilles tendon and the posterior tibial margin (PEER et al. 2002). Here the nerve lies close to the posterior tibial vessels between the flexor hallucis longus and flexor digitorum muscle. In some cases color Doppler may be used to identify the vascular bundle, which provides a fine landmark for localization of the nerve. The nerve is larger than the common peroneal nerve and its fascicular texture is normally better discernible. From this position the nerve is followed downward to the tarsal tunnel with documentation of its bifurcation. The two terminal tibial nerve branches are normally easily followed a certain way along their course to the planta pedis. The flexor retinaculum may normally be identified as a distinct hypoechoic line.

Sonographic findings in patients with TTS depend on the etiology: with the existence of ganglia or posttraumatic changes an external compression is easily confirmed in the same way as in other anatomic regions, with direct nerve compromise and reactive nerve edema representing a common pathway of neuropathy (MARTINOLI et al. 2000; NAGAOKA and SATOU 1999). The latter is the only apparent finding in so-called idiopathic TTS (Fig. 3.27).

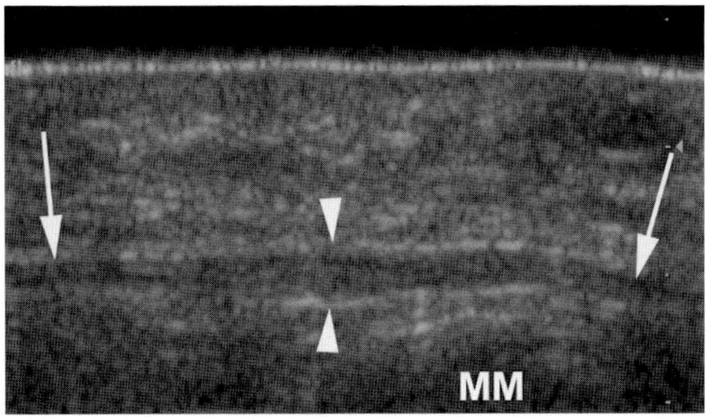

Fig. 3.27. Longitudinal sonogram through tibial nerve (*arrows*) just proximal to medial malleolus (*MM*) in a female patient with idiopathic tarsal tunnel syndrome. A short segment of spindle-shaped edematous enlargement of the nerve (*arrowheads*) is seen proximal to the level of compression

References

Arle JE, Zager EL (2000) Surgical treatment of common entrapment neuropathies in the upper limbs. Muscle Nerve 23:1160–1174

Balogh B, Vass A, Piza-Katzer H (1997) Ist eine Vorverlagerung des N.ulnaris beim Sulcus nervi ulnaris-Syndrom wirklich indiziert. Handchir Mikrochir Plast Chir 29:133–139

Bodner G, Harpf C, Meirer R, et al (2002) Ultrasonographic appearance of supinator syndrome. J Ultrasound Med 21: 1289–1293

Bozentka DJ (1998) Cubital tunnel syndrome pathophysiology. Clin Orthop 351:90–94

Buchberger W, Schoen G, Strasser K, et al (1991) High resolution ultrasonography of the carpal tunnel. J Ultrasound Med 101:531–537

Buchberger W, Judmaier W, Birbamer G, et al (1992) Carpal tunnel syndrome: diagnosis with high resolution sonography. AJR Am J Roentgenol 159:793–798

Bui-Mansfield LT, Williamson M, Wheeler DT, et al (2002) Guyon's canal lipoma causing ulnar neuropathy. AJR Am J Roentgenol 178:1458

Campbell WW (1998) Entrapment neuropathies. In: Gilchrist J (ed) Prognosis in neurology. Butterworth-Heinemann, Boston, pp 307–312

Campbell W (2000) Ulnar neuropathy at the elbow. Muscle Nerve 23:450–452

Campbell WW, Sahni KS, Pridgeon RM, et al (1988) Intraoperative electroneurography: management of ulnar neuropathy at the elbow. Muscle Nerve 11:75–81

Campbell WW, Pridgeon RM, Riaz G, et al (1991) Variations in anatomy of the ulnar nerve at the cubital tunnel: pitfalls in the diagnosis of ulnar neuropathy at the elbow. Muscle Nerve 14:733–738

Campbell WW, Pridgeon RM, Sahni KS (1992) Short segment incremental studies in the evaluation of ulnar neuropathy at the elbow. Muscle Nerve 15:1050–1054

Childress HM (1975) Recurrent ulnar nerve dislocation at the elbow. Clin Orthop 108:168–173

Chiou HJ, Chou YH, Cheng SP, et al (1998) Cubital tunnel syndrome: diagnosis by high resolution ultrasonography. J Ultrasound Med 17:643–648

DeLisa JA, Saeed MA (1983) The tarsal tunnel syndrome. Muscle Nerve 6:664–670

Dellon AL, Hament W, Gittelshon A (1993) Nonoperative management of cubital tunnel syndrome: an 8-year prospective study. Neurology 43:1673–1677

Dilley A, Greening J, Lynn B, et al (2001) The use of cross correlation analysis between high frequency ultrasound images to measure longitudinal median nerve movement. Ultrasound Med Biol 27:1211–1218

Duncan I, Sullivan P, Lomas F (1999) Sonography in the diagnosis of carpal tunnel syndrome. AJR Am J Roentgenol 173:681–684

Eversmann W (1988) Entrapment and compression neuropathies. In: Green DP (ed) Operative hand surgery, vol 2. Churchill Livingstone, New York, pp 1430–1441

Felsenthal G (1977) Median and ulnar distal motor and sensory latencies in the same normal subject. Arch Phys Med Rehabil 58:297–302

Gassner E, Schocke M, Peer S, et al (2002) Persistent median artery in the carpal tunnel – color Doppler ultrasonographic findings. J Ultrasound Med 21:455–461

Goodgold J, Kopell HP, Spieholz NI (1965) The tarsal tunnel syndrome. New Engl J Med 273:742–746

Green DP (1984) Diagnostic and therapeutic value of carpal tunnel injection. J Hand Surg 9:850–854

Jacobson JA, Jebson PJL, Jeffers AW, et al (2001) Ulnar nerve dislocation and snapping triceps syndrome: diagnosis with dynamic sonography – report of three cases. Radiology 220: 601–605

Jamadar DA, Jacobson JA, Hayes CW (2001) Sonographic evaluation of the median nerve at the wrist. J Ultrasound Med 20:1011–1014

Kalb K, Gruber P, Landsleitner B (1999) Die nicht traumatisch bedingte Parese des Ramus profungdus nervi radialis. Aspekte eines seltenen Krankheitsbildes. Handchir Mikrochir Plast Chir 32:26–32

Keck C (1962) The tarsal tunnel syndrome. J Bone Joint Surg 44A:180–182

Kimura J (1979) The carpal tunnel syndrome: localization of conduction abnormalities within the distal segment of the median nerve. Brain 102:619–635

Kleindienst A, Hamm B, Lanksch WR (1998) Carpal tunnel syndrome: staging of median nerve compression by MR imaging. J Magn Reson Imaging 8:1119–1125

Kopell HP, Thompson WA (1960) Peripheral entrapment neuropathies of the lower extremities. N Engl J Med 262:56–60

Kumak D (1987) The facts of Kathmandu: squatters palsy. JAMA 257:28

Kuschner SH, Ebramzadeh E, Johnson D, et al (1992) Tinel's sign and Phalen's test in carpal tunnel syndrome. Orthopedics 15:1297–1302

LeGeyt MT, Ambrose J (1998) Nontraumatic compression of the common peroneal nerve: a case report and review of the literature. Am J Orthop 27:521–523

Lee D, van Holsbeeck MT, Janevski PK, Ganos DL, Ditmars DM, Darian VB (1999) Diagnosis of carpal tunnel syndrome. Ultrasound versus electromyography. Radiol Clin North Am 37:859–872

Liveson JA, Ma DM (1992) Laboratory reference for clinical neurophysiology. Davis, Philadelphia

Lorea P, Schuind F (2000) False aneurysm appearing as delayed ulnar nerve palsy after minor penetrating trauma in the forearm. J Trauma 51:144–145

Martinoli C, Serafini G, Bianchi S, et al (1996) Ultrasonography of peripheral nerves. J Peripher Nerv Syst 1:169–174

Martinoli C, Bianchi S, Gandolfo N, et al (2000) Ultrasound of nerve entrapment in osteofibrous tunnels of the upper and lower limbs. Radiographics 20:199–217

Martinoli C, Bianchi S, Dahmane MH, et al (2002) Ultrasound of tendons and nerves. Eur Radiol 12:44–55

Mazurek MT, Shin AY (2001) Upper extremity peripheral nerve anatomy: current concepts and applications. Clin Orthop 383:7–20

Miller RG (1991) AAEM case report #1: ulnar neuropathy at the elbow. Muscle Nerve 14:97–101

Miller RG, Camp PE (1979) Postoperative ulnar neuropathy. JAMA 242:1636–1639

Miller RG, Hummel EE (1980) The cubital tunnel syndrome: treatment with simple decompression. Ann Neurol 7: 567–569

Monagle K, Dai G, Chu A, et al (1999) Quantitative MR imaging of carpal tunnel syndrome. AJR Am J Roentgenol 172: 1582–1586

Mondelli M, Giannini F, Reale F (1998) Clinical and electrophysiological findings and follow-up in tarsal tunnel syndrome. Electroencephalogr Clin Neurophysiol 109: 418–425

Mumenthaler M, Schliack H, Stoehr M (1998) Läsionen peripherer Nerven und radikuläre Läsionen. Thieme, Stuttgart

Nagaoka M, Satou K (1999) Tarsal tunnel syndrome caused by ganglia. J Bone Joint Surg Br 81:607–610

Nakamichi KI, Tachibana S (2000) Enlarged median nerve in idiopathic carpal tunnel syndrome. Muscle Nerve 23: 1713–1718

O'Driscoll SW, Horii E, Carmichael SW, et al (1992) The cubital tunnel and ulnar neuropathy. J Bone Joint Surg Br 74: 84–94

Ogino T, Minami A, Kato H (1991) Diagnosis of radial nerve palsy caused by ganglion with use of different imaging techniques. J Hand Surg [Am] 16:230–235

Oh SH, Meyer RD (1999) Entrapment neuropathies of the tibial (posterior tibial) nerve. Neurol Clin 17:593–615

Okamoto M, Abe M, Shirai H, et al (2000) Morphology and dynamics of the ulnar nerve in the cubital tunnel: diagnosis by high resolution ultrasonography. J Hand Surg [Br] 25:85–89

Pecina MM, Krmpotic-Nemanic J, Markiewitz AD (eds) (2001) Tunnel syndromes. Peripheral nerve compression syndromes, 3rd edn. CRC-LLC Press, Boca Raton

Peer S, Kovacs P, Harpf C, et al (2002) High resolution sonography of lower extremity peripheral nerves: anatomic correlation and spectrum of pathology. J Ultrasound Med 21: 315–322

Phalen GS (1966) The carpal tunnel syndrome: seventeen years' experience in diagnosis and treatment of six hundred fifty-four hands. J Bone Joint Surg 48A:211–228

Phalen GS, Kendrick JI, Rodriguez JM (1971) Lipomas of the upper extremity. A series of fifteen tumors in the hand and wrist and six tumors causing nerve compression. Am J Surg 121:298–306

Prevel CD, Matloub HS, Zhong Y, et al (1993) The extrinsic blood supply of the ulnar nerve at the elbow: an anatomic study. J Hand Surg 18A:433–438

Puig S, Turkhof E, Sedivy R, et al (1999) Sonographic diagnosis of recurrent ulnar nerve compression by ganglion cysts. J Ultrasound Med 18:433–436

Ritts GD, Wood MB, Linscheid RL (1987) Radial tunnel syndrome. A ten-year surgical experience. Clin Orthop 219: 201–205

Roles NC, Maudsley RH (1972) Radial tunnel syndrome. Resistant tennis elbow as a nerve entrapment. J Bone Joint Surg 54B:499–508

Rosenbaum R (1999) Disputed radial tunnel syndrome. Muscle Nerve 22:960–967

Rosenbaum RB, Ochoa JL (1993) Carpal tunnel syndrome and other disorders of the median nerve. Butterworth-Heinemann, Boston

Sarria L, Cabada T, Cozcolluela R, et al (2000) Carpal tunnel syndrome: usefulness of sonography. Eur Radiol 10:1920–1925

Shea JD, McClain EJ (1969) Ulnar nerve compression syndromes at and bellow the wrist. J Bone Joint Surg 51: 1095–1103

Sidey JD (1969) Weak ankles: a study of common peroneal entrapment neuropathy. BMJ 3:623–626

Spinner M (1968) The arcade of Frohse and its relationship to posterior interosseous nerve paralysis. J Bone Joint Surg 50B:809–812

Spinner RJ, Goldner RO (1998) Snapping of the medial head of the triceps and recurrent dislocation of the ulnar nerve. J Bone Joint Surg Am 80:239–247

Stevens JC (1987) AAEE minimonograph #26: electrodiagnosis of carpal tunnel syndrome. Muscle Nerve 10:99–113

Stevens JC, Sun S, Beard CM, et al (1988) Carpal tunnel syndrome in Rochester, Minnesota, 1961 to 1980. Neurology 38:134–138

Stevens JC, Beard M, O'Fallon WM, et al (1992) Conditions associated with carpal tunnel syndrome. Mayo Clin Proc 67:541–548

Stewart JD (1993) Compression and entrapment neuropathies. In: Dyck PJ, Thomas PK (eds) Peripheral neuropathy, 3rd edn. Saunders, Philadelphia, pp 1354–1379

Stoehr M, Bluthardt M (1993) Atlas der klinischen Elektromyographie und Neurographie. Kohlhammer, Stuttgart

Sturzenegger M, Rutz M (1991) Radial nerve paralysis – causes, site and diagnosis. Analysis of 103 cases. Nervenarzt 62:722–729

Szabo RM, Chidgey LK (1989) Stress carpal tunnel pressures in patients with carpal tunnel syndrome and normal patients. J Hand Surg 14:624–627

Wilhelm A (1985) Das proximale Radialiskompressionssyndrom. Behandlung und Ergebnisse. Handchirurgie 17: 215–224

4 Traumatic Nerve Lesions

G. Bodner and S. Peer

CONTENTS

4.1 Introduction 61
4.2 Primary Evaluation of Traumatic Nerve Lesions in the Extremities
G. Bodner, S. Peer 62
4.2.1 Radial Nerve Trauma 62
4.2.2 Peroneal Nerve Trauma 63
4.3 Traumatic Lesions of the Brachial Plexus
G. Bodner, S. Peer 66
4.3.1 Etiology 66
4.3.2 Clinical Diagnosis 66
4.3.3 Sonography 66
4.3.4 Therapy 68
4.4 The Postoperative Nerve
S. Peer 68
4.4.1 Normal Findings in Postoperative Nerves 68
4.4.2 Postoperative Scarring 71
4.4.3 Neuroma Formation 72
4.5 Iatrogenic Nerve Lesions
S. Peer 72
4.5.1 Nerve Lesions in Association with Head and Neck Surgery 74
4.5.2 Nerve Lesions Associated with Orthopedic Surgery 76
4.5.3 Miscellaneous Postoperative Lesions 79
4.5.4 Nerve Lesions Associated with Anesthesia 79
References 80

4.1 Introduction

Traumatic lesions of peripheral nerves are common. According to the literature a relevant lesion of a peripheral nerve exists in roughly 2% to 3% of patients admitted to Level I trauma centers. If plexus and root injuries are included the incidence rises to about 5% (Noble et al. 1998; Robinson 2000). Besides the medical impact of these lesions, they constitute a major social problem, as recovery is often incomplete (especially in cases of delayed treatment), which may result in long-lasting disability. This is even more troublesome, as patients with these types of injuries belong to a younger and highly productive age group within the trauma population. Institution of adequate and early treatment is the only chance to prevent unfavorable outcomes in these patients, and therefore an exact diagnostic work-up is mandatory. Sonography and other imaging techniques may be helpful in this regard, as they allow direct visualization of the nerve and its surroundings, thus setting the path for early institution of surgery in cases where improvement of nerve function with conservative treatment is not to be expected. The latter is true for completely or partially dissected nerves, nerves compressed by close lying hematomas or bony spurs in the case of coexisting fractures, etc.

The reasons for a traumatic peripheral nerve lesion may be manifold but in our opinion two large groups have to be discerned in general: *direct lesions during the course of trauma* and *iatrogenic nerve lesions*. While the first group implies mainly a medical problem, the latter constitutes a medicolegal problem, due to coexisting issues of malpractice and insurance (Birch et al. 1991; Peer et al. 2001; Wilbourn 1998). Especially in the latter group, exact documentation of the type and extent of a nerve lesion is necessary and the differentiation between a lesion that is truly related to bad medical practice (such as transection of the accessory nerve during neck dissection) and a lesion that is due to some type of unfavorable clinical outcome (development of scar tissue, for example) is of the utmost importance. After an introduction to sonography of primary nerve lesions in sections 4.2 and 4.3, we focus in more detail upon iatrogenic types of lesions in section 4.4.

G. Bodner, MD
Professor, Department of Radiology, Section for Diagnostic and Interventional Sonography, University Hospital Innsbruck, Anichstrasse 35, 6020 Innsbruck, Austria
S. Peer, MD
Professor, Department of Radiology, Section for Diagnostic and Interventional Sonography, University Hospital Innsbruck, Anichstrasse 35, 6020 Innsbruck, Austria

4.2 Primary Evaluation of Traumatic Nerve Lesions in the Extremities

G. Bodner, S. Peer

Traumatic injury to peripheral nerves results in considerable disability across the world. In peace-time, motor vehicle accidents are among the most common reasons, followed by penetrating trauma, falls and industrial injuries (Robinson 2000). In war-time peripheral nerve trauma is much more common, and much of the knowledge about these injuries and their treatment was acquired during the two World Wars and subsequent wars (Seddon et al. 1975; Sunderland 1978). While in the upper limb, the radial nerve is most commonly involved, the sciatic nerve is most frequently injured in the lower limb, but in general lower limb lesions are much less frequent (Noble et al. 1998; Robinson 2000). Nerve lesions often occur in association with fractures of nearby bones, such as radial nerve injuries with humeral shaft fractures. Peripheral nerve injuries may be seen as isolated lesions, but also accompany central nervous system trauma. About 10% to 34% of patients admitted to rehabilitation units have coexisting peripheral nerve injuries (Stone and Keenan 1988). This may cause problems in so far as the detection and classification of a peripheral nerve injury is much more difficult in this patient group.

Among the possible traumatic lesions, radial nerve palsy in traumatic humerus fractures is the most common, reported to be 2% to 18% (Mast et al. 1975; Shah and Bhatti 1983). The general sonographic appearance of nerve pathology in direct trauma is essentially the same irrespective of the nerve involved, which is why we focus on radial nerve lesions as an example of traumatic lesions. As already mentioned, these lesions are most common and therefore also the experience with sonography of these lesions is well settled. In addition we discuss an often-missed type of traumatic peroneal nerve lesion, which occurs in the setting of knee luxation.

4.2.1 Radial Nerve Trauma

4.2.1.1 *Etiology*

The radial nerve has a close anatomic relationship to the humerus in the spiral groove. Owing to this close relationship of the radial nerve with the bone and the low mobility of the nerve at the site, where it pierces the lateral intermuscular septum, fractures with radial nerve paralysis are usually located at the middle or distal third of the humeral shaft. The nerve may be injured by direct contusion or laceration, by fracture fragments piercing the nerve, interposition between fragments or by traction due to dislocation of the bone.

In traumatic humerus fractures associated with radial nerve palsy, we have to distinguish primary lesions, which occur with the trauma event, and secondary lesions, which appear during the operation (squeezing of the nerve or interposition between fracture fragments or implants during closed or open reposition of the fracture) or the healing process of the humerus fracture. The nerve may be impinged upon, partially or completely dissected, or simply become swollen and edematous due to an encasing intrafascicular hematoma. In secondary nerve palsy, the nerve may be surrounded or displaced by callus or even be compromised by metallic implants (Bodner et al. 2001).

4.2.1.2 *Clinical Diagnosis*

Besides a clinical neurological examination, an electrodiagnostic examination is currently the method of choice to indicate the presence and level of nerve damage and to assess functional nerve recovery. In most cases of a radial nerve palsy, conduction studies show some amount of activity and therefore at least partial integrity of the nerve. Follow-up EMG can assess the amount of recovery. Nerve conduction tests, however, are unable to differentiate the cause of the nerve damage, for example if the nerve is partially dissected, impinged upon by fracture fragments or severely encased by callus. It is important to diagnose these underlying reasons for the nerve palsy at an early stage, as irreversible degeneration of the motor end-plate of the muscle may occur after 6 to 12 months. According to the literature, a nerve without signs of recovery within 3 to 4 months has to undergo surgical inspection, but the proper treatment for a humeral fracture with coexisting radial paralysis is still a matter of debate. Spontaneous recovery is reported to occur in 73% to 92% of cases, but this is not to be expected in cases with direct compromise of a nerve by callus or interposition of a nerve within the fracture (see above).

4.2.1.3 *Sonographic Findings*

Sonography performed at the time of trauma helps in the triage of patients with radial palsy into those in whom immediate surgical exploration and nerve reconstruction is indicated and those who will benefit from conservative treatment. Using a 5–12 MHz broadband linear array the radial nerve is easily detected at the lateral aspect of the mid-humerus. In addition color Doppler sonography allows the accompanying deep brachial artery to be visualized, which may serve as a guideline for identification of the nerve. The nerve is best identified in a transverse scan. It consists of four to eight hypoechoic tubular structures surrounded by an echoic rim. The nerves normal transverse diameter ranges from 4.0 to 4.2 mm and the normal anteroposterior diameter ranges from 2.3 to 3.5 mm.

The common finding of a swelling proximal to the damaged segment, which is observed in any injured peripheral nerve, is also an apparent feature of the traumatically injured radial nerve. On sonography the nerve appears hypoechoic with loss of its regular dotted pattern on cross sections. In two of our own cases sonography played an important role in the decision as to whether or not to surgically inspect the nerve. Sonography allows callus encasing the nerve and callus simply displacing the nerve to be differentiated (Figs. 4.1 and 4.2). In the first case surgical removal is needed; in the second case conservative treatment is indicated.

Nerve dissection is best visualized in a longitudinal scan, and the gap between the two dissected parts can be measured. In all cases a differentiation of complete from partial dissection should be attempted by careful evaluation of the integrity of the superficial epineurium, as this will probably change the surgical approach. In this regard sonography also allows exact location of the stumps in complete dissections, which is very important information for the surgeon. On sonography the proximal stump generally appears thicker than the distal stump (Figs. 4.3 and 4.4).

Nerve entrapment between fracture fragments or riding of a nerve on the edge of a fracture fragment are further important sonographic diagnoses, as they will also necessitate surgical intervention (Fig. 4.5).

4.2.1.3
Therapy

Conservative treatment (physiotherapy, antiinflammatory drugs) is the method of choice in radial nerve palsy associated with humerus fracture with resolving neurological symptoms within 1 month and without previous sonographic evidence for a pathology requiring early surgery.

Surgical nerve inspection is required in radial nerve palsy associated with open humeral shaft fracture, in vascular injury or when bone débridement is required. In these cases the nerve is inspected and then embedded between the triceps muscles. When the nerve is dissected or severely damaged, nerve grafting is the method of choice.

4.2.2
Peroneal Nerve Trauma

4.2.2.1
Etiology

Peroneal nerve injury in traumatic knee dislocation is not uncommon and occurs especially in high-

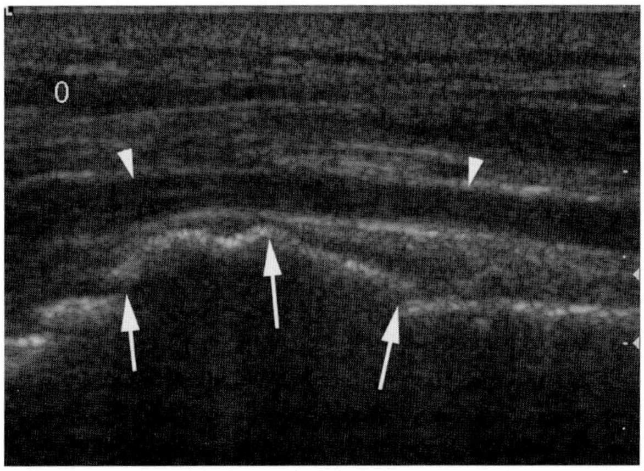

Fig. 4.1. Longitudinal sonogram through radial nerve in a patient after humeral shaft fracture with partial radial nerve palsy shows radial nerve (*arrowheads*) abutted upon by a large callus (*arrows*)

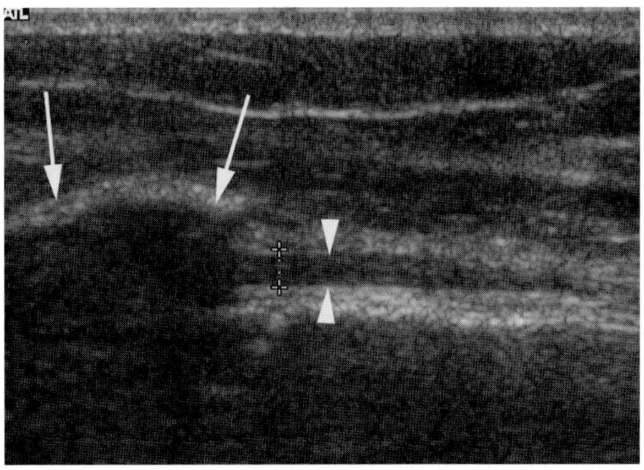

Fig. 4.2. Longitudinal sonogram through radial nerve in a different patient after humeral shaft fracture with radial nerve palsy shows the nerve (*arrowheads*) traversing underneath the callus (*arrows*). The nerve could not be demonstrated beyond the callus in a transverse plane which confirmed encasement

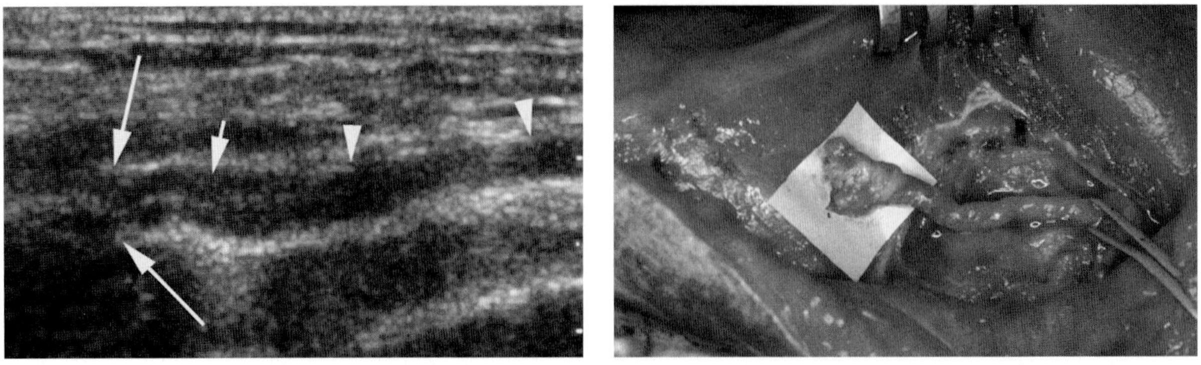

a b

Fig. 4.3a, b. Longitudinal sonogram (**a**) and intraoperative photograph (**b**) of transected radial nerve (**a** *arrowheads*) in a patient with complete radial nerve paralysis after humeral shaft fracture. The distal stump (*long arrows*) is thickened with edematous fascicles (*short arrow*), which was confirmed during surgery (**b**)

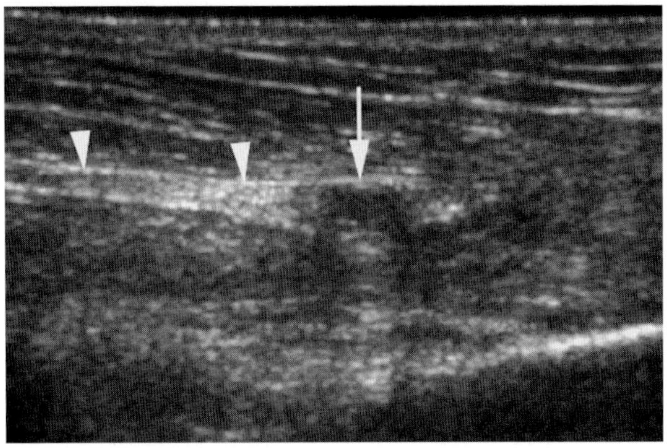

Fig. 4.4. Longitudinal sonogram of transected radial nerve in a patient with complete radial nerve paralysis after humeral shaft fracture (same patient as in Fig. 4.3). The distal stump of the radial nerve is thin (*arrow*), the nerve itself shows a normal caliber (*arrowheads*)

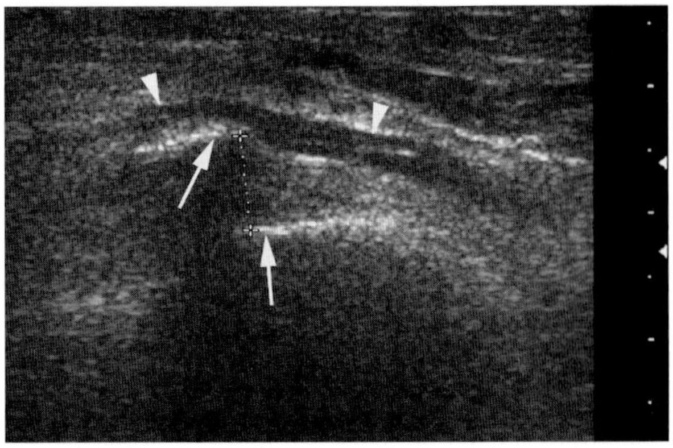

Fig. 4.5. Longitudinal sonogram through radial nerve (*arrowheads*) in a patient with radial nerve palsy after humeral shaft fracture. Sideways compression of the nerve by marked displacement of fracture fragments (*arrows*) is seen

speed accidents or athletic sports injury (Kim and Kline 1996). The common peroneal nerve takes an oblique course in the proximal popliteal fossa after its division from the sciatic nerve. Afterwards it runs in an exposed fibro-osseous tunnel behind the fibular head and, running distally in a very superficial layer, splits into a superficial and a deep branch. Various mechanisms may injure the nerve: overt stretching induced by knee fracture or luxation, complete dissection with or without integrity of the outer nerve sheath (also called neuroma in continuity lesion), penetrating injury or mere contusion.

4.2.2.2 Clinical Considerations

Traumatic peroneal nerve palsy presents with foot drop, pain and sensory deficit at the anterolateral skin surface of the lower leg. In up to 80% of cases, nerve function recovers completely with conservative management, which is monitored with electrodiagnostic testing. When spontaneous regeneration of nerve function does not occur within 6 months, surgical inspection has to be performed. The limitations of electrodiagnosis have already been discussed, but in addition the impossibility of giving an exact estimate of the length of the damaged nerve is especially problematic for peroneal nerve lesions. It has been shown in the literature that, especially in nerve trauma associated with knee dislocation, the damaged nerve segment may reach 20 cm (Tomaino et al. 2000). This was also the case in 4 of 12 patients in our own series of traumatic peroneal nerve palsies. During surgery the stretched nerves in these patients showed a high amount of fibrosis with neuroma formation.

4.2.2.3 Sonography

The easiest access to the peroneal nerve is with the patient lying on the nonaffected side, with the knee in slight extension. After identification of the distal part of the sciatic nerve in a transverse plane, the transducer is moved downward to the division of the tibial and peroneal nerve and further on along the course of the common peroneal around the fibular head. Depending on patient size a 7–12 MHz linear array may be needed for sonography of the sciatic nerve, while a 7–15 MHz linear array is more appropriate for investigation of the common and superficial peroneal nerve.

The normal peroneal nerve is a rather small nerve with just a few fascicles. However, when injured the nerve loses its typical sonographic fascicular pattern due to edema and vasocongestion. In severe nerve damage, the edema may even reach far proximal into the sciatic nerve. In this case the sciatic nerve may only partially show abnormal signal, with normal appearing tibial nerve elements and partial loss of fascicles corresponding to the damaged common peroneal nerve elements (Fig. 4.6).

Neuroma in continuity appears as a long tubular hypoechoic structure with a variable length of up to 20 cm (Fig. 4.7). The sonographic diagnosis of complete nerve dissection is straightforward with apparent discontinuity of the nerve with a hypoechoic, thickened proximal stump. The stump can be embedded in hematoma or in older lesions in scar tissue (Fig. 4.8).

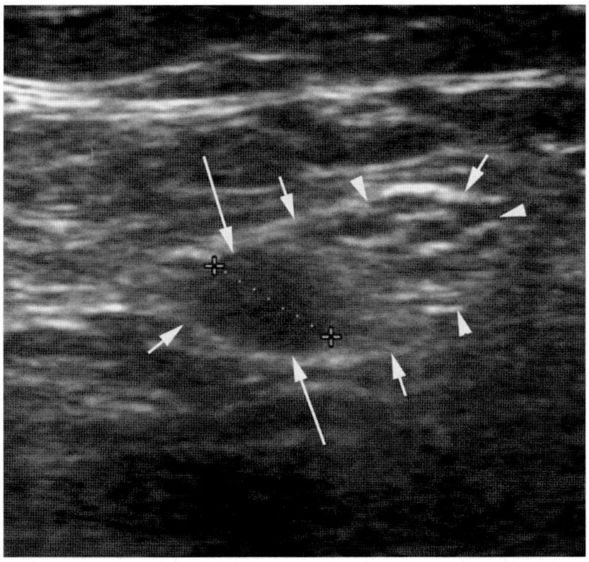

Fig. 4.6. Transverse sonogram through sciatic nerve in a patient with peroneal nerve palsy after knee luxation shows marked edema and loss of fascicular texture of the peroneal elements inside the sciatic nerve (*long arrows*), whereas tibial components (*arrowheads*) are normal. Note normal appearing uninterrupted epineurium (*small arrows*)

4.2.2.4 Therapy

Conservative management includes physiotherapy to strengthen the atrophic muscles, and local steroid infiltration may bring relief in hypertrophic scar formation. However, any external compression of the nerve by scar tissue or callus formation requires surgical intervention. In general, surgical nerve inspection is indicated when electroneurographic testing shows no improvement of nerve function during

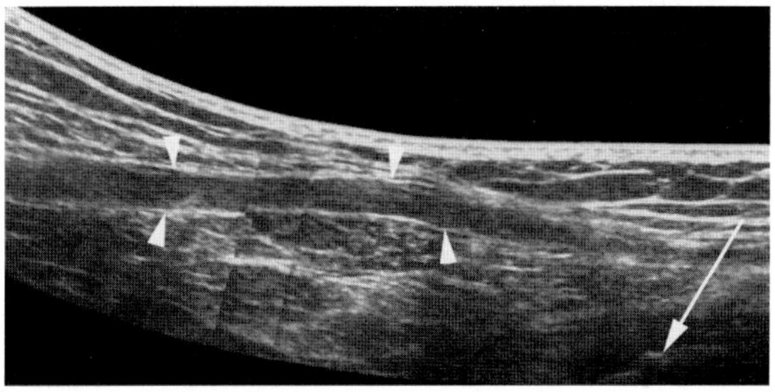

Fig. 4.7. Longitudinal panoramic sonogram along the course of the common peroneal nerve in a patient with peroneal palsy after knee luxation. Marked swelling and edema with loss of fascicular texture of the nerve is seen along a considerable distance (*arrowheads*) consistent with neuroma in continuity (*long arrow* fibular head)

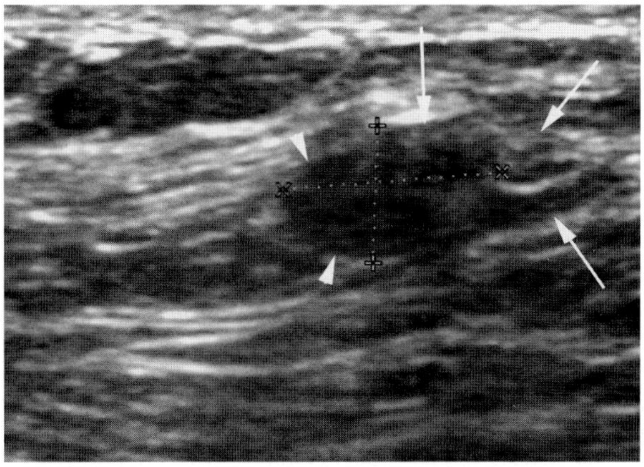

Fig. 4.8. Transverse sonogram through common peroneal nerve in a patient who developed peroneal palsy after knee luxation shows thickened nerve segment (*arrowheads*) impacted by scar tissue (*arrows*)

conservative treatment, or when sonography shows extensive intraneural neuroma formation or complete nerve dissection. The nerve inspection has to be extended to the proximal section of the common peroneal nerve in order not to overlook fibrotic nerve segments caused by traction injury.

4.3 Traumatic Lesions of the Brachial Plexus

G. Bodner, S. Peer

Magnetic resonance imaging and CT myelography are currently considered the techniques of choice for imaging of the brachial plexus. Most centers favor MRI because of the inherent multiplanar capability and high soft-tissue contrast. In a recent study (Doi et al. 2002), a sensitivity of 92% for MRI and CT myelography was found in the diagnosis of nerve root avulsion, and according to Penkert et al., CT myelography and MRI are accurate in 85% and 52%, respectively, in the diagnosis of brachial plexus lesions (Penkert et al. 1999).

Conversely, little is known of the value of sonography for imaging the plexus and reports in the literature mainly center around the possibility of sonography to guide the administration of anesthetics to the plexus fascicles (Sheppard et al. 1998; Yang et al. 1998) (see also Chapter 6). In section 4.3.3 an overview of the possible applications of sonography to imaging of traumatic plexus lesions is given.

4.3.1 Etiology

A variety of traumatic events may result in immediate injuries to the brachial plexus including massive shoulder trauma, head and neck trauma and direct thoracic trauma. Other secondary causes for brachial plexus palsy are fractures of the clavicle with subsequent scarring or callus formation, infiltration by tumors of the thoracic apex or neck, direct neurogenic tumors and iatrogenic injuries. Nerve root avulsion injury occurs in injuries involving severe traction on the upper extremity, most commonly in motorcycle accidents. The injuries can affect the complete extent of the plexus from the cervical roots to the supra- and infraclavicular area. In severe trauma a "chain injury" with involvement of different parts of the brachial plexus is frequently observed.

4.3.2 Clinical Diagnosis

Brachial plexus palsy shows a varying combination of sensory deficits, dysesthesia or hyperesthesia, together with muscle weakness and motor deficiency, depending on the level of injury (C4–Th1). Electroneurographic testing shortly after the injury and in monthly controls can reliably assess the level of injury and show signs of nerve regeneration.

4.3.3 Sonography

Sonography is best performed with a 7–12 MHz linear array. The patient is positioned supine, with the head turned to the side opposite the investigated area. Sonograms should be acquired in a transverse and longitudinal scan, at the level of the intervertebral foramen and in the supra- and infraclavicular region. For identification of the cervical roots it is best to first identify the vertebral artery in a longitudinal scan. From here the scan head should be moved slightly dorsal to the level of the transverse processes. The cervical roots appear as hypoechoic longitudinal and sometimes slightly bulbous structures arising from the intervertebral foramen. Especially in slender patients with a long and thin neck, even the base of the nerve root can be assessed (Fig. 4.9).

The cervical roots from C4 to C7 can always be detected with sonography, whereas the first thoracic root is not always visible, especially in patients with a short neck. Visualization may be improved if the patient is asked to lower the shoulder, and an examination of the lower roots may even be tried with the patient in a sitting position.

After detection of the cervical roots, the scanhead is turned 90° into a transverse plane and moved downwards along the plexus fascicles. In the interscalene region the plexus appears as a cluster of hypoechoic nodules interposed between the scalenus anterior and medius muscles. The formation of the medial, posterior and lateral plexus trunks can also be established scanning in the inferior interscalene region. In a longitudinal plane, these plexus elements are seen as a hypoechoic tubular structure, with occasional thin internal hyperechoic elements resembling a variable amount of interfascicular epineurium. The diameters of each single root and the individual plexus fascicles are documented in comparison with the noninjured opposite side. Access to the infraclavicular part of the brachial plexus is from below the clavicle and

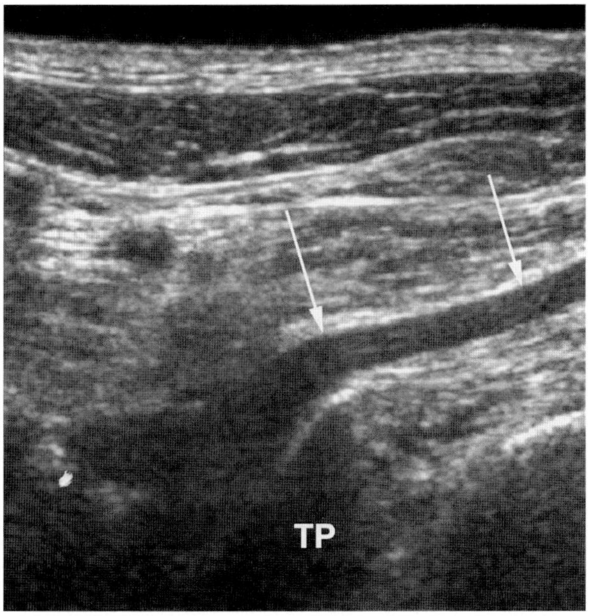

Fig. 4.9. Transverse sonogram through C6 nerve root (*arrows*) in a healthy asymptomatic volunteer demonstrates sonographic visualization of the entire nerve root to the neural foramen (*TP* transverse spinal process)

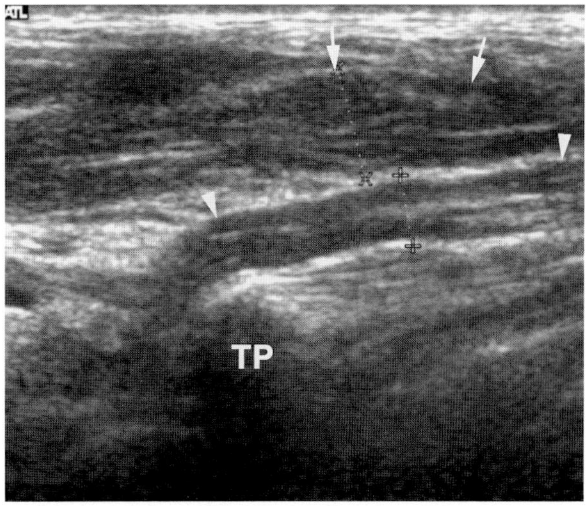

Fig. 4.10. Longitudinal sonogram through paravertebral brachial plexus in a patient after a snowboard accident with evidence of upper plexus palsy. Marked swelling of C5 nerve root (*small arrows*) consistent with traction neuroma but only minimal edema of C6 nerve root (*arrowheads*) consistent with minor traction edema is demonstrated (*TP* transverse spinal process)

an additional axillary approach. While access to the supraclavicular plexus is feasible in almost all patients, the infraclavicular plexus cannot always be visualized sufficiently. As a guiding landmark for identification of the plexus in this region, we use the subclavian artery which is visualized with color Doppler sonography.

Traction neuroma, localized edema (Fig. 4.10) and posttraumatic scarring are the most common traumatic plexus lesions. On sonography traction neuroma has the same appearance as traction neuroma of a peripheral nerve, and shows a hypoechoic enlargement of fascicles proximal to the level of injury (Fig. 4.11).

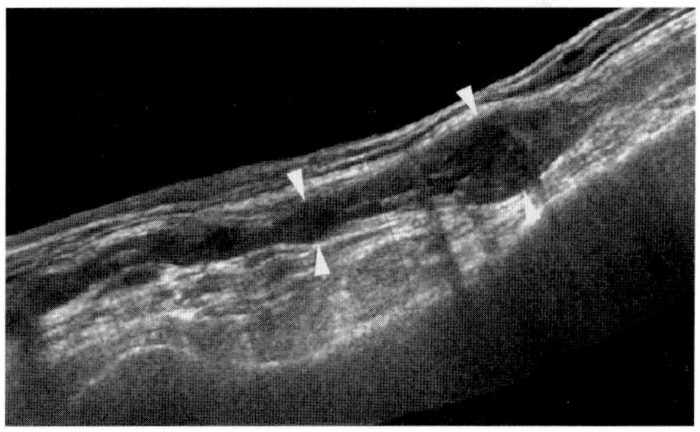

Fig. 4.11. Longitudinal panoramic sonogram in a female patient with severe traction injury of upper extremity in a motor vehicle accident. Bulbous lesions along the plexus fascicle (*arrowheads*) consistent with traction neuromas are demonstrated

Nerve dissection is best demonstrated in a longitudinal scan plane, and in the case of complete transection shows a complete interruption of the fascicles with a variably sized gap (Fig. 4.12), sometimes with demonstration of a thickened proximal nerve stump. The latter finding, however, seems to depend on the delay between the traumatic event and the sonographic examination: in one of our patients with a traumatic brachial nerve palsy sonography was performed within 1 day of trauma. Both dissected nerve stumps were clearly demonstrated without evidence of a bulbous swelling (Fig. 4.13). Two weeks later the proximal stump had changed its shape and appeared bulbous and hypoechoic, which reflects ongoing reparative mechanisms with sprouting of axons.

There are no larger controlled trials on the sensitivity and specificity of sonographic plexus evaluation in traumatic injuries, but according to our experience results are surgically confirmed in most cases. A single study published in the Japanese literature is known to the authors. In this study, sonographic findings in traumatic plexus lesions after motor vehicle accidents were compared with surgical findings, and showed excellent correlations (Hayamizu et al. 1995). The authors especially stress the value of sonography in the preoperative identification of patients in whom surgery is not indicated: those with lesions that favor conservative treatment or lesions with avulsion of the ganglion.

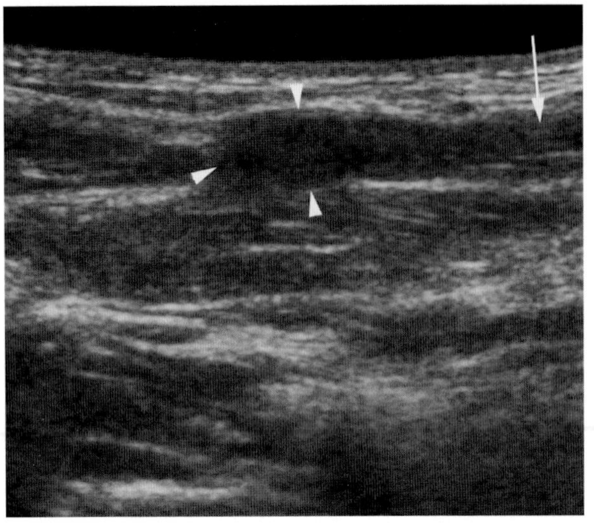

Fig. 4.12. Longitudinal sonogram through C6 nerve root in a patient after a snowboard accident shows complete dissection of nerve root (*arrow*) with swollen stump (*arrowheads*)

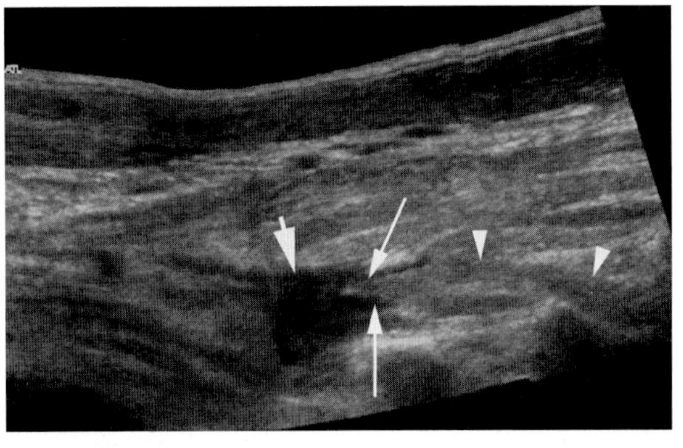

Fig. 4.13. Longitudinal sonogram in another patient with complete dissection of a nerve root (*arrowheads*) acquired on first presentation of the patient to the outpatient department shows a gap with fresh hematoma (*thick arrow*) and proximal stump without thickening (*arrows*)

4.3.4 Therapy

Initial conservative treatment includes physiotherapy and antiinflammatory medication, which is especially indicated in patients with electroneurographic evidence of functional recovery.

If primary evaluation of the plexus shows a lesion, which warrants immediate surgery, such as complete transection of a fascicle, or if no signs of recovery are seen during a trial of conservative treatment, surgical nerve inspection is advocated. The treatment of dissection with nerve grafting is straightforward. In the case of scarring an internal or external neurolysis is performed depending on the extent of damage. Patients who undergo nerve inspection with neurotomy or nerve grafting within 6 month of trauma generally have a better outcome than patients operated upon later than 12 months after the injury (Penkert et al. 1999).

4.4 The Postoperative Nerve

S. Peer

The rationale for sonographic assessment of postoperative nerves is straightforward: incomplete recovery of clinical symptoms after surgical exploration, decompression or microsurgical reconstruction of a peripheral nerve. As is true for other organ systems, typical and transient postoperative findings have to be differentiated from unfavorable development with the need for further intervention. In respect of iatrogenic nerve lesions, it is important to have an adequate knowledge of the postoperative evaluation of a nerve. Typical postoperative changes, such as short-lasting edema and/or hypervascularization of a nerve, the formation of hematomas or scars have to be differentiated from incomplete surgical repair with persistent transection of nerve bundles or development of neuroma.

4.4.1 Normal Findings in Postoperative Nerves

The spectrum of imaging findings in postoperative nerves depends on the type and extent of surgery performed. In external neurolysis a nerve is isolated from surrounding tissues, which in many instances is simply performed to allow direct inspection of the nerve and intraoperative electrodiagnostic testing. In the same way, a nerve known to be surrounded by scar tissue may be released. As the outer sheath of the nerve and the nerve fascicles are not involved in this type of surgery, changes during an uncomplicated postoperative course are only subtle. With only minimal surgical disturbance of the nerve sonographic studies may be normal or show only mild nerve edema with loss of normal fascicular pattern.

The latter is thought to represent a common and nonspecific reaction of a nerve to minor compromise, which may occur in the postsurgical setting, and is most probably caused by transient stretching of the nerve during the operation. The same reaction is also known in nerve compression syndromes such as carpal tunnel disease, nerves subjected to direct blunt trauma and various other pathologies, and represents a disturbance of localized microvascular blood flow in the epineurium and perineurium. There is a gradual transition from mere loss of fascicular pattern to localized swelling of nerve fascicles with an increase in the outer nerve diameter, related to more pronounced edema and hypervascularization. In these more advanced states, differentiation between a self-limited postoperative finding and a persistent impairment of the nerve may be difficult, and the value of sonography lies mainly in the exclusion of external reasons for nerve swelling, such as encasing scars. As a general rule, we may observe a gentle tapering of a nerve to normal size above and below the level of swelling in transient edema and an abrupt change in nerve caliber in nerves hampered by scars (Fig. 4.14).

Persistent nerve edema and swelling of fascicles may commonly be seen as a complication after release and transposition of a nerve, when the extrinsic blood supply of the nerve is severed. As for the ulnar nerve the extrinsic vessels (superior and inferior ulnar collateral artery and posterior ulnar recurrent artery) may be transected during release of the nerve in patients with cubital tunnel syndrome (Balogh et al. 1997; Prevel et al. 1993). Due to a localized disturbance of blood supply in the postoperative nerve a persistent clinical impairment follows and sonographically this may appear as a persistent and pronounced edema of the nerve.

With *internal neurolysis* the nerve and its sheath are directly involved in surgery and this procedure is mainly used for reconstruction of partial nerve lesions requiring a split repair in which functioning nerve fascicles are separated from nonfunctioning transected elements or scarred intraneural tissue. In this procedure, there is the risk of inadvertent damage to still-functioning nerve elements, and postoperative scar formation close to the nerve surface may deleteriously affect nerve recovery (Mackinnon and Dellon 1988) (we comment on the latter in more detail in the next paragraph).

With complete traumatic transection of a nerve or after resection of nerve tumors a more extensive surgical procedure with approximation of the nerve ends is required. The choice of reconstruction depends on the width of the gap between the nerve stumps after resection of all irreversibly traumatized tissue. Given a small gap an end-to-end anastomosis is generally preferred, but significant tension on the approximated ends has to be avoided at all costs. If such end-to-end anastomosis cannot be achieved, then the gap is bridged with interposition of nerve grafts, usually harvested from superficial sensory nerves, such as the sural nerve or the medial brachial and antebrachial cutaneous nerves. In both types of surgical repair the nerve (or nerve and graft) ends are anastomosed with fine monofilament sutures placed within the external or internal epineurium. Despite being only very thin, these sutures are constantly seen on sonographic examinations of reconstructed

a 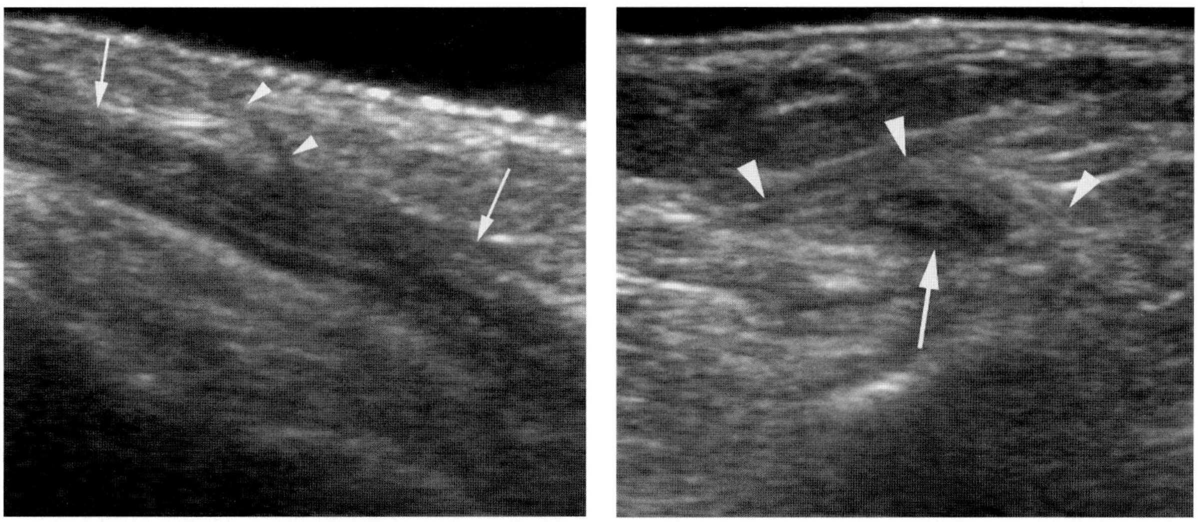 b

Fig. 4.14a, b. Longitudinal (**a**) and transverse (**b**) sonograms in a patient after ulnar nerve decompression because of cubital tunnel disease. A small scar (**a** *arrowheads*) is seen traversing the nerve (*arrows*) and constricting it from above. Note swelling of the nerve distal to the scar (**a** *right side of image*). On the transverse scan the extent of the scar (*arrowheads*) and the encasement of the nerve (*arrow*) are better demonstrated peripheral nerves (Fig. 4.15) and should not be mistaken for pathology, such as fibrotic changes or tiny calcifications in granulation tissue, for example.

The sonographic examination of internal neurolysis or complete nerve reconstruction should always attempt to define the continuity of reconstructed elements. According to our experience with sonography in a large series of patients who received nerve reconstruction after partial or complete traumatic transection, this is only partly achieved. While the integrity of the outer epineurium or the continuity of the nerve in total may be achieved in most cases (Fig. 4.16), an evaluation of the continuity of single fascicles is often not possible. This is most probably due to a somewhat oblique course of the proximal and distal fascicles, which hampers the achievement of a sonographic scan alignment that directly shows both fascicles in continuity. A certain increase in nerve diameter is generally seen at the level of nerve sutures, which is a normal finding as long as it appears mild and fusiform (Fig. 4.17). An irregular bulging of the nerve surface or single nerve elements on one surface, however, should raise a suspicion of partial incomplete fusion of nerve fascicles and neuroma formation (Fig. 4.18). The latter is especially true if an additional hypoechoic fibrous mass lesion exists.

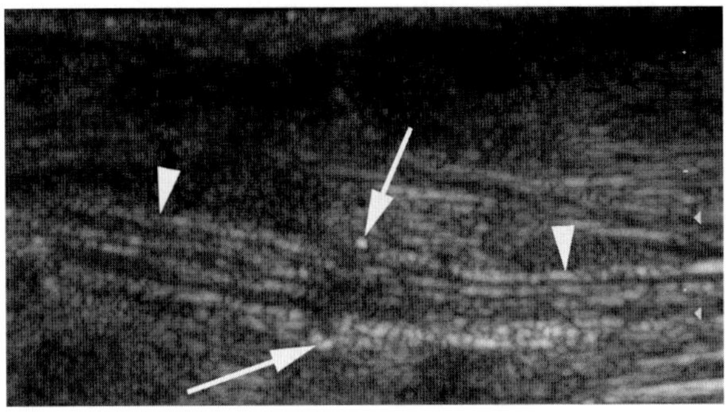

Fig. 4.15. Longitudinal sonogram through median nerve (*arrowheads*) in a patient with forearm amputation and replantation. Tiny echogenic foci caused by suture material are seen on both sides of the site of nerve suture (*arrows*). Note that there is no increase in nerve diameter at the suture site and good continuation of single nerve fascicles in this reconstruction (clinically the patient showed excellent restoration of nerve function)

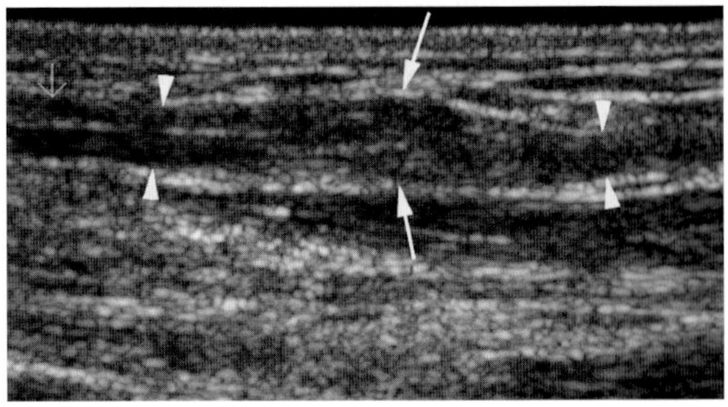

Fig. 4.17. Longitudinal sonogram through ulnar nerve proximal to the elbow in a patient with traumatic ulnar nerve dissection (sharp transection with the edge of a metal plate), who had undergone ulnar nerve repair. Note continuous epineurium (*arrowheads*) and only mild fusiform swelling of the nerve at the site of repair (*arrows*)

a 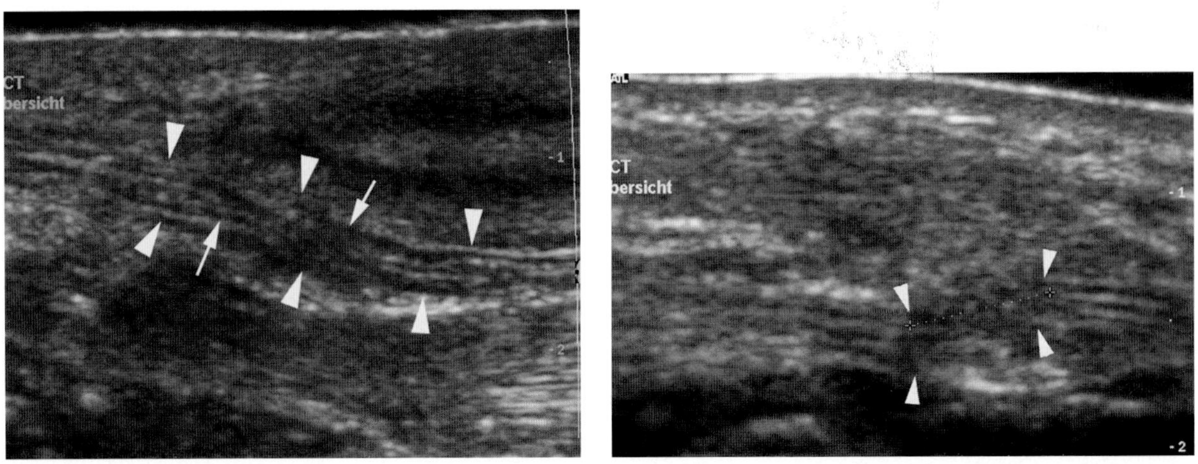 b

Fig. 4.16. a Longitudinal sonogram through ulnar nerve in a patient with forearm amputation and replantation (same patient as in 4.15). While continuity of epineurium (*arrowheads*) is readily identified, an evaluation of the continuity of single fascicles (*small arrows*), however, is not feasible. **b** Longitudinal sonogram through median nerve in another patient who had received primary surgical repair after sharp trauma. Note separation of nerve stumps (*arrowheads*) due to loosening of sutures and subsequent interposition of scar tissue

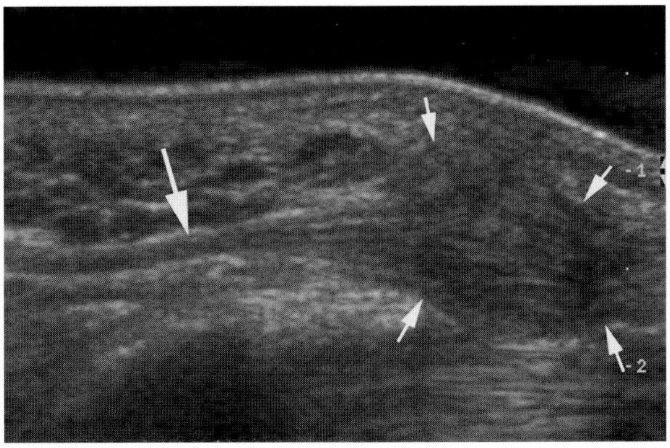

a

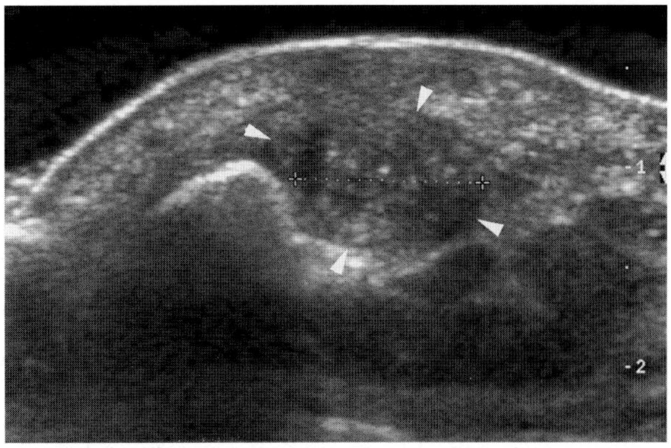

b

Fig. 4.18a, b. Longitudinal (**a**) and transverse (**b**) sonogram in a patient with traumatic transection of the ulnar nerve proximal to the wrist. Normal appearing ulnar nerve (**a** *large arrow*) is seen running into a markedly swollen bundle of irregular nerve elements (**b** *arrowheads*) with indistinct outer surface (**a** *small arrows*), which raised the suspicion of incomplete healing of reconstructed fascicles with superficial scarring and neuroma formation, which were confirmed on subsequent surgical exploration

4.4.2 Postoperative Scarring

Postoperative scarring is a common problem after reconstructive nerve surgery and sonography has proven helpful in early detection of scars in patients with bad recovery after nerve repair (Peer et al. 2001). Scarring may also follow external neurolysis or surgery not primarily directed to a nerve itself (fracture repair, vascular surgery, etc.). While the mechanism of nerve compression by an overlying scar is easily understood, other pathophysiological influences have to be considered, which may lead to a more refined sonographic examination technique. A nerve encased by a scar not only experiences compression with an apparent decrease in nerve diameter on sonography, but may also have tight adhesions between the outer epineurium and the scar tissue. In the case of a close-lying scar, the nerve with an adhesion may even have a fairly normal or even larger diameter (due to edema) compared to more proximal or distal nerve portions (Fig. 4.19).

In this situation scar tissue can cause persistent pain as well as delayed recovery of sensory and motor deficits because of constant traction on the nerve due to the limited possibility for longitudinal translation during movement of an extremity. A functional sonographic examination with close inspection of longitudinal nerve motion at the site of suture during passive or active movement should therefore be attempted in postoperative patients to rule out compromise due to adhesions.

A nerve with too large a gap between nerve stumps following reconstruction by direct anastomosis will react by developing an intraneural scar due to constant traction on the rejoined fascicles. These fibrotic changes must not be confused with neuroma formation, which has a completely different pathophysiological reason. However, intraneural scars and neuromas may hardly be differentiated with sonography based on the echotexture of the pathological tissue elements. Only the shape and course of these lesions may aid in the differential diagnosis. We do not consider the low specificity in this differential a great drawback of sonography, as a second surgical exploration will normally be adequate for treatment of both types of lesions. The mechanism of neuroma formation and its sonographic work-up is discussed in the next section.

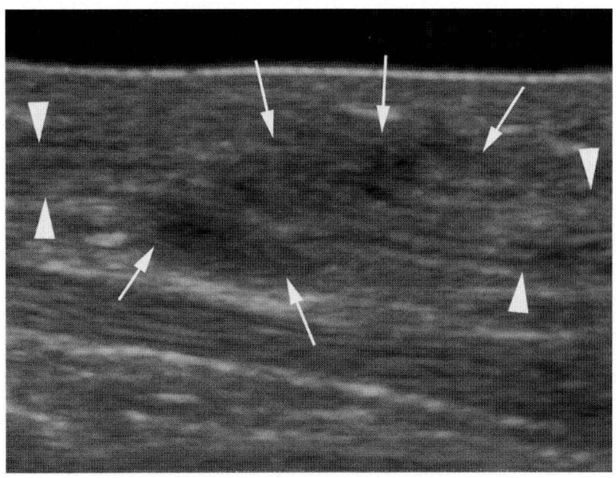

Fig. 4.19. Longitudinal sonogram in a patient after traumatic transection of second median nerve branch just distal to the carpal tunnel, who received primary surgical repair. Extensive scarring (*arrows*) at the site of reconstruction with encasement of the nerve (*arrowheads*) and mild swelling is seen

4.4.3
Neuroma Formation

Neuroma formation is common in traumatic peripheral nerve lesions and may develop in two distinct settings. First it may constitute a direct result of the trauma. If an incomplete nerve lesion undergoes a trial of conservative treatment, there may be partially damaged axons which try to reestablish continuity by sprouting axons and Schwann cells at the proximal stump. The success of this restitutional mechanism depends on the integrity of the axonal or fascicular outer sheath. If this is also impaired, axonal overgrowth results, as sprouting axons and Schwann cells lack a pathway to reach their distal target. A typical example for this type of injury is traction neuroma, which – as the name suggests – is a consequence of excessive stretching of a nerve. Traction neuroma is easily visualized with sonography, and constitutes an ovoid or spindle shaped mass inside a peripheral nerve. This mass is of variable size depending on the number of nerve elements involved. With only single fascicles involved, the outer diameter of the nerve may appear fairly normal or only slightly enlarged, due to coexisting edema. Inside the nerve a hypoechogenic bulbous mass can be detected (Fig. 4.20). If the whole nerve is involved, normal fascicular echotexture is replaced by a mass enlarging the nerve diameter, but the outer nerve sheath if not impaired may appear normal (Fig. 4.21). The latter type of injury is commonly seen in traction injuries of the brachial plexus (motor vehicle accidents).

The second mechanism for the development of neuroma is postsurgical. Focal external or intraneural scarring may impair the reestablishment of nerve continuity and result in neuroma formation. In this regard neuroma is a major complication of surgical interventions, and research on surgical techniques to help reduce the incidence of postsurgical neuroma is still going on. In this regard resection of nerve stumps to functioning neural tissue, microsurgical adaptation of fascicles and epineural sheaths (with or without grafting) and the avoidance of traction are the main concerns. The sonographic appearance of this type of neuroma is fairly similar to posttraumatic neuroma. According to our own hitherto unpublished experience, the sensitivity of sonography in the detection of posttraumatic and postsurgical neuroma is very high. Definition of the extent of nerve involvement, and determination of the exact localization and size of the neuroma in respect of further surgical intervention is straightforward.

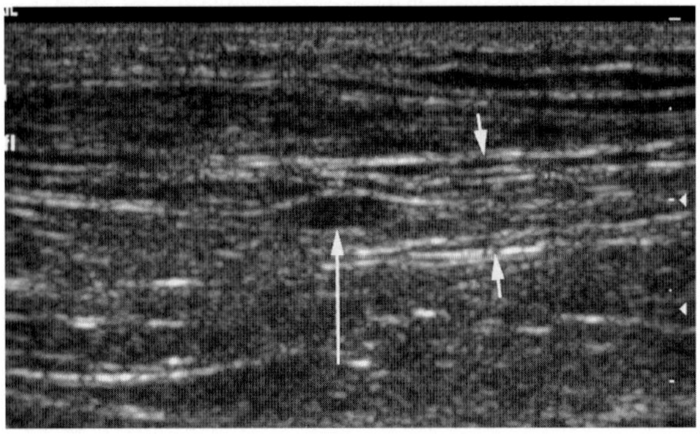

Fig. 4.20. Longitudinal sonogram through sciatic nerve (*small arrows*) in a female patient after total hip arthroplasty with neurological evidence of a sciatic nerve lesion. A small spindle shaped mass (*long arrow*) consistent with intraneural traction neuroma is seen

4.5
Iatrogenic Nerve Lesions

S. Peer

Peripheral nerve lesions secondary to various surgical procedures are not uncommon. Some of these lesions may occur during surgical procedures not primarily directed towards the nerve itself. Dissection of the nerve, traction, or insertion of retractors are the most common causative agents for this type of injury. Another large group of patients sustain peripheral nerve lesions in the course of surgery of the nerve itself, for example for the release of a nerve encased in a narrow osteofibrous tunnel, or nerve suturing after traumatic dissection. In addition, secondary neural damage due to excessive scar formation or compression by hematomas has to be considered. While the first kind of nerve injury has to be considered as truly iatrogenic, the second type may be regarded as an unfavorable postoperative result due to complications occurring.

As mentioned in the introduction to this chapter, true iatrogenic peripheral nerve lesions are a clinical as well as medicolegal problem, as the causal relationship between medical intervention and the nerve lesion is frequently not easily established. Furthermore, detailed information about the type and extent of neural damage is crucial for the selection of adequate treatment.

The diagnosis of peripheral nerve lesions and the decision towards surgical or conservative treatment is normally achieved with the use of clinical and electrodiagnostic tests. Electrodiagnosis may precisely differentiate low-grade lesions without axonal loss ("neurapraxia" according to the Seddon/Sunderland

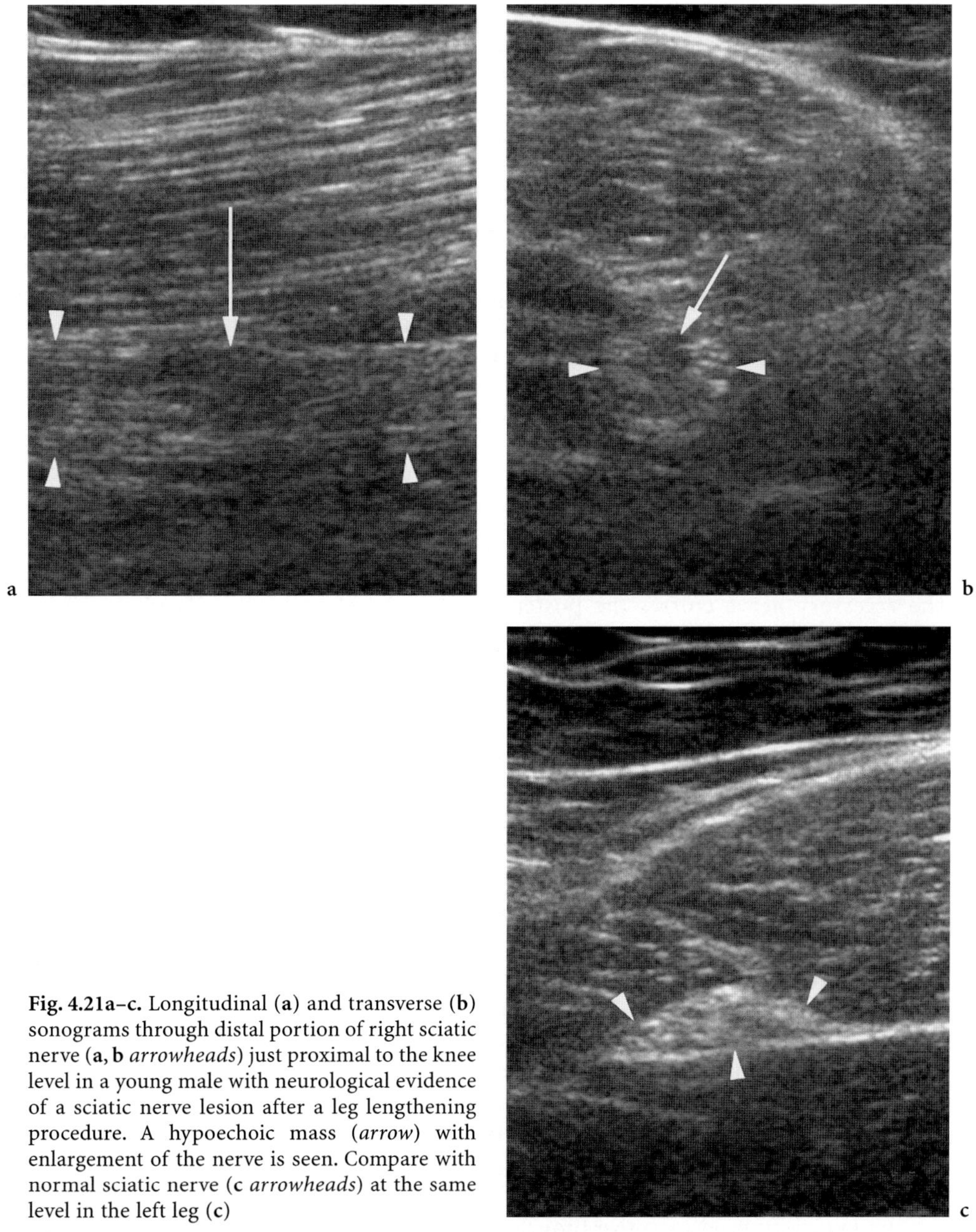

Fig. 4.21a–c. Longitudinal (**a**) and transverse (**b**) sonograms through distal portion of right sciatic nerve (**a, b** *arrowheads*) just proximal to the knee level in a young male with neurological evidence of a sciatic nerve lesion after a leg lengthening procedure. A hypoechoic mass (*arrow*) with enlargement of the nerve is seen. Compare with normal sciatic nerve (**c** *arrowheads*) at the same level in the left leg (**c**)

classification) from higher-grade lesions which involve axon loss and some damage to one or more of the nerve sheath elements ("axonotmesis/neurotmesis") (Seddon 1975; Sunderland 1978). As far as localization of lesions is concerned, there are a variety of pitfalls in electromyography and nerve conduction studies, which therefore may often not yield reliable information about the precise site of nerve involvement. In the same way, electrodiagnostic tests do not give precise information to help in deciding whether to proceed with conservative or surgical therapy. Often a trial of conservative treatment is instituted. If the nerve does not show recovery on follow-up examinations, surgery is performed. Nevertheless, early surgery would be more appropriate even in purely neurapraxic lesions if the nerve is encased by scar tissue, in which case it may not recover during conservative treatment. This diagnosis, however, is beyond the scope of electrodiagnosis and may only be accomplished with direct imaging of the nerve itself, and here sonography may be helpful (Peer et al. 2001).

In the next paragraphs we present an overview of common postoperative/iatrogenic nerve lesions and typical sonomorphological findings.

4.5.1 Nerve Lesions in Association with Head and Neck Surgery

Various surgical procedures in the neck are associated with a potential risk for iatrogenic peripheral nerve damage. The nerve most commonly involved, which allows sonographic assessment, is the accessory nerve. Surgical damage to other nerves in the neck region is either rare or the involved nerves are not easily examined by sonography, which is why we focus on sonography of the accessory nerve only.

4.5.1.1 Accessory Nerve Lesions

4.5.1.1.1 Clinical Considerations

The accessory nerve crosses the posterior cervical triangle in a superficial course, which makes it rather susceptible to injury. Historically, iatrogenic injury of this nerve has been one of the leading causes of trapezius paralysis. As early as the 1940s, accessory nerve injury in association with removal of tuberculous lymph nodes was reported (Wulff 1941). In general, any kind of surgery in the posterior cervical triangle can injure the nerve, for example cervical lymph node biopsy, excision of benign masses or radical neck dissection for malignancy (Woodhall 1952; Harpf et al. 1999; Remmler et al. 1986). Even though iatrogenic injury is still the most common cause of trapezius paralysis, the nerve may rarely be injured in blunt or penetrating trauma to the neck during contact sports, or indirectly with traction injury to the upper extremity (Kauppila and Vastamaki 1996; Vastamaki and Solonen 1984).

The accessory nerve, or cranial nerve IX, is the only motor nerve innervating the trapezius muscle, but it may be joined by proprioceptive branches from the second, third or fourth cervical nerve. Bearing in mind this peculiar anatomical situation, the leading clinical symptom of accessory nerve lesions is impaired trapezius muscle function. Patients typically have an asymmetric neck line because of the atrophic trapezius and drooping of the shoulder girdle. Pain with prolonged use of the shoulder, or a constant feeling of a dull ache or heaviness about the shoulder are common complaints. Patients have difficulty with overhead movements, heavy lifting, prolonged writing or driving a car (Wiater and Bigliani 1999). During active elevation of the arm winging of the scapula is observed as it is displaced laterally, rotating downward and outward. Characteristic findings are difficulty abducting the extremity above the horizontal plane and weakness during elevation against resistance.

Conventional imaging studies such as radiography of the cervical spine and/or shoulder are not generally diagnostic but are almost always carried out and serve the purpose of excluding coexisting bony pathology. Computed tomography and MRI are only indicated in cases where mass lesions with direct compromise of the nerve are suspected, but even in this situation sonography may serve as a primary imaging study.

4.5.1.1.2 Sonography

Sonographic access to the accessory nerve is easy if some basic anatomical considerations are observed. The nerve is best identified at the lateral cervical triangle. After identification of the trapezius muscle and the sternocleidomastoideus muscle, which aid as guiding structures, the scanhead is moved upwards towards the location of the nerve, which lies superficially just underneath the skin. After identification of the nerve it is easily followed in its upward course to the spine and downwards along the trapezius muscle.

As the accessory nerve is a small nerve, its sonographic appearance may not typically resemble the commonly known dotted pattern characteristic of larger peripheral nerves, but may be more like a single hypoechogenic tubular structure (Fig. 4.22) (Bodner et al. 2002).

In the case of complete transection, a gap in the continuity of the nerve may directly be shown with

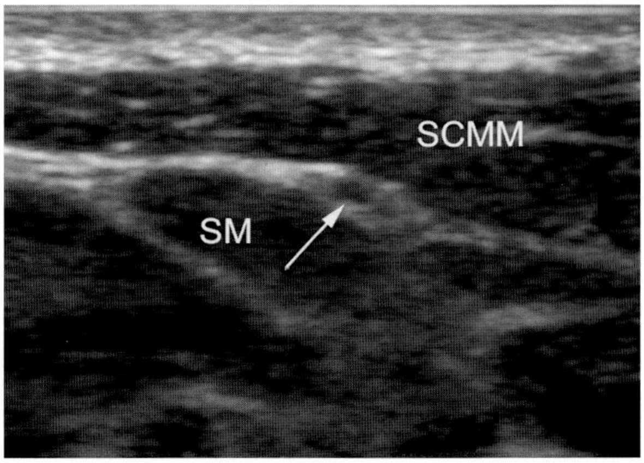

Fig. 4.22. Transverse sonogram acquired at lateral neck triangle showing normal sonographic appearance of accessory nerve (*arrow*) (*SCMM* sternocleidomastoideus muscle, *SM* scalenus muscle)

sonography (Fig. 4.23), but this will sometimes be overshadowed by postoperative scar tissue which impairs direct visualization of a gap within the nerve (Fig. 4.24). A loss of the normal nerve texture and outer diameter is nevertheless observed in these situations (BODNER et al. 2002).

While the existence of such a complete nerve transection is readily diagnosed with electrodiagnostic tests, the value of sonography in this situation is to establish the exact localization of the nerve interruption, which is important information for planning surgical reconstruction. In particular, the distance between the nerve stumps and the shape of the stumps, and the presence of additional scarring or neuroma formation in older nerve lesions are to be examined thoroughly during sonography (Fig. 4.25). The examinations provide important information for the decision towards primary nerve anastomosis or nerve grafting.

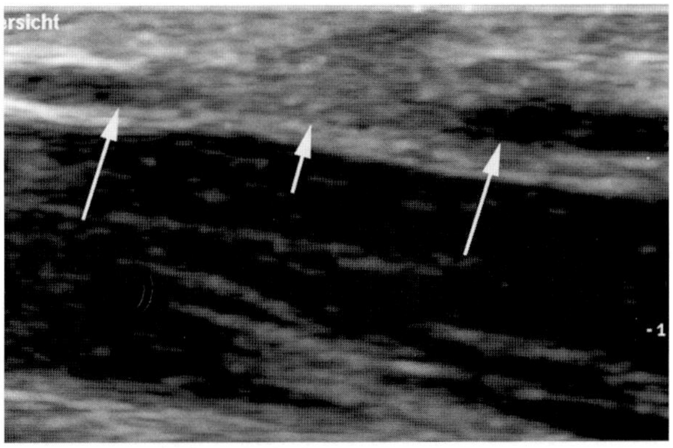

Fig. 4.23. Longitudinal sonogram through accessory nerve in a patient who had undergone lateral cervical lymphadenectomy. Complete transection of accessory nerve with demonstration of a small gap (*short arrow*) and separated and swollen nerve stumps (*long arrows*)

While the therapy of complete transection is straightforward, incomplete nerve lesions may pose a clinical and therapeutic problem. In general, surgery is advocated by some authors if a nerve lesion does not show any clinical or electrodiagnostic signs of recovery within 3 months (PERLMUTTER and APRUZZESE 1998), whereas others advise exploration at 6 to 12 months after injury. Another approach, especially with accessory nerve lesions, is to perform early microsurgical nerve repair (WIATER and BIGLIANI 1999), which may be particularly appropriate in patients in whom sonographic studies indicate that recovery with conservative management is not to be expected, such as in those with injuries with interposition of scar tissue or organized hematoma (GRANT et al. 1999; PEER et al. 2002). An early reconstruction spares the patient from long-lasting, and in this case, fruitless physical therapy and improves postoperative outcome in a situation where the function of the trapezius is still good, with no muscular atrophy (NORDEN 1946; WIATER and BIGLIANI 1999).

In chronic lesions of the accessory nerve sonography may not only be useful for evaluation of the nerve itself, but also for direct evaluation of trapezius muscle thickness (Fig. 4.26). Again this is critical information for surgical planning. With long-lasting trapezius muscle dysfunction, results of microsurgical nerve reconstruction will mostly depend on the state of the trapezius muscle (BIGLIANI et al. 1996). With severe muscular atrophy detected during sonographic examinations a decision to perform an extensive muscle transfer, such as the Eden-Lange procedure,

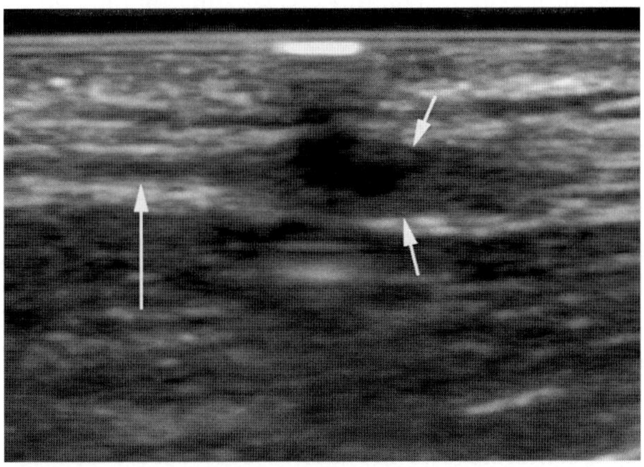

Fig. 4.24. Longitudinal sonogram through accessory nerve in a patient with iatrogenic accessory nerve palsy shows nerve (*long arrow*) impacted in scar tissue (*small arrows*). The continuity of the nerve was not reliably assessed in this patient

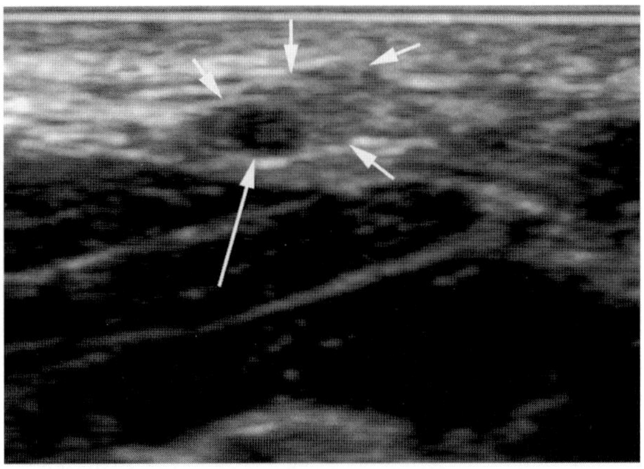

Fig. 4.25. Transverse sonogram through accessory nerve in a patient with accessory nerve palsy after lateral cervical lymphadenectomy. A swollen, edematous nerve stump (*long arrow*) is seen covered by scar tissue (*small arrows*)

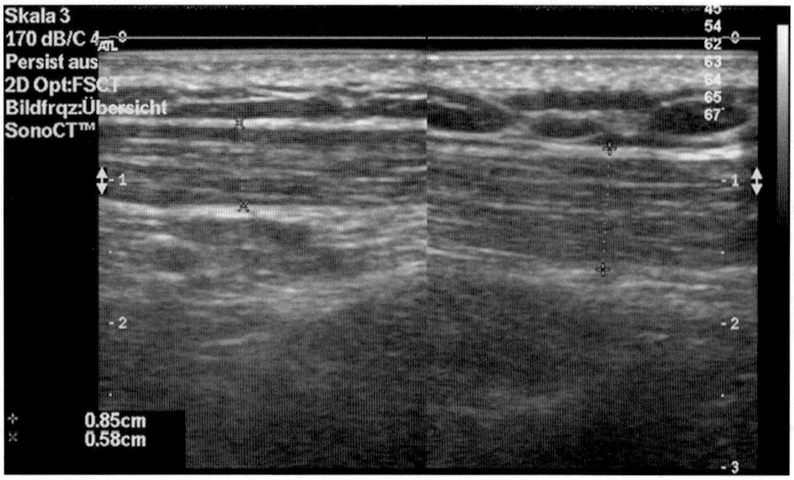

Fig. 4.26. Comparative measurement of trapezius muscle thickness in a patient with iatrogenic accessory nerve palsy showing reduction of muscle diameter in affected side (*left half of image*)

will be more appropriate to receive good restoration of shoulder motion (Bigliani et al. 1996).

4.5.2 Nerve Lesions Associated with Orthopedic Surgery

Various orthopedic procedures (hip surgery, shoulder surgery, leg lengthening, etc.) may be potentially harmful for peripheral nerves. Compared with nerve lesions in association with hip surgery, however, postoperative lesions to other peripheral nerves are less frequent. Therefore we concentrate mainly on lesions associated with hip surgery and comment only briefly on the less-frequent entities.

4.5.2.1 Total Hip Arthroplasty

4.5.2.1.1 Clinical Considerations

The clinical incidence of nerve palsy after primary total hip replacement (THR) is reported to range from 0.08% to 3.7% (Eggli et al. 1999). However, electrodiagnostic studies indicate that nerve damage may occur in up to 70% of cases (Weber et al. 1976). Revision arthroplasty, lengthening of the leg by more than 4 cm, dislocation of the hip during the operation, hemorrhage, direct injury by a retractor, the duration of the operation, the heat of polymerization and intrapelvic extrusion of cement have all been implicated, but the cause of the injury is uncertain in most cases. Several reports suggest that revision arthroplasty and leg lengthening are the most significant factors (Eggli et al. 1999; Oldenburg and Müller 1997). In the orthopedic literature there is also some dispute about an increased incidence of nerve lesions with various surgical approaches to the hip (i.e. direct lateral or posterior approach). The direct lateral approach, or Charnley transtrochanteric procedure, has been found to be more likely to lead to the development of nerve injury (Weale et al. 1996). The reason for this lies in the use of sturdy self-retaining retractors positioned anteriorly and posteriorly in this procedure, which may exert a considerable amount of traction on the soft tissues. Besides direct compromise of a nerve with the retractor, an indirect type lesion may develop with excessive stretching of a nerve. Stretching of the nerve reduces the cross-sectional area of the fascicles and increases intrafascicular pressure thus impairing blood flow in the perineural vascular plexus. Sunderland found that even though nerves are quite elastic structures, stretching by only 20 to 35% is able to cause a functional nerve injury (Sunderland 1978), but this may occur in lengthening of the hip or with excessive stretching of soft tissues.

The nerves most commonly injured during hip surgery are the sciatic and femoral nerve, but also the obturator nerve may be involved. Clinical findings range from causalgic pain in the distribution of the nerve to impairment of walking ability. In the postoperative situation the early clinical diagnosis of a nerve lesion is often difficult, as postoperative pain may be attributed to the procedure itself and the significance of the incidence of nerve injury reported in the literature is masked as only severe damage presents as a clinical complication. Nerve injury may vary from transient blocks in conduction to irreversible damage secondary to transection of the axons. While according to our experience complete lesions are very rare, most patients experience nerve damage to a certain bundle of fascicles within the sciatic or femoral nerve trunk. The latter type of lesions pose the biggest problems as far as differential diagnosis and treatment decisions are considered.

4.5.2.1.2 Sonography

In general sonography may help in the diagnostic work-up of nerve lesions after THR in so far as direct evaluation of the nerve and its surroundings is feasible, thus enabling direct evaluation of hematomas or scars compressing a nerve, direct visualization of transected nerve bundles or localized nerve edema. However, visualization of the sciatic and femoral nerves with sonography is limited to certain anatomical regions, where the nerve is lying superficially with sufficient sonographic access.

Access to the sciatic nerve is normally possible along the whole course of the nerve along the posterior thigh, where it lies on top of the adductor magnus muscle after having entered the thigh at the lower border of the gluteus maximus muscle. The more proximal course from the greater sciatic foramen underneath the gluteal muscles may only be examined with low-frequency scanheads allowing adjustment of the scan to the deep-lying nerve. This necessary compromise in examination technique results in limited resolution, which is why subtle lesions of the nerve may be missed in this region, especially in obese patients. In these cases MR neurography may be used for imaging of the more proximal portions of the sciatic nerve, and this technique has been shown to yield reliable results if specially optimized MR sequences are applied (Maravilla et al. 1998). The second commonly injured nerve during THR is the femoral nerve, which is much more readily accessible with sonography.

Lesions of the sciatic and femoral nerves attributed to THR may include the whole range of sonographically detectable nerve impairment known from other injuries, ranging from localized swelling of single fascicles, to partial interruption with neuroma formation (Fig. 4.27) and compression by scar tissue or hematoma (Fig. 4.28).

4.5.2.2 Shoulder Surgery

There are various reports of postsurgical damage of the axillary nerve or brachial plexus (De Laat et al. 1994; Boardman and Cofield 1999), but despite shoulder surgery being a frequent procedure, these lesions are rare and there is only limited experience with sonographic assessment of the axillary nerve. While the axillary nerve may be identified with sonography at the back of the shoulder – where it appears at the dorsal aspect of the humerus entering from beneath the lower border of the teres minor muscle – it is not as easily assessed on its course through the axilla (see also Chapter 2). A good guiding structure for identification of the axillary nerve is the posterior

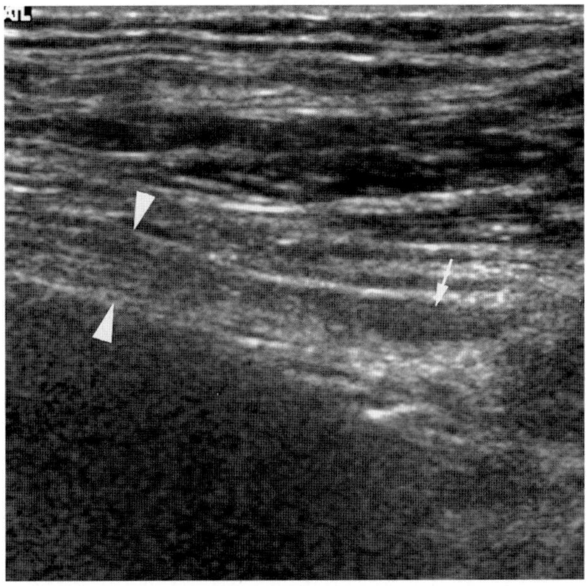

Fig. 4.27. Longitudinal sonogram through femoral nerve (*arrowheads*) in a patient after total hip arthroplasty. A small intraneural traction neuroma (*arrow*) is identified in the distal portion of the femoralis main stem

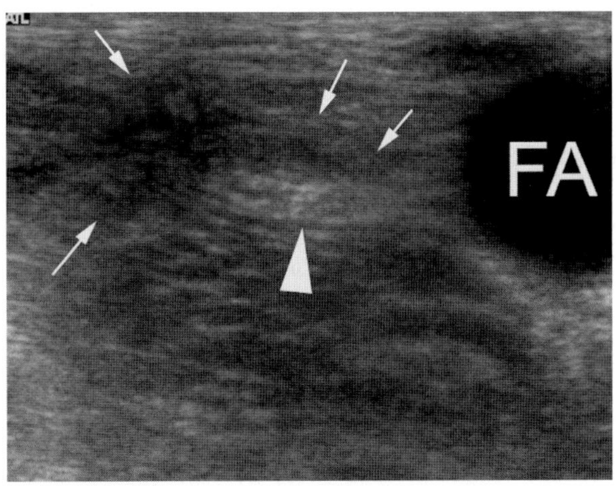

Fig. 4.28. Transverse sonogram through femoral nerve in a patient after total hip arthroplasty. A flattened femoral nerve (*arrowhead*) is seen lying on top of the iliopsoas muscle. The nerve is compressed by a tight close-lying scar (*small arrows*) (*FA* femoral artery)

circumflex artery of the humerus. We aim for examination of this nerve following its course from the back of the shoulder to the axilla and upward to its origin from the posterior plexus fascicle, but in many cases it is not seen in its complete extent. This necessitates a cautious interpretation of results, but pathology such as hematomas after shoulder dislocation with possible compromise to the nerve may be identified.

4.5.2.3
Peroneal Nerve Lesions

Direct surgical damage to the peroneal nerve is possible during leg lengthening procedures or correction osteotomies at the lower leg. Depending on the type of surgical procedure this may involve the common peroneal nerve or one of the peroneal nerve branches. While the common peroneal nerve is easily assessed with sonography (PEER et al. 2002), and the superficial branch may be followed almost down to the ankle, identification of the deep peroneal nerve is especially difficult in the postsurgical patient. Localized scarring or diffuse swelling of the leg with edema leads to sonographic artifacts with degradation of image quality, which especially affects visualization of the deep peroneal nerve on its course underneath the peroneus muscles. Typical peroneal nerve lesions include compression by scars or direct nerve damage due to inadvertent transection or traction injury (Figs. 4.29 and 4.30).

4.5.2.4
Tibial Nerve Lesions

Lesions to the tibial nerve following orthopedic operations are rare, but we have encountered lesions associated with removal of osteosynthetic material, or external fixation of tibiotalar fractures (Fig. 4.31).

The rationale for sonography in these cases is to differentiate direct nerve damage from a so-called posttraumatic tarsal tunnel syndrome. The latter is a condition similar to the idiopathic tarsal tunnel syndrome, and is due to reduction of space in the tarsal tunnel because of abutting periosteal callus, malpositioned fractures or organized hematoma.

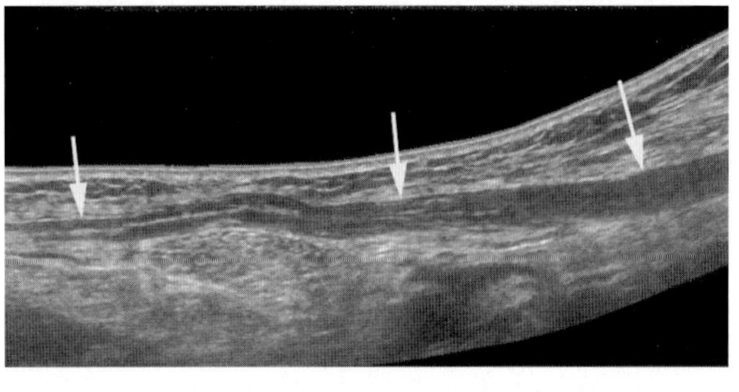

Fig. 4.29. Longitudinal panoramic sonogram of peroneal nerve in a patient with trauma to the lateral aspect of the knee and clinical evidence of peroneal nerve lesion (muscle weakness, paresthesia). Marked swelling of peroneal nerve (*arrows*) with loss of fascicular echotexture is seen in the distal course of the nerve (note normal-appearing fascicles in proximal part of nerve)

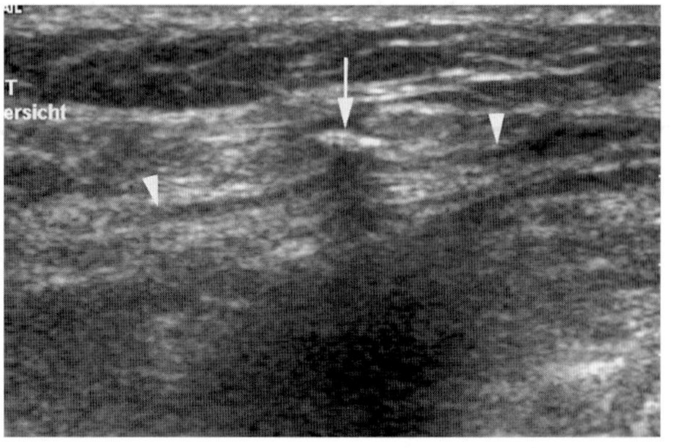

Fig. 4.30. Longitudinal sonogram of peroneal nerve (*arrowheads*) in a patient with peroneal palsy after knee joint luxation. A small calcification with posterior acoustic shadowing and direct contact with the somewhat displaced epineurium is revealed, which may most probably be related to a small, organized hematoma

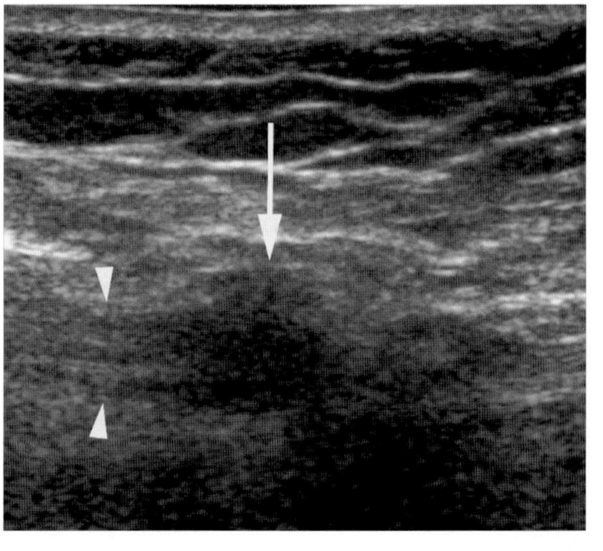

Fig. 4.31. Transverse sonogram through tibial nerve (*arrowheads*) just proximal to the medial malleolus in patient after a distal tibial fracture and osteosynthesis. The patient developed partial paralysis of the tibial nerve after removal of osteosynthetic implants. Tight scar tissue encasing the nerve (*arrow*) was revealed during sonography

4.5.3 Miscellaneous Postoperative Lesions

Various other operative procedures may result in peripheral nerve lesions. General surgical procedures on the lower abdominal or inguinal region may result in damage to the ilioinguinal, iliohypogastric or genitofemoral nerve. During cardiac surgery median sternotomy is associated with a considerable risk of perioperative damage to the brachial plexus, possibly due to excessive traction on the brachial plexus or compression of its medial cord by the first rib (Fig. 4.32).

The harvesting of bone grafts from the iliac crest may be followed by meralgia paresthetica due to injury of the lateral femoral cutaneous nerve. Simonetti and coworkers reported on sural nerve lesions in association with stripping of the small saphenous vein (Simonetti et al. 1999). Furthermore, lesions to the sciatic and femoral nerve may follow various gynecological operations (Fig. 4.33).

In many of the aforementioned situations direct sonographic visualization of the involved nerve – even if it has a superficial course – is possible in certain circumstances only because of the small size of some nerves involved such as the iliohypogastric or ilioinguinal nerve. A sonographic evaluation of the site of postsurgical cutaneous scars is nevertheless useful in many situations, especially if neuroma formation is suspected in patients with operations dating back some weeks or months. The ability of sonography to image neuromas has been shown in various studies (Graif 1995; Peer et al. 2001), and the sonographic features of these types of lesions are discussed in more detail in the section on postoperative findings.

4.5.4 Nerve Lesions Associated with Anesthesia

Perioperative nerve lesions can spoil an otherwise successful operation. The patient may be handicapped with some amount of functional disability and the medical team will possibly face litigation. The true incidence of perioperative nerve damage remains still unclear and is probably under-reported. In direct surgical nerve injury, the leading neurological symptom may appear minor to the attending physician compared with the clinical disorder that led to the surgery, and therefore may be dismissed. The belief that such a minor lesion may be self-limited

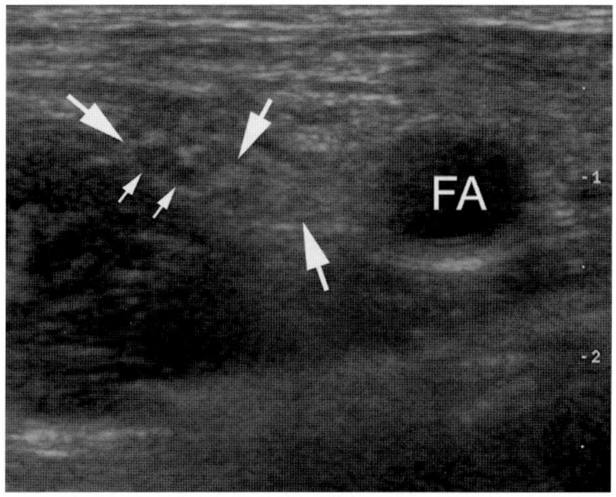

Fig. 4.33. Transverse sonogram through the femoral nerve at the level of the inguinal canal in a patient after total hysterectomy and reconstructive surgery of pelvic floor. Inside the otherwise normal femoral nerve (*large arrows*) two distinct hypoechoic nodules consistent with traction neuromas (*small arrows*) are demonstrated (*FA* femoral artery)

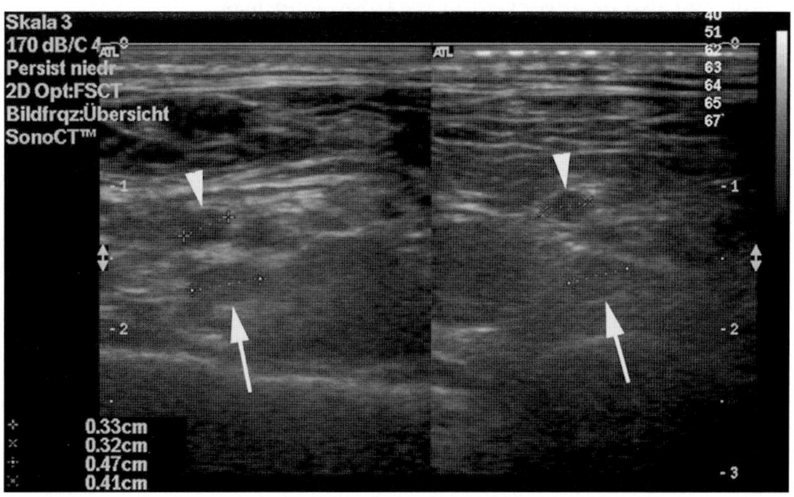

Fig. 4.32. Comparative transverse sonograms of brachial plexus (*right side* left image, *left side* right image) in a patient who had undergone medial sternotomy for cardiac surgery and developed partial radial paralysis thereafter. In side-by-side comparison enlargement with edema of the right-sided posterior plexus fascicle is seen (47 versus 41 mm, *short arrows*), while the medial fascicles show equal caliber (33 versus 32 mm, *arrowheads*)

with full spontaneous recovery is widespread, but often this is not the case.

Malpositioning of the patient on the operation table with subsequent stretching and/or compression of a nerve is today considered the most frequent cause of this type of injury, with direct needle trauma or chemical irritation being rare (Sawyer et al. 2000). With the first type of injury the ulnar nerve is most commonly involved. The ulnar nerve is rather susceptible to compression against the operating table, especially when the forearm is extended and pronated. Another nerve which is frequently injured is the common peroneal nerve, which may be compressed between the head of the fibula and the operating table, or against a leg fixation device with the patient in the lithotomy position. Rarely also other peripheral nerves such as the median nerve may be compressed with the patient in a prone position (Fig. 4.34).

Direct peripheral nerve lesions in association with regional anesthesia are reported in the literature but are relatively rare and may be avoided with meticulous technique and choice of material (Sawyer et al. 2000). In this regard, we want to stress the value of sonography as a guide for regional nerve blocks, which is discussed in more detail in Chapter 6 (Yang et al. 1998).

Sonographic features in these types of nerve lesions are the same as in other types of traumatic nerve injury: localized swelling of nerve fascicles, complete or partial transection of a nerve or secondary nerve compromise due to hematomas or scars. The nerves commonly involved in association with anesthesia such as the ulnar or peroneal nerve are normally easy to assess with sonography due to their superficial course. As a general rule, it is beneficial to compare the possibly damaged nerve with the unimpaired contralateral side, as findings with minor nerve lesions may only be subtle. A comparative study may also be advocated in regard to later legal issues, where exact documentation of site and extent of lesions is of the utmost importance.

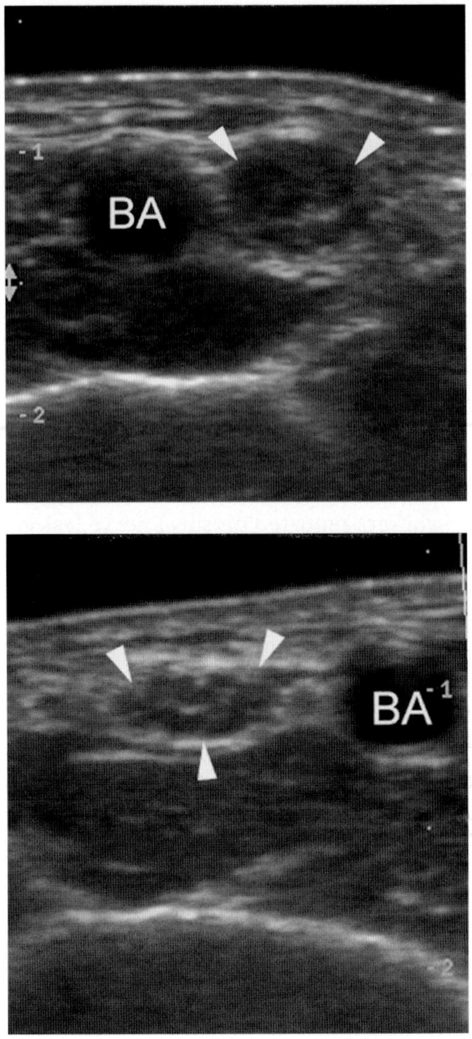

a

b

Fig. 4.34. Comparative transverse sonogram through median nerve at the level of the elbow in a postsurgical patient with partial postoperative neurological deficit (paresthesia in thumb and index finger, with muscle weakness). Note normal-appearing median nerve (*arrowheads*) with distinct fascicular echotexture on normal side (**b**), while in the affected side (**a**) the nerve (*arrowheads*) is markedly enlarged with loss of internal definition (*BA* brachial artery)

References

Aagaard BD, Maravilla KR, Kliot M (1998) MR neurography – imaging of peripheral nerves. Magn Reson Imaging Clin N Am 6:179–194

Balogh B, Vass A, Piza-Katzer H (1997) Ist eine Vorverlagerung des N.ulnaris beim Sulcus nervi ulnaris-Syndrom wirklich indiziert. Handchir Mikrochir Plast Chir 29:133–139

Bigliani LU, Compito CA, Dualde XA, et al (1996) Transfer of the levator scapulae, rhomboid major, and rhomboid minor for paralysis of the trapezius. J Bone Joint Surg Am 78:534–540

Birch R, Bonney G, Dowell J, et al (1991) Iatrogenic injuries of peripheral nerves. J Bone Joint Surg Br 73:280–285

Boardman ND, Cofield RH (1999) Neurologic complications of shoulder surgery. Clin Orthop 368:44–52

Bodner G, Buchberger W, Schocke M, et al (2001) Radial nerve palsy associated with humeral shaft fracture: evaluation with US – initial experience. Radiology 219:811–816

Bodner G, Harpf C, Gardetto A, et al (2002) Ultrasonography of the accessory nerve: normal and pathologic findings in cadavers and patients with iatrogenic accessory nerve

palsy. J Ultrasound Med 21:1159–1163
De Laat EA, Visser CP, Coene LN, et al (1994) Nerve lesions in primary shoulder dislocations and humeral neck fractures. A prospective clinical and EMG study. J Bone Joint Surg Br 76:381–383
Doi K, Otsuka K, Okamoto Y, et al (2002) Cervical nerve root avulsion in brachial plexus injuries: magnetic resonance imaging classification and comparison with myelography and computerized tomography myelography. J Neurosurg 96:277–284
Eggli S, Hankemayer S, Müller ME (1999) Nerve palsy after leg lengthening in total replacement arthroplasty for developmental dysplasia of the hip. J Bone Joint Surg Br 81:843–845
Graif M (1995) Peripheral nerves. In: Fornage BD (ed) Musculoskeletal ultrasound. Churchill Livingston, New York, pp 73–98
Grant GA, Goodkin R, Kliot M (1999) Evaluation and surgical management of peripheral nerve problems. Neurosurgery 44:825–840
Harpf C, Rhomberg M, Rumer A, et al (1999) Iatrogenic lesion of the accessory nerve in cervical lymph node biopsy. Chirurg 70:690–693
Hayamizu K, Naito K, Ito K (1995) Ultrasonography for traction injuries of the brachial plexus. Nippon Igaku Hoshasen Gakkai Zasshi 55:873–877
Kauppila LI, Vastamaki M (1996) Iatrogenic serratus anterior paralysis: long term outcome in 26 patients. Chest 109: 31–34
Kim DH, Kline DG (1996) Management and results of peroneal nerve lesions. Neurosurgery 39:312–319
Mackinnon SE, Dellon AL (1988) Nerve repair and nerve grafts. In: Mackinnon SE, Dellon AL (eds) Surgery of the peripheral nerve. Thieme, New York, pp 89–129
Mast JW, Spiegel P, Harvey JP (1975) Fracture of the humeral shaft – a retrospective study of 240 adult fractures. Clin Orthop 118:254–257
Noble J, Munro CA, Vannemredy SSV, et al (1998) Analysis of upper and lower extremity peripheral nerve injuries in a population of patients with multiple injuries. J Trauma 45: 116–122
Norden A (1946) Peripheral injuries to the spinal accessory nerve. Acta Chir Scand 94:515–532
Oldenburg M, Müller RT (1997) The frequency, prognosis and significance of nerve injuries in total hip arthroplasty. Int Orthop 21:1–3
Peer S, Bodner G, Meirer R, et al (2001) Evaluation of postoperative peripheral nerve lesions with high resolution ultrasound. AJR Am J Roentgenol 177:415–419
Peer S, Kovacs P, Harpf C, et al (2002) High resolution sonography of lower extremity peripheral nerves: anatomic correlation and spectrum of pathology. J Ultrasound Med 21: 315–322
Penkert G, Carvalho GA, Nikkhah G, et al (1999) Diagnosis and surgery of brachial plexus injuries. J Reconstr Microsurg 15:3–8
Perlmutter GS, Apruzzese W (1998) Axillary nerve injuries in contact sports: recommendations for treatment and rehabilitation. Sports Med 26:351–361
Prevel CD, Matloub HS, Zhong Y, et al (1993) The extrinsic blood supply of the ulnar nerve at the elbow: an anatomic study. J Hand Surg [Am] 18:433–438
Remmler D, Byers R, Scheetz J, et al (1986) A prospective study of shoulder disability resulting from radical and modified neck dissections. Head Neck Surg 8:280–286
Robinson LR (2000) Traumatic injury to peripheral nerves. Muscle Nerve 23:863–873
Sawyer RJ, Richmond MN, Hickey JD, et al (2000) Peripheral nerve injuries associated with anaesthesia. Anaesthesia 55: 980–991
Seddon HJ (1975) Surgical disorders of the peripheral nerves, 2nd edn.. Churchill Livingstone. New York
Shah JJ, Bhatti NA (1983) Radial nerve paralysis associated with fracture of the humerus. A review of 62 cases. Clin Orthop 172:171–176
Sheppard DG, Iyer RB, Fenstermacher MJ (1998) Brachial plexus: demonstration at US. Radiology 208:402–406
Simonetti S, Bianchi S, Martinoli C (1999) Neurophysiological and ultrasound findings in sural nerve lesions following stripping of the small saphenous vein. Muscle Nerve 22: 1724–1726
Sunderland S (1978) Nerves and nerve injury, 2nd edn. Churchill Livingstone, New York
Stone L, Keenan MA (1988) Peripheral nerve injuries in the adult with traumatic brain injury. Clin Orthop 233: 136–144
Tomaino M, Day C, Papageorgiou C, et al (2000) Peroneal nerve palsy following knee dislocation: pathoanatomy and implications for treatment. Knee Surg Sports Traumatol Arthrosc 8:163–165
Vastamaki M, Solonen KA (1984) Accessory nerve injury. Acta Orthop Scand 55:296–299
Weale AE, Newman P, Ferguson IT, Bannister GC (1996) Nerve injury after posterior and direct lateral approaches for hip replacement. J Bone Joint Surg Br 78:899–902
Weber ER, Daube JR, Coventry MB (1976) Neural and vascular injury in total hip arthroplasty. J Bone Joint Surg Am 58: 66–69
Wiater JM, Bigliani LU (1999) Spinal accessory nerve injury. Clin Orthop 368:5–16
Wilbourn AJ (1998) Iatrogenic nerve injuries. Neurol Clin 16: 55–82
Woodhall B (1952) Trapezius paralysis following minor surgical procedures in the posterior cervical triangle. Ann Surg 136:375–380
Wulff HB (1941) Treatment of tuberculous cervical lymphoma: late results in 230 cases treated partly surgically. Acta Chir Scand 84:343–366
Yang WT, Chui PT, Metreweli C (1998) Anatomy of the normal brachial plexus revealed by sonography and the role of sonographic guidance in anesthesia of the brachial plexus. AJR Am J Roentgenol 171:1631–1636

5 Tumors and Tumor-Like Lesions

S. Peer and G. Bodner

CONTENTS

5.1 Introduction 83
5.2 Benign Peripheral Nerve Tumors
G. Bodner, S. Peer 84
5.2.1 Schwannoma (Neurilemmoma) 84
5.2.2 Neurofibroma 85
5.3 Malignant Peripheral Nerve Tumors
G. Bodner, S. Peer 86
5.4 Tumor-Like Lesions
S. Peer 88
5.4.1 Nerve Sheath Ganglion 88
5.4.2 Morton's Neuroma 89
5.4.3 Neuroma 92
5.4.4 Neural Fibrolipoma 93
References 94

5.1 Introduction

Peripheral nerve tumors are uncommon and their clinical signs and symptoms often nonspecific, which is why they may pose a diagnostic problem (this is particularly true for the neck, where a palpable mass is often mistaken for an enlarged lymph node by the referring clinician). Several neurogenic tumors can affect the musculoskeletal system, including traumatic neuroma, Morton's neuroma, neural fibrolipoma, nerve sheath ganglia, neurilemmoma, neurofibroma and malignant peripheral nerve sheath tumors (Murphey et al. 1999). In general the diagnosis of such a lesion is based on the detection of a mass in association with neurological signs. It is important, however, to differentiate musculoskeletal lesions with secondary nerve involvement from lesions directly derived from neurogenic tissue. In this regard imaging may be helpful, but only if the applied method has the potential to establish the diagnosis by demonstration of a lesion in direct continuity with a peripheral nerve (Fig. 5.1).

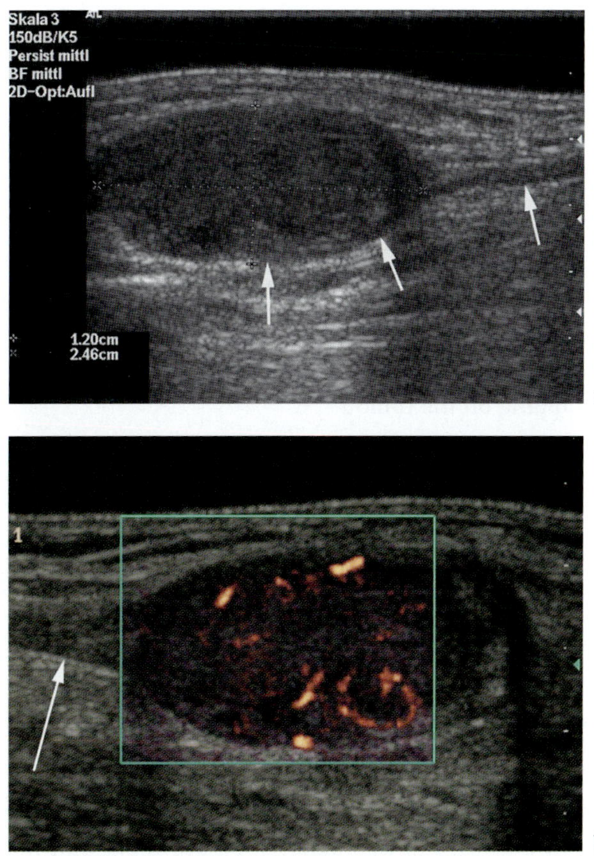

Fig. 5.1a, b. Longitudinal sonogram (**a**) and color Doppler sonogram (**b**) in a patient with a firm palpable mass distal to the proximal tibiofibular joint. A well-defined lesion with hypoechoic echotexture is seen, which shows direct continuity with common peroneal nerve (*arrows*), the lesion arising from the surface of the nerve. Color Doppler sonography reveals multiple tumor vessels. The combination of findings is characteristic of schwannoma

S. Peer, MD
Professor, Department of Radiology, Section for Diagnostic and Interventional Sonography, University Hospital Innsbruck, Anichstrasse 35, 6020 Innsbruck, Austria
G. Bodner, MD
Professor, Department of Radiology, Section for Diagnostic and Interventional Sonography, University Hospital Innsbruck, Anichstrasse 35, 6020 Innsbruck, Austria

Further an exact description of the intrinsic imaging appearance and location of a lesion is necessary, as these may present clues for the final differential diagnosis (Fig. 5.1). According to our experience, sonography is a valuable diagnostic tool for these purposes, as it is a generally available and cheap method, which allows direct evaluation of these mostly superficially lying tumors. In most cases the association with a peripheral nerve is easily established and with the application of color Doppler, power Doppler and spectral wave analysis a lesion's malignant potential may even be realized (Bodner et al. 2002).

5.2 Benign Peripheral Nerve Tumors

G. Bodner, S. Peer

Classically, benign peripheral nerve tumors have been divided into schwannoma (neurilemmoma) and neurofibroma, which constitute the most frequent benign nerve tumors (Weiss 2001). While these tumors are similar in appearance and contain cellular elements related to normal Schwann cells, some distinguishing clinical and pathological features exist. Other rare benign neural tumors include granular cell tumor, nerve sheath myxoma and extracranial meningiomas. Clinically all benign tumors present as a slow growing mass, with or without pain. Sometimes a Tinel's sign can be shown by tapping on the tumor.

5.2.1 Schwannoma (Neurilemmoma)

5.2.1.1 Clinical Introduction

Schwannoma most commonly affects patients 20 to 30 years of age (but may also appear in the older age group) and constitutes approximately 5% of all benign soft tissue neoplasms (Murphey et al. 1999). It occurs equally in both genders. Areas of predilection are the flexor surface of the upper and lower limbs and the neck. It mainly appears as a solitary lesion, rarely presenting in a plexiform or multinodular form. The lesion shows nonaggressive features including slow growth and small size, pain and neurological symptoms are unusual except in larger tumors. On clinical examination the lesion is freely mobile to palpation except at the site of nerve attachment.

On pathological analysis the schwannoma has a size of 2 to 5 cm and shows a true capsule – which allows easy surgical enucleation – and a fusiform shape, because of the nerve entering and exiting the mass. In larger nerves the mass has an eccentric location in relationship to the involved nerve, which is an important sonographic criterion for its differentiation from neurofibroma. Histologically the lesion derives from the nerve sheath, and may appear in a solid and myxoid form. It is distinguished on immunohistochemical analysis from neurofibroma by intense staining for S-100 protein. A large schwannoma (also called ancient schwannoma) may show a high amount of cystic degeneration, central hemorrhage and calcification, which is attributed to its slow growth. Malignant transformation in a schwannoma is extremely rare.

The treatment of schwannoma is usually surgical enucleation of the lesion after incision of the epineurium, which because of the eccentric location of the tumor in contrast to neurofibroma normally allows the native nerve to be spared.

5.2.1.2 Sonography

Sonographic visualization of benign peripheral nerve tumors depends on the location of the tumor. Deep lying tumors at a depth of more than 3 cm below the skin surface are better visualized with a 4–7 MHz linear probe, whereas superficially lying tumors are best investigated with 5–12 or 15 MHz linear probes.

Many reports in the literature describe the sonographic appearance of peripheral nerve tumors in various locations (Martinoli 2000; Peer et al. 2002; Beggs 1999), and in fact the earliest reports on the application of sonography for imaging of peripheral nerves focused on the evaluation of nerve tumors (Hughes and Wilson 1986; Fornage 1988).

The typical sonographic appearance of a peripheral nerve tumor in general is a well-defined mass with an oval or fusiform shape (Fig. 5.1). This shape is considered to be the number one imaging feature, which should raise the suspicion for a peripheral nerve tumor – as it is caused by the tubular entering and exiting of a nerve in a typical nerve distribution (Murphey et al. 1999). In superficial nerve tumors, however, the sonographic demonstration of a connection to a nerve is unlikely due to the small size of the affected nerve.

Because of the uniform cellular pattern of schwannoma a homogeneous echotexture is found in most tumors. In general they show a medium to low echogenicity, but schwannomas with a hyperechoic echotexture have also been reported in the literature (Simonovsky 1997). In tumors with a more myxoid matrix, real cystic internal changes may be seen. The advantage of sonography for the differential diagnosis of schwannoma and neurofibroma is the demonstration of the tumor originating at an eccentric location relative to the nerve, which is typical for schwannoma (Fig. 5.1). This is especially true for tumors larger than 2 cm. Just like other neurogenic tumors affecting the peripheral nerve schwannomas may demonstrate high vascularity on color Doppler studies.

5.2.2 Neurofibroma

5.2.2.1 Clinical Introduction

Neurofibromas share the same features as schwannomas as far as predilection for age and gender are concerned. They are classically divided into three groups depending on their appearance: localized, diffuse and plexiform. The plexiform and sometimes also the diffuse form are closely associated with Recklinghausen's disease (neurofibromatosis type I).

The *localized neurofibroma* is the most common, accounting for approximately 90% of lesions, and mainly affects young patients of either gender. Macroscopically it has a fusiform appearance with entering and exiting of a nerve. Often it affects rather superficially lying small nerves of the extremities. Histologically neurofibroma shows wavy, elongated cells within bands of collagen. Tumor vascularity is usually rich. Rarely myxoid cells appear within the tumor, but they are never as prominent as in schwannoma. Treatment of neurofibroma is normally surgical and, in contrast to schwannoma, implies reconstruction with nerve grafting if a deep nerve is involved.

The *diffuse form of neurofibroma* primarily affects children and young adults and most frequently is found in the subcutis of the neck region. In most cases (up to 90%) this is a solitary lesion not associated with neurofibromatosis.

Neurofibromatosis, first described by von Recklinghausen, is an inherited autosomal dominant genetic disease and affects one in 3000 births, which is why it is one of the most common genetic disorders. The classic clinical triad consists of cutaneous lesions, skeletal deformities and mental deficiency. The first characteristic signs appear in early childhood: café au lait spots, pigmented hamartomatous lesions of the iris (Lisch nodule) and osseous lesions. Neurofibromas can be found in virtually any part of the body including visceral organs (Roos and Muckway 1995) and constitute the hallmark of neurofibromatosis.

All three types of neurofibromas may appear in neurofibromatosis, but only the *plexiform neurofibroma* is pathognomonic and it usually appears in an early stage, even before other cutaneous signs of neurofibromatosis may occur. This tumor has a tortuous internal appearance, with separation of single nerve fascicles by endoneural tumor material. The lesion may induce a massively hypertrophic and disfigured limb, called elephantiasis neuromatosa, which is probably caused by the hypervascular condition of the tumor. Neurofibromas in association with neurofibromatosis type I (Recklinghausen's disease) may undergo malignant transformation in 2–29%. Treatment of patients with neurofibromatosis is often nonsurgical because of the multiplicity of lesions or surgery is reserved for symptomatic lesions.

5.2.2.2 Sonography

The sonographic appearance of localized solitary neurofibromas is more or less the same as in neurofibromatosis. In patients with neurofibromatosis type I, small tumors without any clinical relevance are frequently detected along peripheral nerves. The individual tumors have an oval shape with mostly hypoechoic texture (Fig. 5.2) and may either be well defined or also somewhat ill-defined (Simonovsky 1997). The plexiform neurofibroma invariably shows a pathognomonic appearance with multiple large fascicles, separated by isoechoic tissue (Fig. 5.3). Fast-growing and especially malignant neurofibromas may show central necrosis, or cystic formation and ill-defined margins (Fig. 5.4).

In a recent report the target sign known as a distinct MRI feature of neurofibroma on T2-weighted sequences has also been reported for sonography (Lin et al. 1999). This finding, however, has to date not been confirmed in a larger series. Despite rather typical sonographic criteria of neurofibroma, which were also apparent in our own series of six patients with neurofibromatosis type I, there is considerable overlap of sonographic features. Grey-scale sonography alone is therefore not considered reliable enough to correctly differentiate benign from malignant nerve tumors, and sonographically guided needle biopsy should be performed.

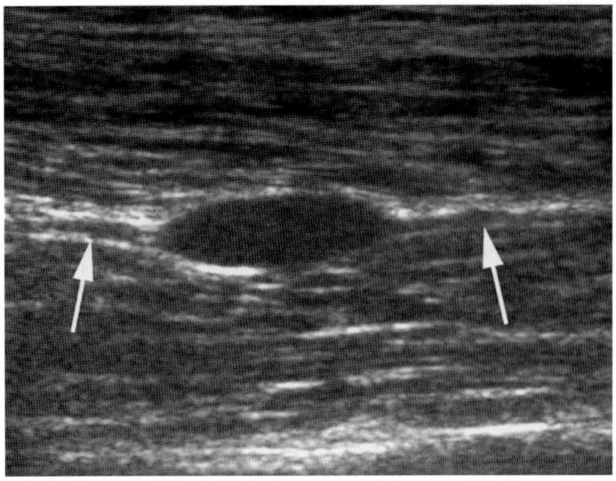

Fig. 5.2. Longitudinal sonogram acquired at the proximal thigh in a female patient with neurofibromatosis type I. A small hypoechoic spindle-shaped mass is demonstrated in continuity with a tiny femoral nerve branch (*arrows*), consistent with a small neurofibroma

a

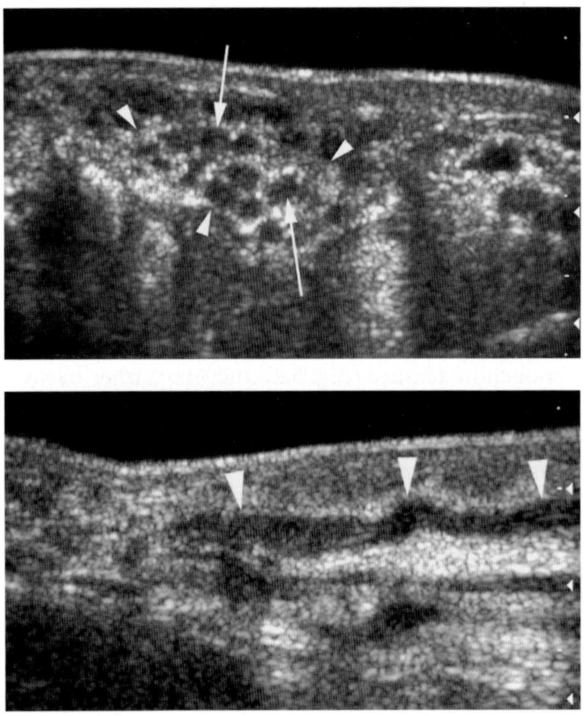

b

Fig. 5.3a, b. Transverse (**a**) and longitudinal (**b**) sonograms acquired at the right hand in a patient with plexiform neurofibroma. The median nerve (**a** *arrowheads*) is enlarged with multiple, enlarged, hypoechoic fascicles (**a** *arrows*). Single fascicles are elongated and distorted (**b** *arrowheads*)

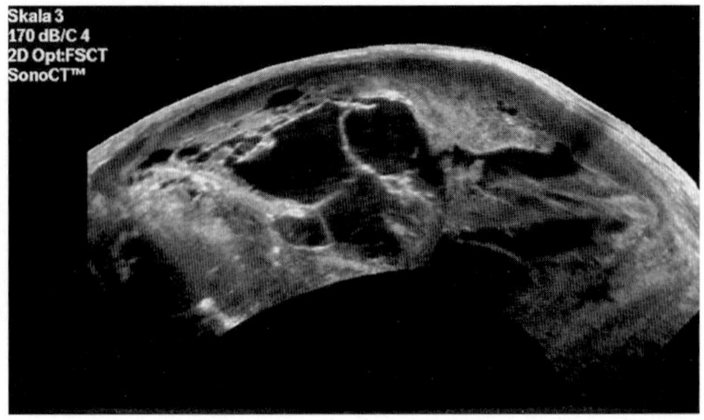

Fig. 5.4. Malignant neurofibroma in neurofibromatosis type I. Panoramic view of a huge tumor at the right shoulder with a maximum outer diameter of 35 cm. The echotexture appears very inhomogeneous with multiple cystic necrotic areas

Most peripheral nerve tumors show a high vascularity, which can be assessed with color Doppler sonography and spectral wave analysis. In a study regarding differentiation of malignant and benign soft tissue tumors we were able to differentiate malignant from benign tumors by analyzing the vascular architecture and spectral wave form (Bodner et al. 2002). In a series of 79 soft-tissue tumors we investigated 7 nerve tumors. Grey-scale information such as echogenicity or echo pattern did not have any significant value for differential diagnosis, but color Doppler sonography was able to demonstrate an anarchic vascular architecture in malignant neurogenic tumors (Fig. 5.5), containing stenosed and occluded vessels, self loops and trifurcations. Especially stenosed vessels showed a high systolic velocity of more then 100 cm/s; a flow velocity below 20 cm/s indicated a distally occluded tumor vessel. The combination of anarchic vessel architecture with these spectral characteristics resulted in a sensitivity of 94% and specificity of 93% in the differentiation of malignant from benign tumors.

5.3 Malignant Peripheral Nerve Tumors

G. Bodner, S. Peer

Malignant peripheral nerve tumors account for 5% to 10% of all soft-tissue sarcomas, they may arise from the nerve sheath, perineural cells and fibroblasts. Lesions mainly affect major nerve trunks such as the sciatic nerve or brachial plexus. Patients with malignant tumors more frequently present with local pain or neurological symptoms than those with

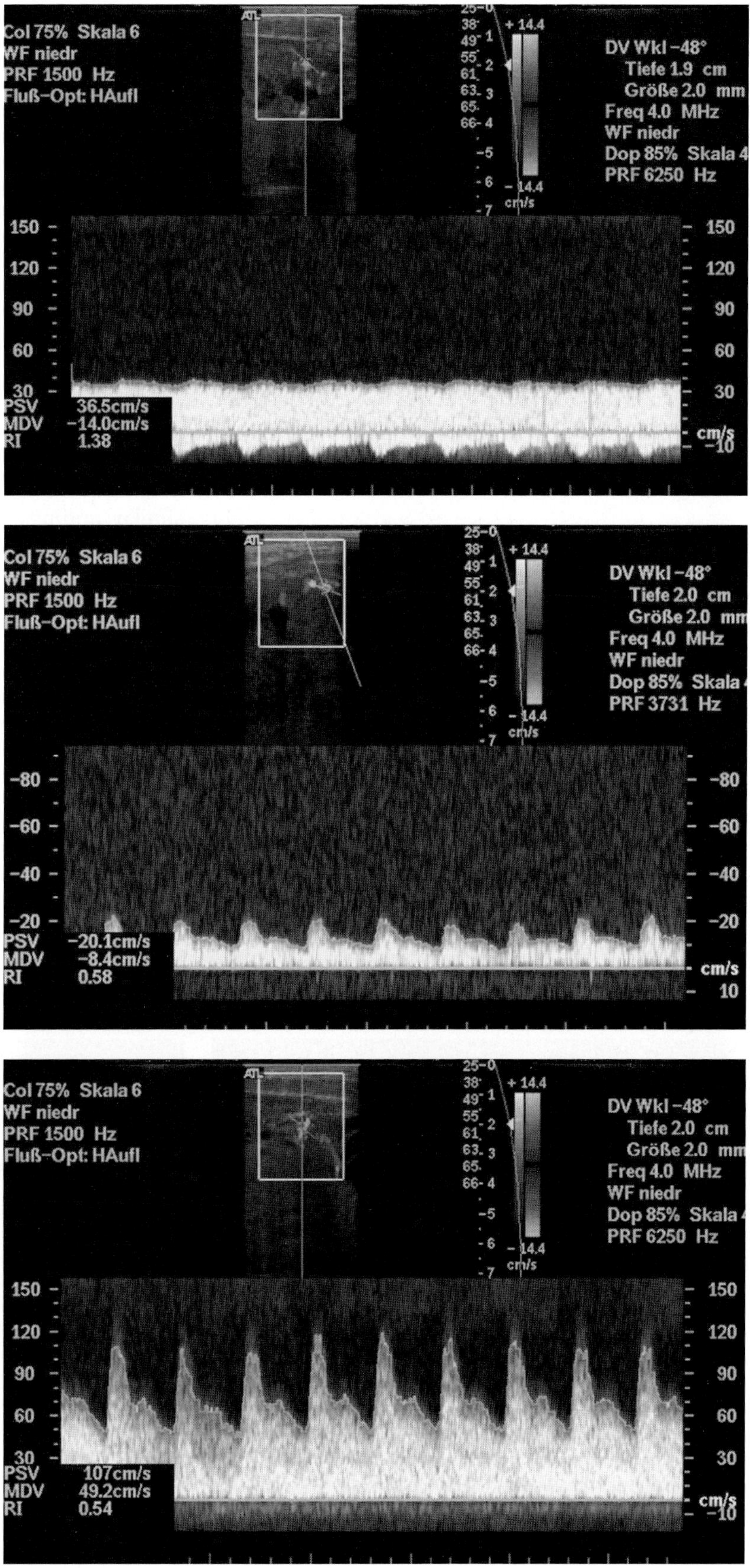

Fig. 5.5a–c. Color Doppler sonograms and spectral wave analysis in a patient with malignant neurofibroma. **a** An arteriovenous shunt with high velocity undulating waveform is demonstrated. **b** Inside the same lesion an arterial vessel with low velocity is demonstrated. **c** Several vessels with high-velocity "stenotic" waveforms are demonstrated

benign tumors. Some of these lesions are secondary tumors which appear after local radiotherapy. Typically these tumors grow fast and reach a large size. Local recurrence after surgical removal is about 40%. Metastatic spread, especially to the lung occurs in up to 68% and the overall 5-year survival rate is 43.7% (Wanebo et al. 1993), depending on the size and location of the tumor.

The sonographic experience with imaging of malignant peripheral nerve tumors is limited, a distinction based on gray-scale imaging alone is practically impossible except with the demonstration of malignant features such as invasive growth. The concept of color Doppler and spectral wave analysis for the differentiation of benign and malignant lesions has been discussed in the previous paragraph..

5.4 Tumor-Like Lesions

S. Peer

5.4.1 Nerve Sheath Ganglion

Intraneural ganglia are rare lesions, most frequently affecting the large nerves about the knee (mainly the common peroneal nerve) (Leijten et al. 1992; Masciocchi et al. 1992; Yamazaki et al. 1999). Involvement of the sciatic nerve, the tibial nerve at the ankle and the ulnar nerve at the elbow has also been reported (Peer et al. 2002; Puig et al. 1998). There is still no agreement on the exact pathogenesis of these lesions. While some may be extensions of ganglions related to joints (most commonly the proximal tibiofibular joint) with secondary nerve involvement (Katz and Lenobel 1970; Yamazaki et al. 1999), others may originate in the nerve itself (Barrett and Cramer 1963) (Figs. 5.6 and 5.7).

Bearing in mind these two pathogenic possibilities, intraneural ganglia may well be two essentially distinct entities. All these lesions, however, share common clinical symptoms resulting from raised intraneural pressure, and stretching or compression of a nerve. The last of these is the most probable mechanism in common peroneal nerve ganglia, where the space-occupying ganglion results in encasement of the nerve between the fibular head and the tight peroneus longus muscle and fascia (Yamazaki et al. 1999). We have reported similar findings in a case with compression of the tibial nerve inside the tarsal tunnel by a tibiotalar joint ganglion (Peer et al. 2002) (Fig. 5.8).

Depending on the size of the ganglion, patients present either with a palpable mass or with neurological symptoms only. From a histological viewpoint these lesions show myxoid changes together with a peripheral fibrotic lining. Their location is often eccentric between the nerve sheath and the nerve which results in displacement or even gross distortion of the nerve (Murphey et al. 1999). Sonography typically reveals a cystic well-defined globular lesion, sometimes septate with anechoic echotexture and posterior acoustic shadowing. If the content of the lesion is more of a myxoid nature, it shows a hypoechoic granular center.

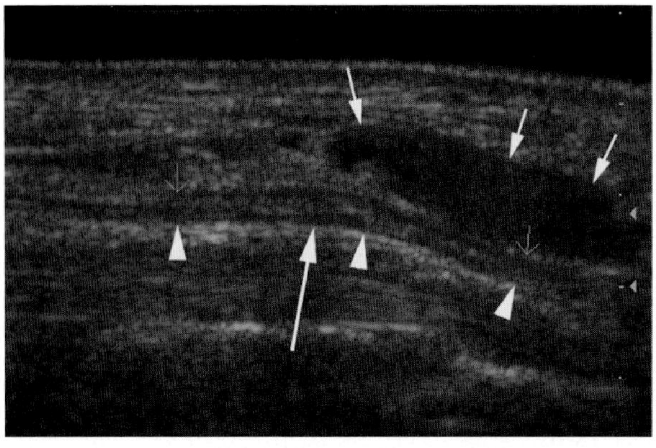

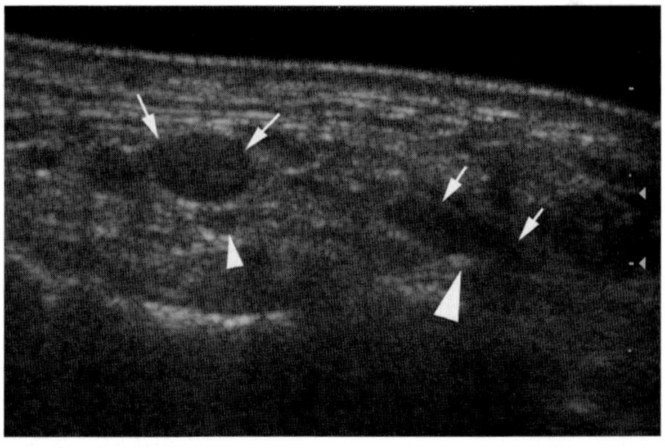

Fig. 5.6a, b. Longitudinal (**a**) and transverse (**b**) sonograms of the tibialis nerve in a patient with paresthesia. On the longitudinal scan the tibialis nerve (*arrowheads*) shows a bowing course just proximal to the medial tibiotalar joint. At the right margin of the image a spindle-shaped hypoechoic lesion with well-defined margins (*small arrows*) lies close to the nerve surface. The nerve diameter is slightly enlarged due to congestive edema (compression by the ganglion) just proximal to the upper pole of the ganglion (**a** *long arrow*). Part of the ganglion (**b** *small arrows*) is visualized in close connection to the distal margin of the tibial metaphysis (**b** *large arrowhead*) confirming its articular extension

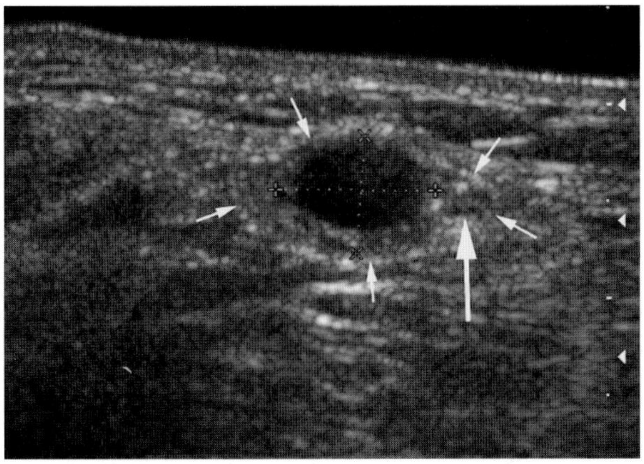

Fig. 5.7. Transverse sonogram of common peroneal nerve in a patient with a palpable popliteal mass, pain and numbness in the dorsal aspect of the foot and muscle weakness in the peroneus as well as tibialis anterior muscles. A round hypoechoic mass with well-defined margins and posterior acoustic enhancement and close relationship to the nerve (*long arrow*) is revealed by sonography. A thin hyperechoic line (the outer nerve sheath) shows direct continuity with the outer layer of the ganglion (*small arrows*) confirming a nerve sheath ganglion. No articular extension of the ganglion to the proximal tibiofibular joint is present

For true intraneural ganglia, surgical enucleation is the most appropriate treatment. For external ganglia with secondary compression of a nerve, a resection of the ganglion plus its articular connection is mandatory to prevent recurrence.

5.4.2 Morton's Neuroma

5.4.2.1 *Clinical Introduction*

Morton's neuroma is not a neoplasm in the true sense. The entity was first described by Thomas Morton in 1876, who reported on 12 patients with "a peculiar and painful affection of the fourth metatarsophalangeal articulation" (Morton 1876). The exact pathophysiological mechanism for this entity is still undetermined, but suggested reasons include repetitive microtrauma and nerve entrapment. While Morton himself favored a mechanical pathomechanism with squeezing of the nerve between the metatarsal heads, Mulder and others suggested an influence of abnormal metatarsal mobility with subsequent enlargement of the intermetatarsal bursa (Mulder 1951; Bossley and Cainey 1980). The latter replaces the plantar nerve and accompanying vessels, which results in a state more prone to pinching of these structures (Bossley and Cainey 1980).

Morton's neuroma, which clinically represents a fusiform enlargement of a digital branch of the medial or lateral plantar nerve, consists of perineural fibrosis, local vascular proliferation, edema of the endoneurium and axonal degeneration (Shereff and Grande 1991). Most commonly the digital nerve in the third intermetatarsal space is involved, the second intermetatarsal space being affected less

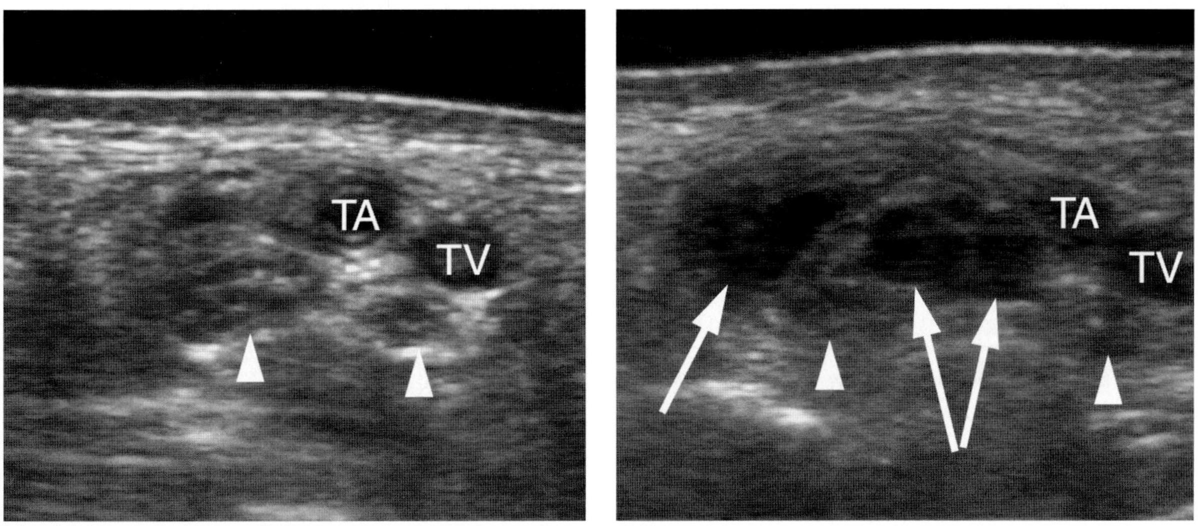

Fig. 5.8. Transverse sonograms through the tibialis nerve bifurcation just distal to the tibial malleolus. The bifurcation of the tibialis nerve in a larger and smaller portion is seen (*arrowheads*), and in addition the proximity of the tibial artery (*TA*) and vein (*TV*) is noted. Just between the two tibial nerve branches there lies a septate globular mass (*arrows*) with a well-defined wall consistent with a complex ganglion abutting the two nerves

frequently and involvement of other digital nerves being rare. There is enlargement of the digital nerve just proximal to its terminal bifurcation and just distal to the level of the intermetatarsal ligament (Fig. 5.9).

Patients typically suffer from a sharp, burning pain originating at the level of the metatarsal heads and radiating to the toes. Tingling sensations and paresthesias in the same distribution are common. Symptoms are worsened by walking and relieved by rest. During physical examination typical signs, such as a positive Tinel's sign (tingling sensations in the distal distribution of a nerve with light taping on the affected part of the nerve trunk) and Mulder's sign (a palpable click when the metatarsals are squeezed together with simultaneous application of pressure to the sole of the foot) may be seen (Mulder 1951). Dorsiflexion of the toes results in worsening of pain, while plantar flexion causes some relief. Morton's neuroma is palpable in one-third of patients only, but associated synovial cysts may be clinically evident. Women are more commonly affected, which is attributed to the more flexible state of the female foot and the habit of wearing high heels (Morton 1876). Asymptomatic lesions are common with a prevalence of 33% reported in an MRI study of 57 patients (Bencardino et al. 2000). The only observable difference between symptomatic and asymptomatic patients is the size of the lesion, with neuromas less than 5 mm in diameter considered asymptomatic (Zanetti et al. 1997).

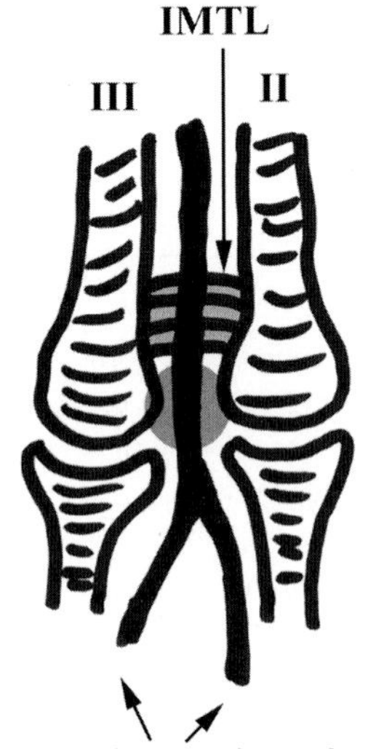

Fig. 5.9. Schematic drawing of the second intermetatarsal space at the level of the metatarsophalangeal joint. Note the position of the intermetatarsal ligament (*arrow*) and its relationship to the terminal bifurcation of the digital nerve. The *gray circle* marks the typical location of Morton's neuroma

The treatment of Morton's neuroma ranges from the use of orthotic devices and local steroid injections to surgical resection in cases resistant to conservative management (Llanos et al. 1999).

5.4.2.2 Sonography

Redd and coworkers first reported the potential of sonography for the detection of Morton's neuroma (Redd et al. 1989). Meanwhile various clinical studies have confirmed their initial experience with reported sensitivities for the sonographic detection of neuromas between 93% and 98% (Quinn et al. 2000; Redd et al. 1989; Shapiro and Shapiro 1995).

Recommendations on the best sonographic examination technique vary among authors. While the initial results of Redd and coworkers were achieved with the patient in a sitting position scanning from the dorsal aspect of the foot, recent studies more commonly favor a plantar approach with the patient lying prone on the examination couch. The reasoning for the dorsal approach may derive from the commonly favored dorsal approach in surgery for Morton's neuroma, and was thought to yield better image quality, as the thick fibrotic plantar pad resulting in some amount of sonographic artifacts can be avoided. However, the dorsal approach is only effective with vigorous plantar flexion of the toes, which enables delivery of the neuroma into the intermetatarsal space. Like other researchers, we use the dorsal approach only in cases where the plantar approach results in equivocal findings. With the plantar approach we use a good amount of transmission gel together with a stand-off pad, which substantially improves image quality. With the nonimaging finger, pressure is exerted on the dorsal aspect of the scanned intermetatarsal space splaying the metatarsals, which allows better sonographic access to the intermetatarsal tissues. A 12 MHz or higher linear array transducer is recommended.

The typical sonographic appearance of Morton's neuroma is a well-defined, hypoechoic, fusiform mass in association with the plantar neurovascular bundle classically of the third digital interspace. As the plantar digital nerve courses plantar to the intermetatarsal ligament, the typical location for neuroma is in the lower aspect of the intermetatarsal space and in between the metatarsal heads (Figs. 5.10 and 5.11) (Peer et al. 2002; Quinn et al. 2000).

However, according to Quinn and coworkers there is some variation in the localization of intermetatarsal

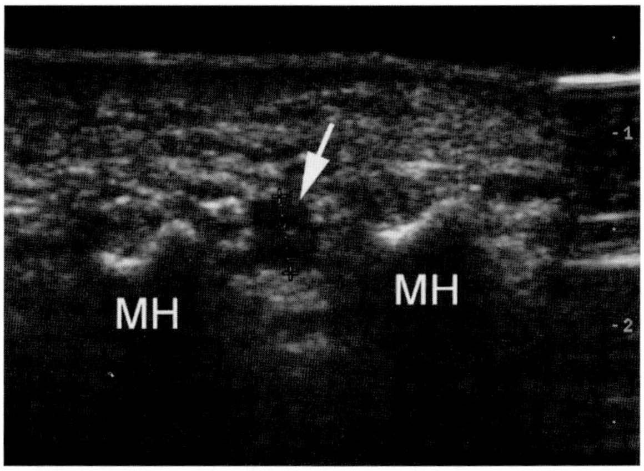

Fig. 5.10. Transverse sonogram in a patient with typical symptoms for Morton's neuroma. At the level of the metatarsal heads (*MH*) a small 0.6 cm globular mass with hypoechoic echotexture is seen, consistent with a small Morton's neuroma (*arrow*)

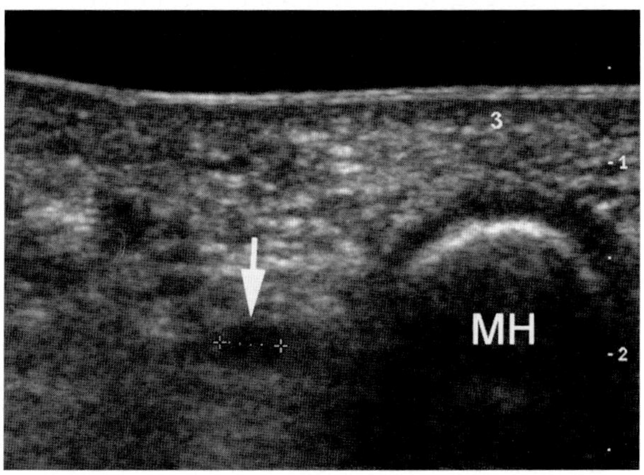

Fig. 5.11. Transverse sonogram in another patient with symptoms suggestive of Morton's neuroma reveals a small nodular lesion of only 4 mm diameter (*arrow*) adjacent to the third metatarsal head (*MH*). Despite its small size this lesion was symptomatic

mass lesions found with sonography (Quinn et al. 2000). In their sonographic study on 27 patients with surgically confirmed neuromas, they detected a mass either located plantar with dorsal extension or in a completely dorsal location in 18 patients. Only nine surgically confirmed neuromas where entirely plantar. This seems anatomically counterintuitive at first sight, given the location of the neurovascular bundle. Two possible explanations for this finding have to be considered. First, according to the early work of Mulder, a neuroma may be located more dorsally because of coexisting abnormal metatarsal mobility with subsequent splaying of the metatarsals and widened digital interspaces (Mulder 1951). Second, the dorsally extending mass may be an enlarged intermetatarsal bursa, which because of its equal echotexture is sometimes difficult to distinguish from a neuroma. This bursa is present in each interspace dorsal to the deep transverse intermetatarsal ligament and is found to be intimately associated with Morton's neuroma during surgery. Inflammation of the bursa has also been proposed as a causative factor in the pathogenesis of Morton's neuroma and associated clinical symptoms (Mulder 1951; Bossley and Cainey 1980).

According to Shapiro the enlarged fluid-filled bursa may be discerned if a lesion with an anechoic center and posterior acoustic enhancement is revealed in the dorsal compartment of an intermetatarsal space (Shapiro and Shapiro 1995). Shapiro and coworkers found an association between an enlarged bursa and a small 2–4 mm diameter neuroma in 10% of patients. So we have to keep in mind that a hypoechoic mass in the intermetatarsal space visualized with sonography in a patient suspected of having Morton's neuroma may in fact be (a) a true neuroma, (b) a neuroma with an associated enlargement of the intermetatarsal bursa, or (c) an enlarged bursa in association with a small neuroma (less than 5 mm), which is not distinguished separately from the bursa. For the sonographer this has some implications for examination technique:

- Always try to establish continuity between the neuroma and a digital nerve, as this will increase the specificity of the sonographic examination. However, this is not always accomplished due to the small size of the plantar nerves (in 55% of true neuromas in the study of Quinn et al.), but with state of the art equipment (i.e. high-frequency transducers) this will probably be achieved in a higher percentage of patients.
- Give close inspection to the echotexture of an intermetatarsal mass and search for liquid components, or posterior acoustic enhancement suggesting a fluid-filled bursa. In contrast, the neuroma itself is of a hypoechoic or mixed echotexture, and sometimes it may even show hyperechoic areas consistent with interspersed fat.
- A larger mass should always raise the suspicion of an enlarged bursa (normally a neuroma only rarely exceeds 20 mm in length) (Quinn et al. 2000).
- Because of the intimate relationship between Morton's neuroma and an enlarged intermetatarsal bursa, the actual size of the neuroma may be overestimated.

In conclusion sonography is valuable for the diagnosis of Morton's neuroma, with a sensitivity close to MR imaging, if a tailored examination is performed.

Besides its diagnostic capabilities, sonography may also serve as a tool for the guidance of local corticoid instillation.

5.4.3 Neuroma

5.4.3.1 Clinical Introduction

Depending on their pathogenesis neuromas may be divided into *posttraumatic* and *postsurgical* lesions (see also Chapter 4). Traumatic neuromas develop after complete or partial transection of a peripheral nerve, and regarding their location this group may further be divided into intraneural or terminal neuromas. While intraneural traumatic neuromas develop in an otherwise intact nerve trunk because of minor trauma (mainly traction injuries), or as a result of chronic irritation and friction, terminal neuromas are always a result of severe trauma with partial avulsion, disruption or total transection of a nerve. Postsurgical neuromas most commonly appear in the lower extremities after leg amputation and in the head and neck region related to tooth extraction, or after surgical nerve reconstruction. Neuromas develop within 1 to 12 months of the initial event, and vary in size depending on the size of the involved nerve and the amount of impaired nerve tissue.

The typical clinical findings in patients with neuroma are a localized soft-tissue mass and pain, which is in most cases reproduced with tapping on the mass (positive Tinel's sign). On histological analysis neuromas show a mixture of various cellular elements including Schwann cells, axons, endoneural and perineural elements, wrapped in dense collagenous, fibrotic tissue (Kransdorf and Murphey 1997). The disorganization of the neural tissue allows histological differentiation of neuroma from neurofibroma.

5.4.3.2 Sonography

Given a patient's history, the sonographic diagnosis of neuroma is straightforward and the differential diagnosis hardly problematic. In the typical clinical setting, a bulbous mass in association with a nerve stump (Fig. 5.12) or arising from the lateral aspect of a nerve with partially discontinuous fascicles (Fig. 5.13), or a spindle-shaped mass inside a nerve (Fig. 5.14) is consistent with neuroma. The diagnostic clue is the demonstration of a nerve in direct continuity with the mass.

The echotexture of neuromas is hypoechoic and more or less homogeneous, lesion margins are generally well defined, but some irregularity, which is probably due to multidirectional cell proliferation, has been reported (Martinoli et al. 1996). Based on the nonspecific intrinsic echotexture of neuromas alone, a differentiation against other lesions is hardly possible, which is why the demonstration of continuity with a nerve and knowledge of patient history is of utmost importance. The latter, however, may sometimes be difficult if very small nerves at the fingers or toes are involved.

Sonography is especially helpful in patients with phantom pain after amputation, because of its ability

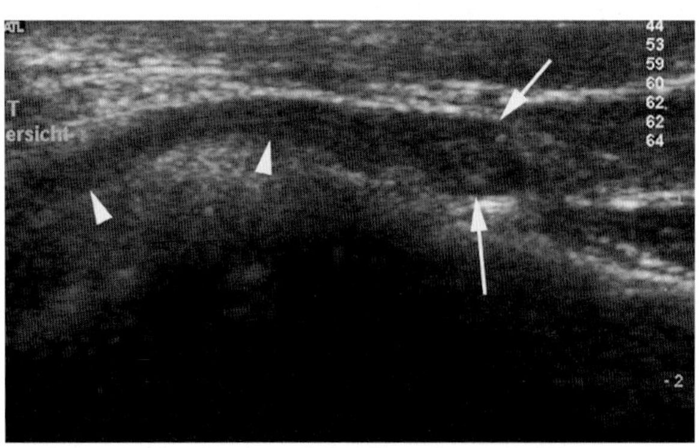

a

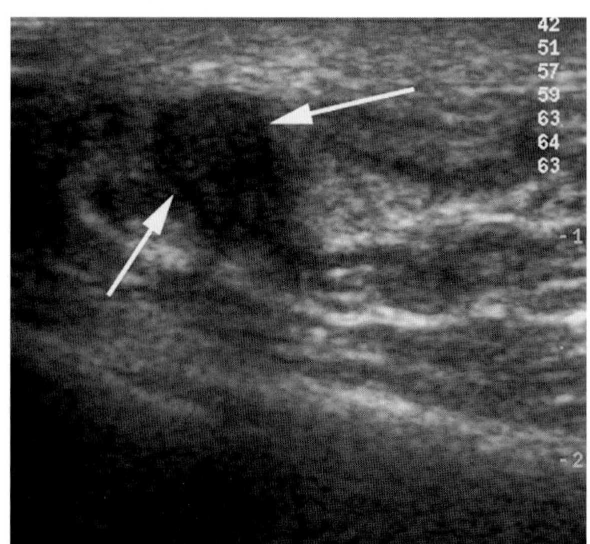

b

Fig. 5.12a, b. Longitudinal (**a**) and transverse (**b**) sonograms in a patient with traumatic amputation of the arm in a motor vehicle accident. The ulnar nerve (**a** *arrowheads*) tapers from a bulbous hypoechoic mass consistent with stump neuroma. In the transverse plane the diagnosis is not readily established, but a localized enlargement of the nerve is seen (**b** *arrows*)

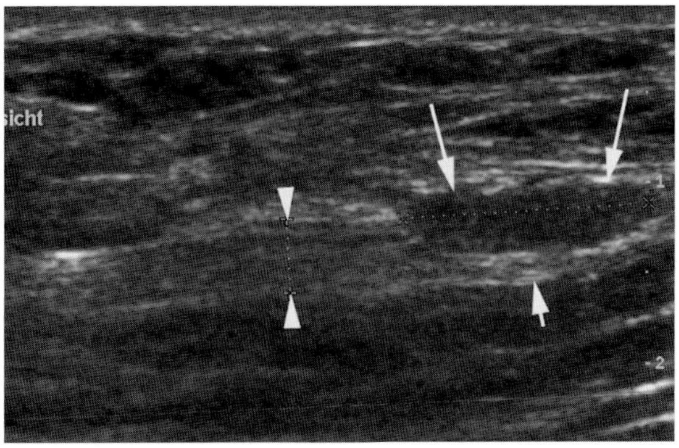

Fig. 5.13. Longitudinal sonogram through the distal portion of the sciatic nerve in a patient with a femoral shaft fracture and traumatic lesion of the sciatic nerve. A spindle-shaped neuroma (*long arrows*) is seen located in the lateral bundle of the sciatic nerve (*arrowheads*) with otherwise continuous nerve fascicles in the lower aspect of the nerve (*short arrow*)

to identify an underlying neuroma and thus rule out other reasons for the development of phantom pain, such as recurring tumor and localized inflammation or abscess formation among others. In addition, sonography may guide local therapy with instillation of corticoids, analgesics or phenol (see also Chapter 6).

5.4.4
Neural Fibrolipoma

Neural fibrolipoma was initially described by Mason in 1952 (Mason 1953), and various synonyms, such as fibrolipomatous hamartoma of nerve, and perineural and intraneural lipoma, have been used for this rare lesion (Silverman and Enzinger 1985). Hypertrophy of fatty tissue and fibroblasts in the epineurium of a nerve are considered the most

a

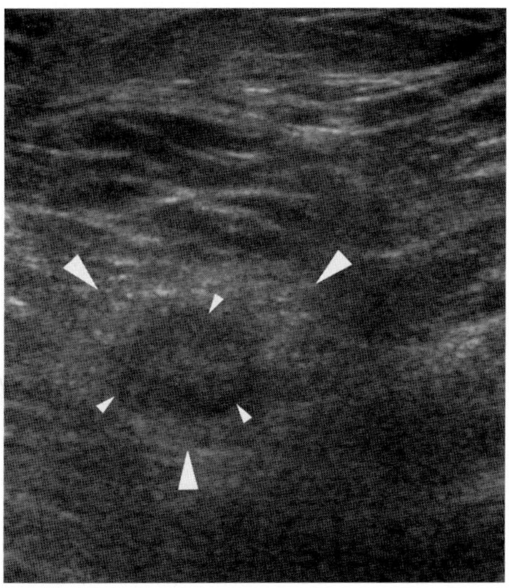

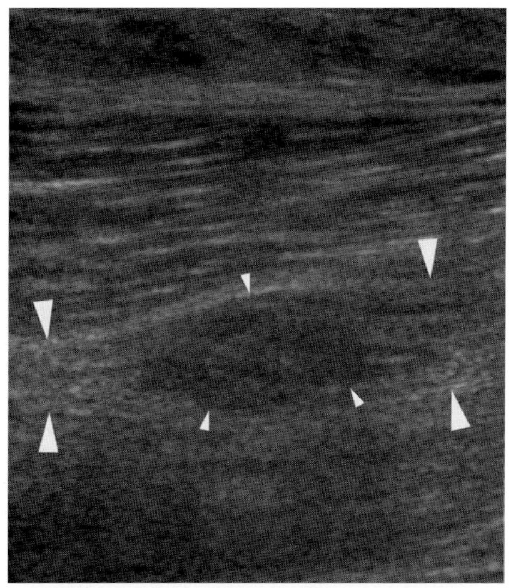

b

Fig. 5.14a–c. Transverse (**a**) and longitudinal (**b**) sonograms through the lower thigh in a female patient who had undergone resection of a sciatic nerve neurofibroma with end-to-end anastomosis of nerve stumps. The patient suffered from burning pain in the lateral aspect of the foot and the fifth toe with hypesthesia, and electrophysiological testing revealed a lesion of the suralis portion of the sciatic nerve. There is marked enlargement of the sciatic nerve (**a, b** *large arrowheads*) due to a fusiform, hypoechoic intraneural mass (**a, b** *small arrowheads*) consistent with postoperative neuroma. Compare normal appearing sciatic nerve proximal to the lesion (**c**) (*GM* gluteus muscle, *AMM* adductor magnus muscle)

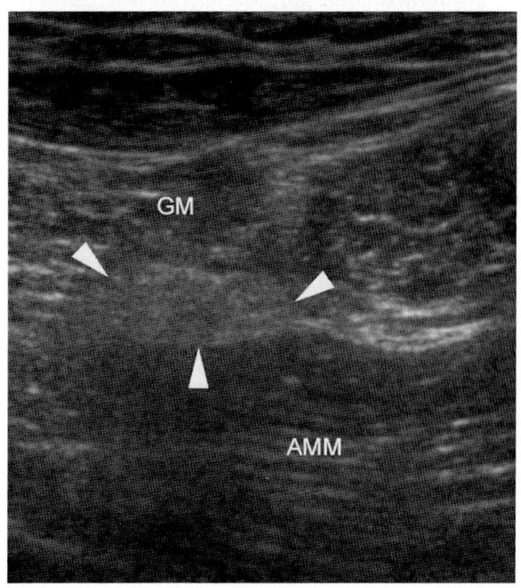

c

probable causes of the development of fibrolipoma, but the exact pathogenesis is still unclear.

The typical presentation is in a patient less than 30 years of age, often at birth or in early childhood. The upper extremity is most commonly involved (78–96% of cases) with a predilection for the median nerve. Involvement of the lower extremity, ulnar or radial nerve, or the brachial plexus is rare. A localized soft, slowly enlarging mass in the wrist or forearm, with or without accompanying pain is usually present. Neurological symptoms consistent with carpal tunnel disease may be the leading finding in lesions involving the median nerve. About one-third to two-thirds of patients have coexisting macrodactyly.

On sonographic examination, the involved nerve is grossly enlarged, with a cable-like appearance on transverse scans, which is caused by the hypoechoic bands resembling the fascicles embedded in hyperechoic surrounding fatty tissue (Murphey et al. 1999). We believe that based on intrinsic features alone the sonographic differentiation of neural fibrolipoma and plexiform neurofibroma may hardly be possible, but experience with sonography in larger series is lacking.

References

Barrett R, Cramer F (1963) Tumors of the peripheral nerves and so called ganglia of the peroneal nerve. Clin Orthop 27:153–146

Beggs I (1999) Sonographic appearances of nerve tumors. J Clin Ultrasound 27:363–368

Bencardino J, Rosenberg ZS, Beltran J, et al (2000) Morton's neuroma: is it always symptomatic. AJR Am J Roentgenol 175:649–653

Bodner G, Schocke M, Rachbauer F, et al (2002) Differentiation of malignant and benign musculoskeletal tumors: combined color Doppler ultrasonography, power Doppler ultrasonography and spectral wave analysis. Radiology 223:410–416

Bossley CJ, Cainey PC (1980) The intermetatarsophalangeal bursa: its significance in Morton's metatarsalgia. J Bone Joint Surg Br 62:184–187

Fornage BD (1988) Peripheral nerves of the extremities: imaging with ultrasound. Radiology 167:179–182

Hughes DG, Wilson DJ (1986) Ultrasound appearances of peripheral nerve tumors. Br J Radiol 59:1041–1043

Katz MR, Lenobel MI (1970) Intraneural ganglion cyst of the peroneal nerve. J Neurosurg 32:692–694

Kransdorf M, Murphey MD (1997) Imaging of soft tissue tumors. WB Saunders, Philadelphia, pp 235–273

Leijten FS, Arts WF, Puylaert JB (1992) Ultrasound diagnosis of an intraneural ganglion cyst of the peroneal nerve. J Neurosurg 76:538–540

Lin J, Jacobson JA, Hayes CW (1999) Sonographic target sign in neurofibroma. J Ultrasound Med 18:513–517

Llanos LF, Vila J, Nunez-Samper M (1999) Clinical symptoms and treatment of the foot and ankle entrapment syndromes. Foot Ankle Surg 5:211–218

Martinoli C, Serafini G, Bianchi S, et al (1996) Ultrasonography of peripheral nerves. J Periph Nerv Syst 1:169–174

Martinoli C, Bianchi S, Derchi LE (2000) Ultrasonography of peripheral nerves. Semin Ultrasound CT MR 21:205–213

Masciocchi C, Innacoli M, Cisternino S, et al (1992) Myxoid intraneural cysts of external popliteal ischiadic nerve. Eur Radiol 14:52–55

Mason ML (1953) Presentation of cases. Proceedings of the American Society for Surgery of the Hand. J Bone Joint Surg Am 35:273–275

Morton TG (1876) A peculiar and painful affection of the fourth metatarsophalangeal articulation. Am J Med Sci 71:37–45

Mulder JD (1951) The causative mechanisms in Morton's metatarsalgia. J Bone Joint Surg Br 33:74–95

Murphey MD, Smith WS, Smith SE, et al (1999) From the archives of the AFIP: imaging of musculoskeletal neurogenic tumors: radiologic-pathologic correlation. Radiographics 19:1253–1280

Peer S, Kovacs P, Harpf C, et al (2002) High resolution sonography of lower extremity peripheral nerves: anatomic correlation and spectrum of pathology. J Ultrasound Med 21: 315–322

Puig S, Turkof E, Sedivy R, et al (1998) Sonographic diagnosis of recurrent ulnar nerve compression by ganglion cysts. J Ultrasound Med 18:433–436

Quinn TJ, Jacobson JA, Craig JG, et al (2000) Sonography of Morton's neuromas. AJR Am J Roentgenol 174:1723–1728

Redd RA, Peters VJ, Emery SF, et al (1989) Morton neuroma: sonographic evaluation. Radiology 171:415–417

Roos KL, Muckway M (1995) Neurofibromatosis. Dermatol Clin 13:105–111

Shapiro PP, Shapiro SL (1995) Sonographic evaluation of interdigital neuromas. Foot Ankle Int 16:604–606

Shereff MJ, Grande DA (1991) Electron microscopic analysis of the interdigital neuroma. Clin Orthop 271:296–299

Silverman TA, Enzinger FM (1985) Fibrolipomatous hamartoma of nerve: a clinicopathologic analysis of 26 cases. Am J Surg Pathol 9:7–14

Simonovsky V (1997) Peripheral nerve schwannoma preoperatively diagnosed by sonography: report of three cases and discussion. Eur J Radiol 25:47–51

Wanebo JE, Malik JM, Vandenberg SR, et al (1993) Malignant peripheral nerve sheath tumors: a clinicopathological study of 28 cases. Cancer 71:247–252

Weiss SW, Goldblum JR (eds) (2001) Enzinger Weiss's soft tissue tumors, 4th edn. Mosby, St Louis

Yamazaki H, Saitoh S, Seki H (1999) Peroneal nerve palsy caused by intraneural ganglion. Skeletal Radiol 28:52–56

Zanetti M, Strehle JK, Zollinger H, et al (1997) Morton neuroma and fluid in the intermetatarsal bursae on MR images of 70 asymptomatic volunteers. Radiology 203:516–520

6 Interventional Techniques

P. Kovacs, H. Gruber, G. Bodner

CONTENTS

6.1 Sonographically Guided Phenol Instillation 95
6.1.1 Therapeutic Agents 95
6.1.2 Sonographically Guided Techniques 96
6.2 Sonographically Guidance for Regional Anesthesia 96
6.2.1 Regional Anesthesia of the Upper Limb 97
6.2.2 Regional Anesthesia of the Lower Limb 100
References 104

6.1 Sonographically Guided Phenol Instillation

The formation of neuromas is part of the normal regeneration process after nerve injury. After amputations stump neuromas may lead to pain, such as stump pain or phantom limb pain. These painful neuromas may be treated by surgical intervention or by instillation of therapeutic agents.

There are a wide range of possible surgical techniques for treatment of neuroma including nerve-to-nerve repair after nerve dissection or transection. After amputations the stump neuroma may be surgically exposed and capped with some inert material, but according to the literature, implantation of the resected nerve stump into the adjacent muscle or even between muscle and bone is considered to be the most efficient treatment option (Dellon et al. 1984; Dellon and Mackinnon 1986).

The therapeutic agents used for instillations include steroids, phenol, alcohol and glycerol.

P. Kovacs, MD; H. Gruber, MD
Department of Radiology, University Hospital Innsbruck, Anichstrasse 35, 6020 Innsbruck, Austria
G. Bodner, MD
Professor, Department of Radiology, Section for Diagnostic and Interventional Sonography, University Hospital Innsbruck, Anichstrasse 35, 6020 Innsbruck, Austria

6.1.1 Therapeutic Agents

6.1.1.1 Steroids

Steroids decrease inflammatory reactions at the site of neuroma formation and help to loosen the connective tissue surrounding the nerve, thereby reducing compression of the nerve by encasing fibrotic tissue. Steroid injections may be used to treat painful lesions in large nerves, such as the sciatic nerve (Hanania and Kitain 1998), but also for painful neuromas of small nerves, such as in the treatment of Morton's neuroma of interdigital nerves (Rasmussen et al. 1996). Despite local administration at the site of neuroma formation, steroid injections may nevertheless cause systemic reactions, or local problems, such as atrophy of fat tissue.

6.1.1.2 Phenol

Besides type A botulinum toxin, phenol is used to treat muscle spasticity with intramuscular injections and pain with perineural and intraneural injections. In a rat model, Lu et al. showed that phenol produces focal swelling of the nerve after intrafascicular and extrafascicular intraneural injection. It further causes severe demyelination, axonal degeneration, edema and hemorrhage leading to complete architectural disruption visible 1 week after injection (Lu et al. 1998). Due to denaturing axonal proteins (Mooney et al. 1969) and a dissolving type of degeneration within the Schwann cell tubes (Westerlund et al. 2001) even extraneural administration of phenol leads to damage of peripheral nerve fibers.

In summary, phenol damages the nerve fibers in a combined toxic and ischaemic way, which is more severe after intraneural than extraneural administration (Westerlund et al. 2001). Despite these profound reactions to phenol instillation, signs of nerve regeneration are detected after 2 weeks, when axonal sprouts become visible (Westerlund et al. 2001). In a similar setting Tsukazaki et al. have reported a significant increase in neuronal recovery at 4 weeks after phenol injection followed by total recovery at 8 weeks (Tsukazaki et al. 1993). This fast and complete recovery may be the reason for the only transient effect of neurolytic block with phenol (Mooney et al. 1969).

On the other hand the development of neuromas is avoided when axons sprout through the nerve lesion (Myers and Katz 1988). Westerlund et al. have reported that treatment with phenol leads to broken basal laminae (Westerlund et al. 2001). Axonal sprouts seem to be guided by the fragments of basal laminae and the lesion recovers without significant misrouting of the sprouts.

In the treatment of painful stump neuromas the damage to the peripheral nerve following phenol injection plays the most important role. The tendency towards nerve recovery has to be determined in follow-up studies.

6.1.1.3 Glycerol

Compared with phenol, glycerol causes similar effects on the nerve fibers, but never produces ischaemia with hemorrhagic necrosis and is less effective in breaking the basal laminae (Westerlund et al. 2001). Due to its viscosity it is difficult to inject with a fine needle and, therefore, is more difficult to handle.

6.1.1.4 Alcohol

In comparison with phenol, alcohol has a slower action, is more irritating to adjacent tissues and is more likely to cause painful neuritis (Myers and Katz 1988). Due to its sclerosing effect alcohol is used to reduce pain in patients with Morton's neuroma. Dockery used a 4% solution of alcohol administered three to seven times every 5–10 days. Of 100 treated patients, 89 showed an improvement and 82 had complete resolution of symptoms (Dockery 1999). Masala et al. reported similar results with sonographically guided administration of a 30% solution (Masala et al. 2001).

6.1.2 Sonographically Guided Techniques

Sonography is able to detect neuromas smaller than 1 cm, which is the critical size for detection by MR or CT. Thomas et al. administered local anesthetic around neuromas under sonographic control to confirm that the neuroma was the reason for stump pain. They then marked the neuroma with breast localization wires to allow minimally invasive surgical resection of the lesion (Thomas et al. 1999).

Our group went a step further and administered phenol directly into the painful stump neuroma under sonographic control. According to their reported procedure a local anesthetic is first infiltrated into the soft tissues surrounding the neuroma to release pain. Then the needle is advanced into the nerve proximal to the neuroma and 0.3 to 0.5 ml of phenol is injected under direct sonographic control. During injection, swelling of the nerve fascicles or injected air within the nerve can be delineated confirming successful administration (Fig. 6.1). After injection the syringe should be flushed with saline to avoid spreading phenol into the adjacent tissue when pulling back the needle. If necessary, the procedure can be repeated after several days. Six months after treatment there was no recurrence or a marked decrease in pain in all patients included in the study. Long-term follow-up will show whether persistent relief can be obtained.

6.2 Sonographic Guidance for Regional Anesthesia

Anesthetists primarily use anatomical landmarks and nerve stimulators to perform regional anesthesia. According to the motto "no paraesthesia, no anesthesia" (Moore 1954) the needle is advanced as close as possible to the nerve. Nerve stimulators are an important tool to control advancement of the needle to the nerve. However, they are only applicable for anesthesia of nerves with sensory elements; stimulation of motor nerves without sensory function, such as the femoral nerve, will not produce paraesthesia. That is the reason why anatomical guidance and the use of nerve stimulators are both associated with the risk of intraneural injection in certain situations. The potential harmful effect on the nerve fibers is the reason why Moore's motto is still under debate (Graf and Martin 2001).

Sonographically guided regional anesthesia can be performed on any nerve that can be localized with sonography. The clinical use of sonographic guidance for regional anesthesia, however, is not well known among anesthetists and is often considered

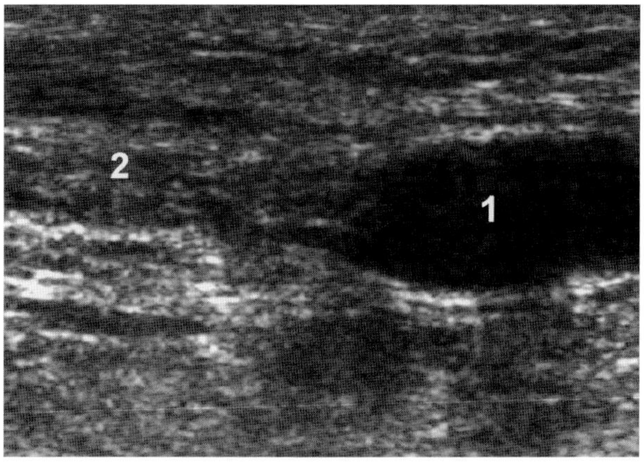

a

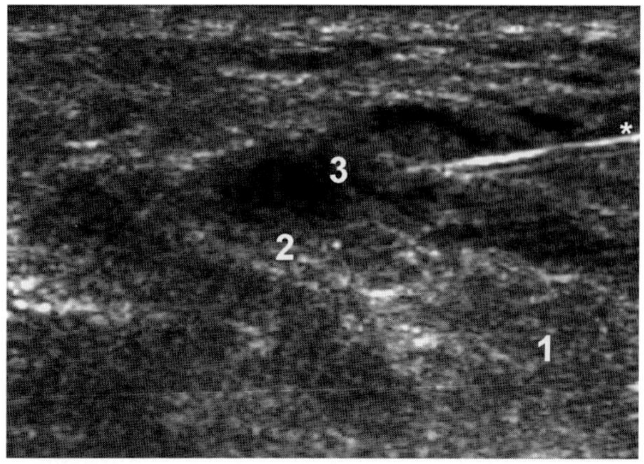

b

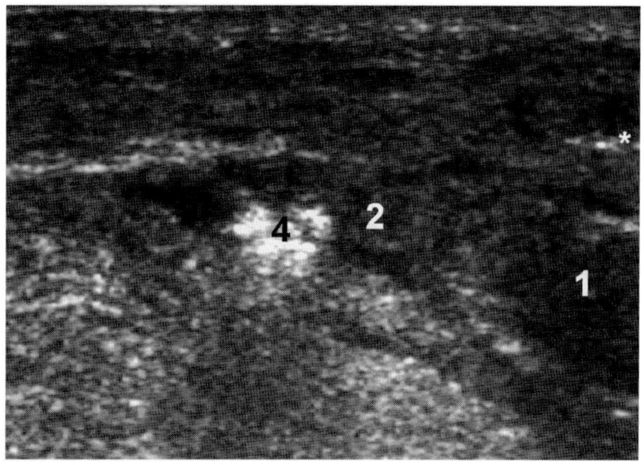

c

Fig. 6.1a–c. Intraneural injection of phenol for treatment of painful neuroma. **a** A stump neuroma (*1*) at the end of the sciatic nerve (*2*) in a 56-year-old male patient. **b** A needle (*asterisk*) is advanced to the nerve proximal to the neuroma and 5 ml of local anesthetic (*3*) is administered. **c** The needle is advanced further into the nerve and 0.5 ml phenol (with air bubbles *4*) is injected directly into the nerve

too difficult or time consuming. Therefore, sonographic guidance is limited to regional anesthesia in locations with a complex anatomy. In these locations sonography is used to delineate the nerve structures themselves to allow administration of anesthetic under direct visual control, or simply to depict the area of injection to avoid unintended complications, such as puncture of vessels or organs.

The type of transducer used depends on the region of concern and the depth of the nerve to be anesthetized. The needle may be inserted in two ways: at the small side of the transducer and advanced parallel to the sonographic section plain, which results in good visualization of the needle path along a greater distance, or perpendicular to the transducer, which needs more experience, because the needle tip comes into view just before reaching the target unless the transducer is continuously tilted in relation to the tip of the needle (Fig. 6.2). To avoid unintended puncture of vessels, muscles or organs, a deposit of local anesthetic or saline can be injected between these structures and the nerves. This deposit allows the needle to be advanced without causing harm to reach all parts of the nerve or plexus.

In addition to better technical results related to needle guidance, reports in the literature show that, in comparison with nonguided blocks, the amount of local anesthetic can be reduced using sonographic guidance. This is because the distribution of the anesthetic around the nerve can be watched directly during injection (Marhofer et al. 1998; Yang et al. 1998). Common beds of connective tissue or compartments favor natural distribution of the anesthetic around the elements of a plexus and even to other nerves. Nevertheless, in some regions this may be less effective than commonly assumed (Marhofer et al. 2000).

6.2.1 Regional Anesthesia of the Upper Limb

Complications of brachial plexus anesthesia performed without sonographic guidance include, besides intraneural injection, puncture of the subclavian artery resulting in hematoma (25.7%), pneumothorax (0.6–5%), and block of the recurrent laryngeal or phrenic nerve as well as the stellate ganglion (1.3%)

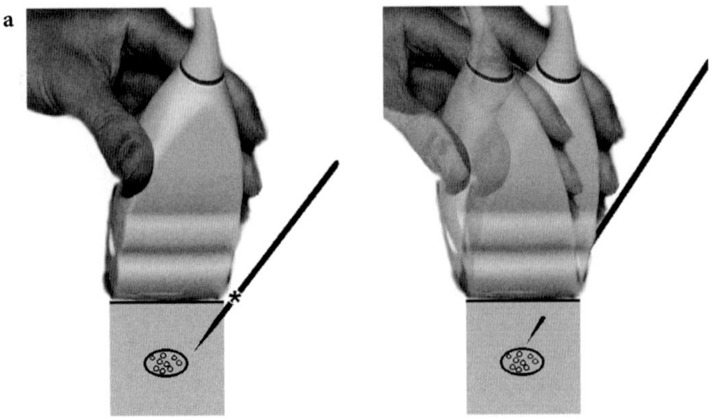

Fig. 6.2a, b. Injection techniques. **a** The needle is inserted at the small side of the transducer (*asterisk*) and advanced diagonally within the sonographic section plain. **b** If the needle is inserted perpendicular to the transducer, it needs to be tilted continuously following the tip of the needle

(Bridenbaugh 1988). The success rate for complete block is between 70% and 80% depending on the technique used and the type of local anesthetic chosen (Goldberg et al. 1987; Bedder et al. 1988).

According to Winnie et al. (1993) the nonguided brachial plexus block can be performed in four regions:

- In the interscalene region (interscalene perivascular brachial plexus block)
- In the supraclavicular region (supraclavicular perivascular brachial plexus block)
- In the infraclavicular region (infraclavicular perivascular brachial plexus block)
- In the axillary region (axillary perivascular brachial plexus block)

6.2.1.1 Interscalene Perivascular Brachial Plexus Block

For sonographically guided interscalene block the brachial plexus is imaged between the anterior and middle scalene muscles where in transverse sections it appears as a chain of hypoechoic nodules (Kapral et al. 1994) representing the spinal roots in the superior interscalene region and the trunks of the plexus in the inferior interscalene region (Yang et al. 1998). The position of the transducer for sonographic access to this region is depicted in Fig. 6.3. The success rate for complete block under sonographic guidance ranges from 95% (Kapral et al. 1994) to 100% (Ting and Sivagnanaratnam 1989) without any complications reported. Compared with the nonguided technique, sonographic guidance succeeds more frequently (98% vs 77%) includes C8 and T1 in a more pronounced way, and allows prolonged anesthesia (Jandrasits et al. 1998). Yang et al. (1998) reported incomplete block in 6 of 15 patients, but achieved postoperative analgesia in all patients, whereas nonguided techniques had a success rate of only 75% for postoperative anesthesia (Tuominen et al. 1989).

6.2.1.2 Supraclavicular Perivascular Brachial Plexus Block

In the supraclavicular region the hypoechoic nodules representing the fascicles of the plexus accompany the subclavian artery craniodorsally (Fig. 6.4). For the approach to the plexus, the patient is positioned supine with the arm resting at the side and the head turned to the contralateral side (Kapral et al. 1994). In contrast to nonguided techniques with a success rate of 72% (Moorthy et al. 1991), sonographic guidance succeeds in 95% of patients (Kapral et al. 1994).

6.2.1.3 Infraclavicular Perivascular Brachial Plexus Block

For infraclavicular block the brachial plexus is scanned by placing the transducer just below the clavicle (Ootaki et al. 2000) and depicting the fascicles surrounding the axillary artery (Fig. 6.5). Ootaki et al. have reported success for complete block in 95% of patients. Complete sensory and motor block was achieved in 100% at the musculocutaneous and medial antebrachial cutaneous nerves, in 96.7% at the median nerve and in 90% to 95% at the ulnar and radial nerve, respectively. Subtotal blocks may be due to variations in the anatomy of the brachial plexus, concerning formation and branching of the nerves.

6.2.1.4 Axillary Perivascular Brachial Plexus Block

A low risk of complications is reported in general for the nonguided axillary perivascular approach to the

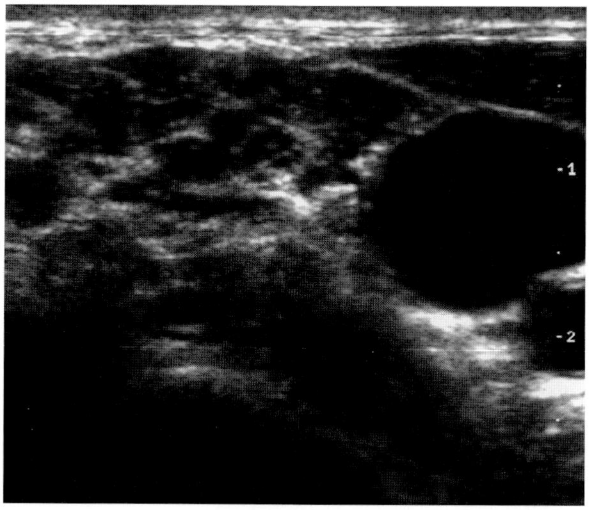

a

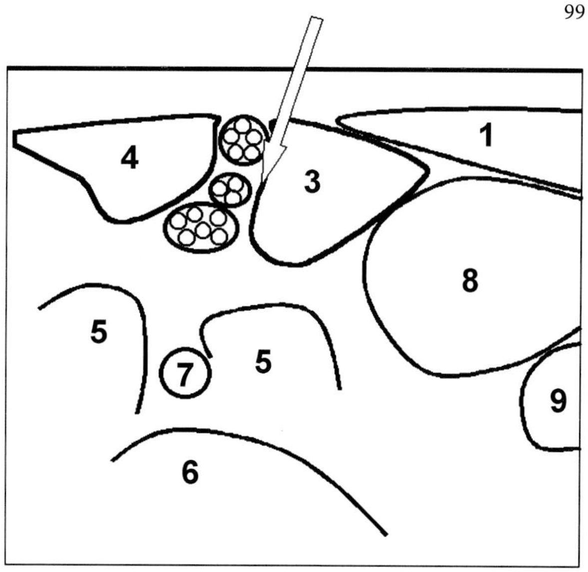

b

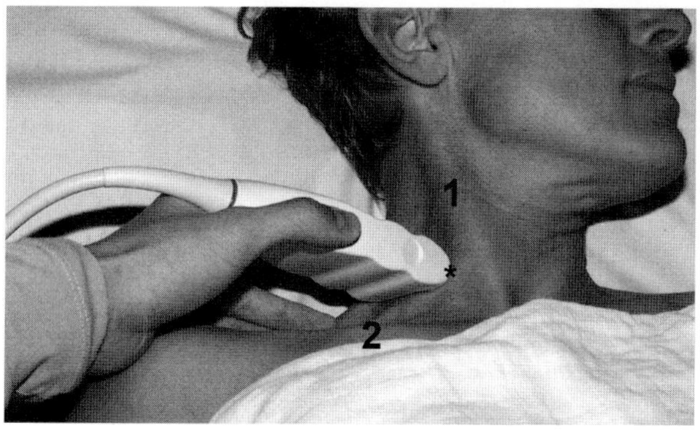

c

Fig. 6.3a–c. Sonographically guided interscalene brachial plexus block. **a** Sonogram with (**b**) corresponding line drawing and recommended position of the needle (*arrow*). **c** Position of the transducer in the transverse plane with the site of needle insertion medial to the transducer (*asterisk*). Posterior to the sternocleidomastoideus muscle (*1*) and proximal to the clavicle (*2*), the brachial plexus is depicted between the anterior (*3*) and the middle scalene muscle (*4*). The roots forming the plexus appear between the tubercles of the transverse process (*5*) of the cervical vertebra (*6*) (*7* vertebral artery, *8* internal jugular vein, *9* common carotid artery)

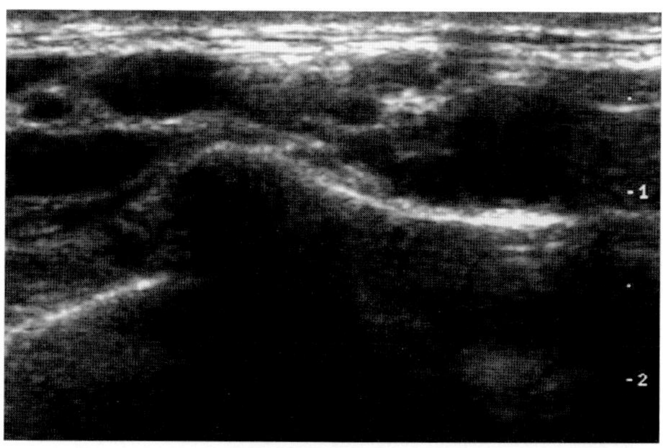

a

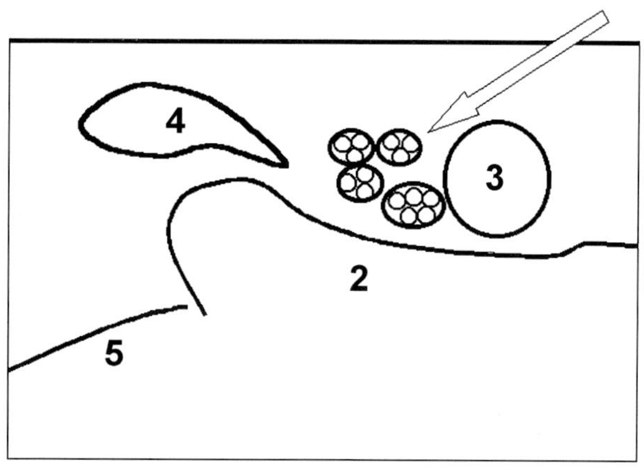

b

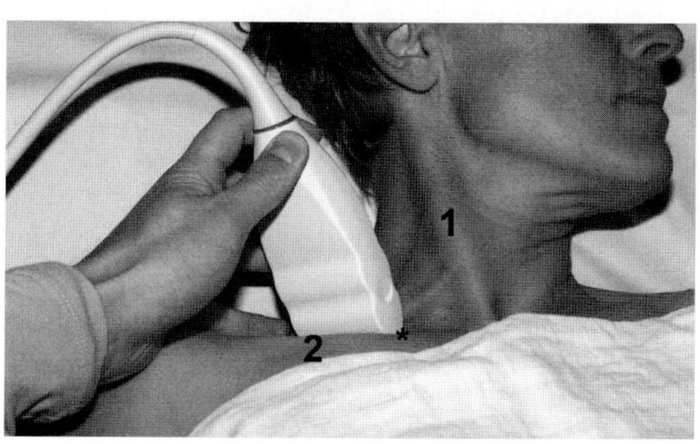

c

Fig. 6.4a–c. Sonographically guided supraclavicular brachial plexus block. **a** Sonogram with (**b**) corresponding line drawing and recommended position of the needle (*arrow*). **c** Position of the transducer in the transverse plane with the site of needle insertion medial to the transducer (*asterisk*) (*1* sternocleidomastoideus muscle). Just above the clavicle (*2*) the forming fascicles of the brachial plexus are accompanied by the subclavian artery (*3*) (*4* ventral border of the trapezius muscle, *5* parietal pleura)

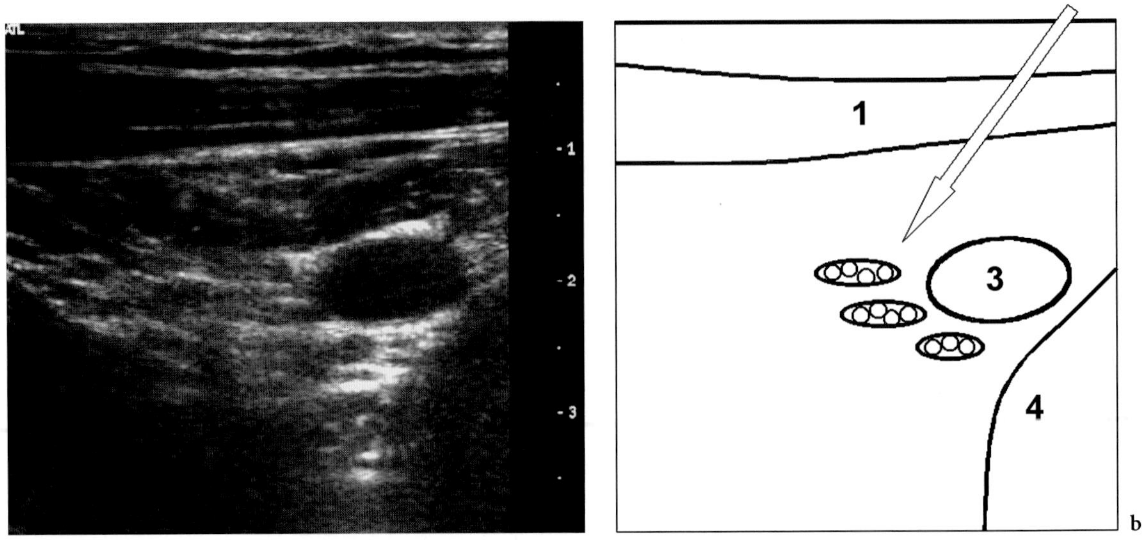

a b

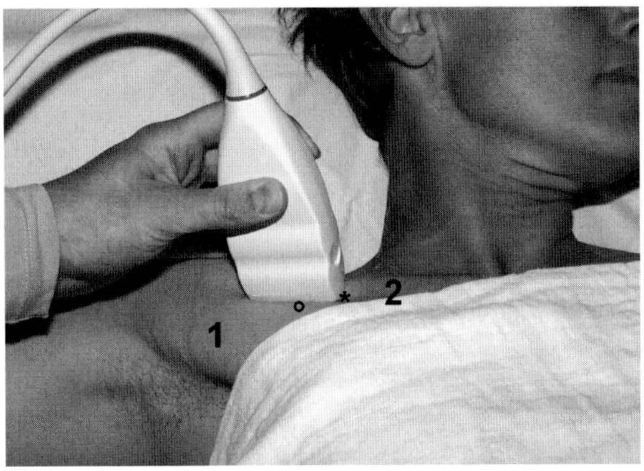

c

Fig. 6.5a–c. Sonographically guided infraclavicular brachial plexus block. **a** Sonogram with (**b**) corresponding line drawing and recommended position of the needle (*arrow*). **c** Position of the transducer in the transverse plane with the site of needle insertion medial to the transducer (*asterisk*) or in the middle of the transducer (*circle*) (*1* pectoralis major). Just below the clavicle (*2*) the axillary artery (*3*) is the landmark to locate the fascicles of the brachial plexus. Orientation is more difficult in this region because the clavicle interferes with tilting of the transducer to gain scanning plains perpendicular to the fascicles (*4* parietal pleura)

brachial plexus (Winnie et al. 1979; Bridenbaugh 1988). The most common disadvantage to this technique is incomplete block because the musculocutaneous and axillary nerves often leave the plexus proximal to the site of the block (Winnie et al. 1979) and the median, radial and ulnar nerves begin to move apart from each other after passing the lateral edge of the minor pectoralis muscle (Retzl et al. 2001). For the sonographically guided axillary block, the patient is positioned supine with the upper arm abducted to 90°, the shoulder rotated externally, and the elbow flexed at 110° (Fig. 6.6). It has to be kept in mind, that abduction to 90° may lead to compression of the axillary vessels and the brachial plexus, which results in insufficient spread of anesthetic. Then slight adduction of the upper arm is recommended to improve spreading (Kapral et al. 1994). Kapral et al. in their series reported no complications and a complete block in 95% of the patients.

6.2.2 Regional Anesthesia of the Lower Limb

At the lower limb sonographic guidance is described for only three regions:

- Psoas compartment block (Kirchmair 2001; Kirchmair et al. 2002)
- Three-in-one block in the inguinal region (Marhofer et al. 1997, 1998)
- Pudendal nerve block in the gluteal region (Gruber et al. 2001; Kovacs et al. 2001)

6.2.2.1 Psoas Compartment Block

The psoas compartment block is used to reach the spinal nerve roots forming the lumbar plexus within the psoas major muscle and is most often performed at the level of L4–L5, because nonguided anesthe-

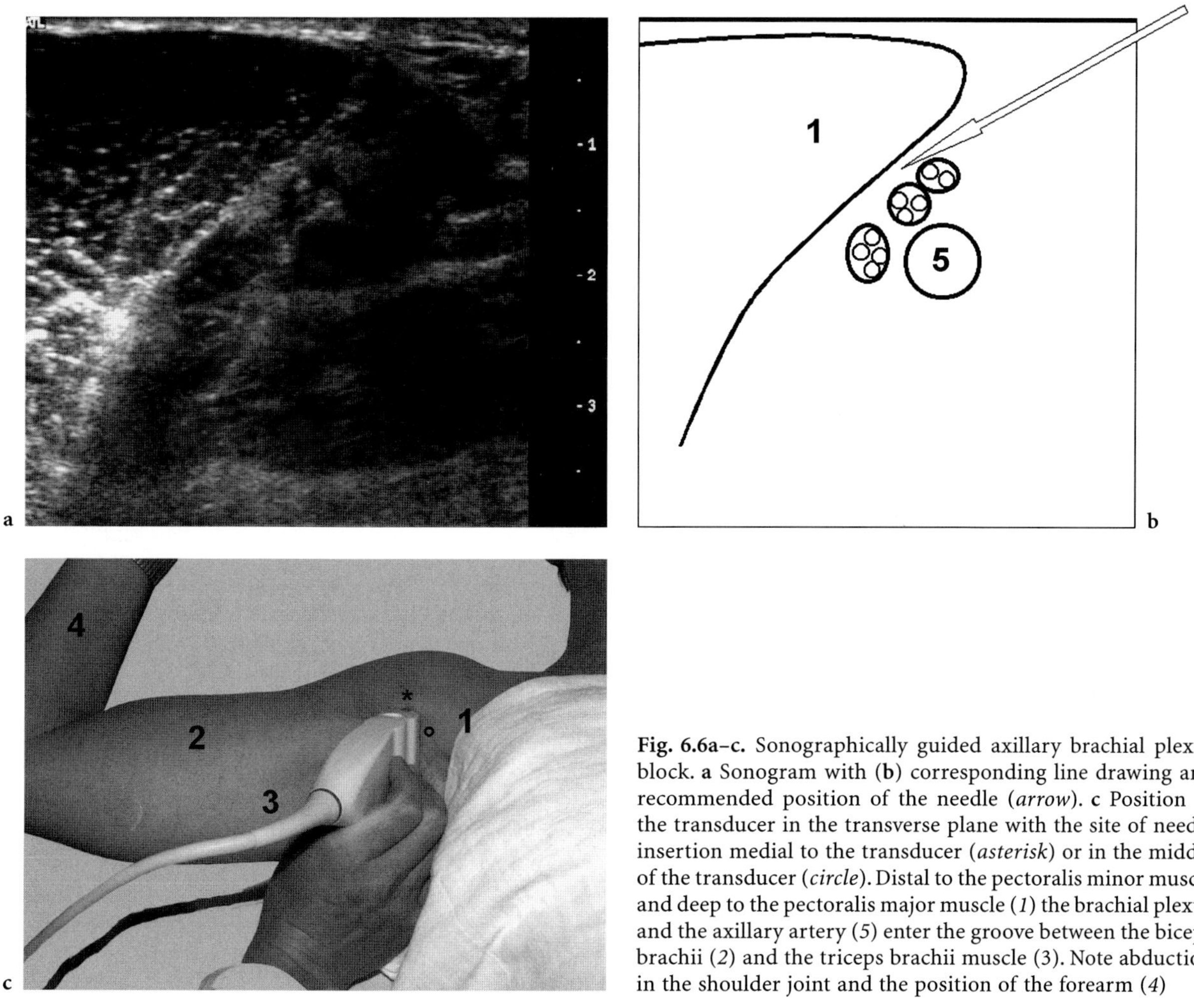

Fig. 6.6a–c. Sonographically guided axillary brachial plexus block. **a** Sonogram with (**b**) corresponding line drawing and recommended position of the needle (*arrow*). **c** Position of the transducer in the transverse plane with the site of needle insertion medial to the transducer (*asterisk*) or in the middle of the transducer (*circle*). Distal to the pectoralis minor muscle and deep to the pectoralis major muscle (*1*) the brachial plexus and the axillary artery (*5*) enter the groove between the biceps brachii (*2*) and the triceps brachii muscle (*3*). Note abduction in the shoulder joint and the position of the forearm (*4*)

sia at levels L2–L3 and L3–L4 may result in renal puncture and a subcapsular hematoma (AIDA et al. 1996). Kirchmair et al. showed that sonographically guided advancement of the needle into the psoas major muscle is possible without risk at the L2–L3 to L4–L5 level (KIRCHMAIR et al. 2002). The patient is seated prone and the needle is inserted 4–5 cm lateral to the spinous processes, guided through the erector spinae muscle into the posterior part of the psoas major muscle (Figs. 6.7 and 6.8). In cadaveric specimens only 1 out of 48 approaches failed and in the one case the needle was advanced insufficiently.

6.2.2.2 Three-in-one Block

The so-called three-in-one block is used to administer a single injection of local anesthetic in the inguinal region resulting in a block of the femoral, the lateral femoral cutaneous and the obturator nerves (WINNIE et al. 1973). The sonographically guided block is performed with the patient positioned supine and the leg rotated externally (15°). The needle is inserted 2 cm distal to the inguinal ligament and advanced as close as possible to the nerve within the fascial space underneath the iliopectineal fascia (MARHOFER et al. 1997, 1998), which separates the femoral nerve and the iliopsoas muscle from the femoral vessels (Fig. 6.9). In contrast to the nonguided technique using a nerve stimulator (success rate lower than 80%), sonographic guidance succeeds in 95% of patients and allows the administration of less local anesthetic (MARHOFER et al. 1998) because it facilitates the optimal positioning of the needle tip in relation to the femoral nerve and allows direct visualization of the spread of the anesthetic (MARHOFER et al. 1997). Nevertheless, only the femoral nerve is infiltrated directly, whereas the lateral femoral cutaneous nerve

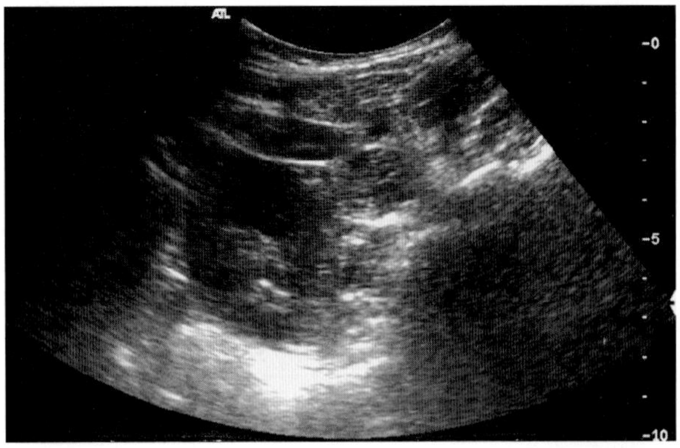

a

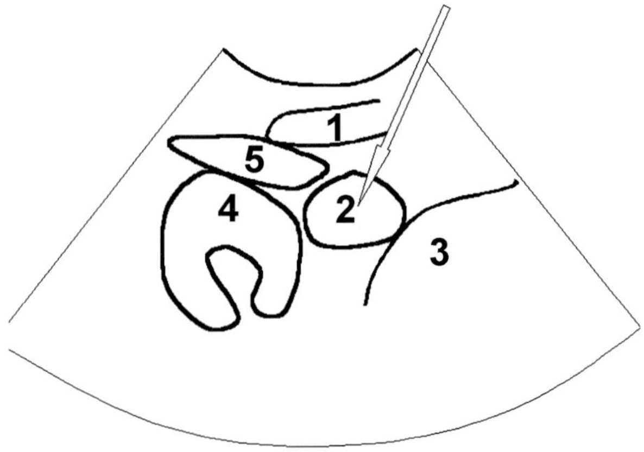

b

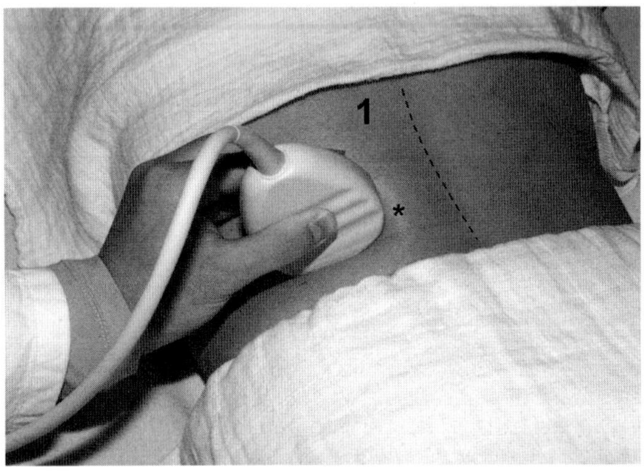

c

Fig. 6.7a–c. Sonographically guided psoas compartment block (L2–L3). **a** Sonogram with (**b**) corresponding line drawing and recommended position of the needle (*arrow*). **c** Position of the transducer in the transverse plane with the site of needle insertion medial to the transducer (*asterisk*) (*dotted line* through spinous processes). Through the erector spinae muscle (*1*) the posterior part of the psoas major muscle (*2*) is reached lateral to the third lumbar vertebra (*3*). Note the close relationship to the kidney (*4*) (*5* quadratus lumborum muscle)

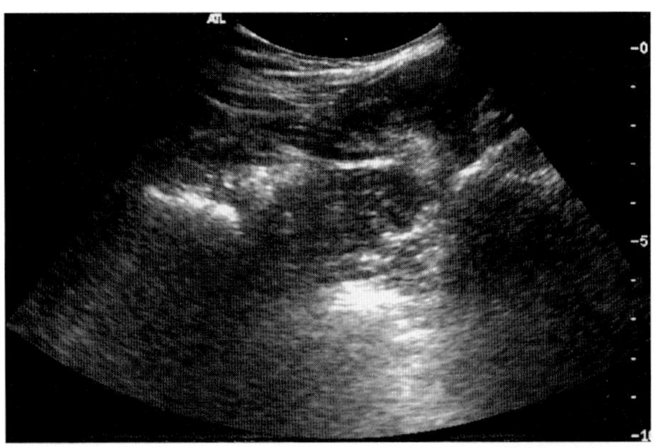

a

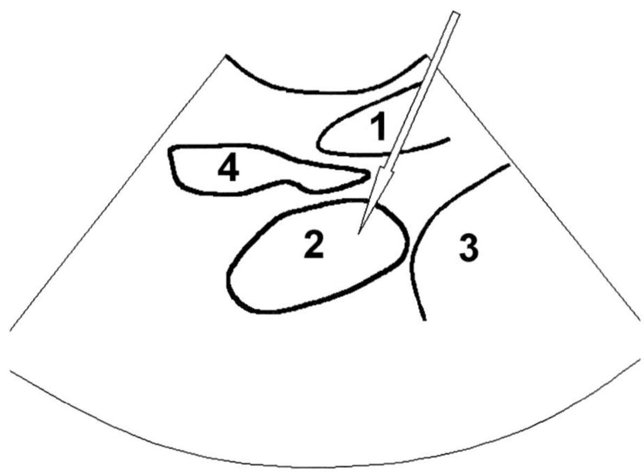

b

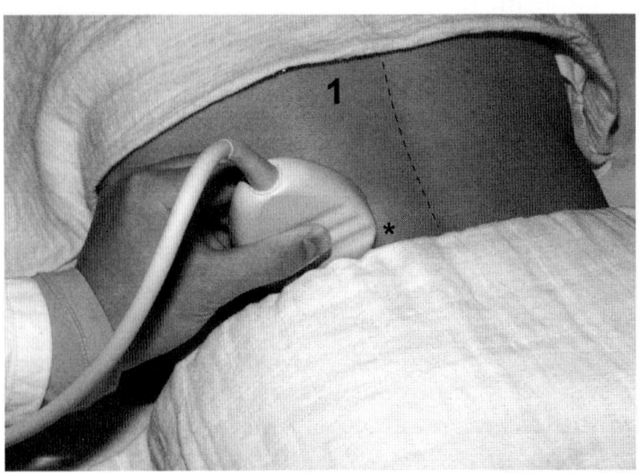

c

Fig. 6.8a–c. Sonographically guided psoas compartment block (L4–L5). **a** Sonogram with (**b**) corresponding line drawing and recommended position of the needle (*arrow*). **c** Position of the transducer in the transverse plane with the site of needle insertion medial to the transducer (*asterisk*) (*dotted line* through spinous processes) (*1* erector spinae muscle, *2* psoas major muscle, *3* fifth lumbar vertebra, *4* quadratus lumborum muscle)

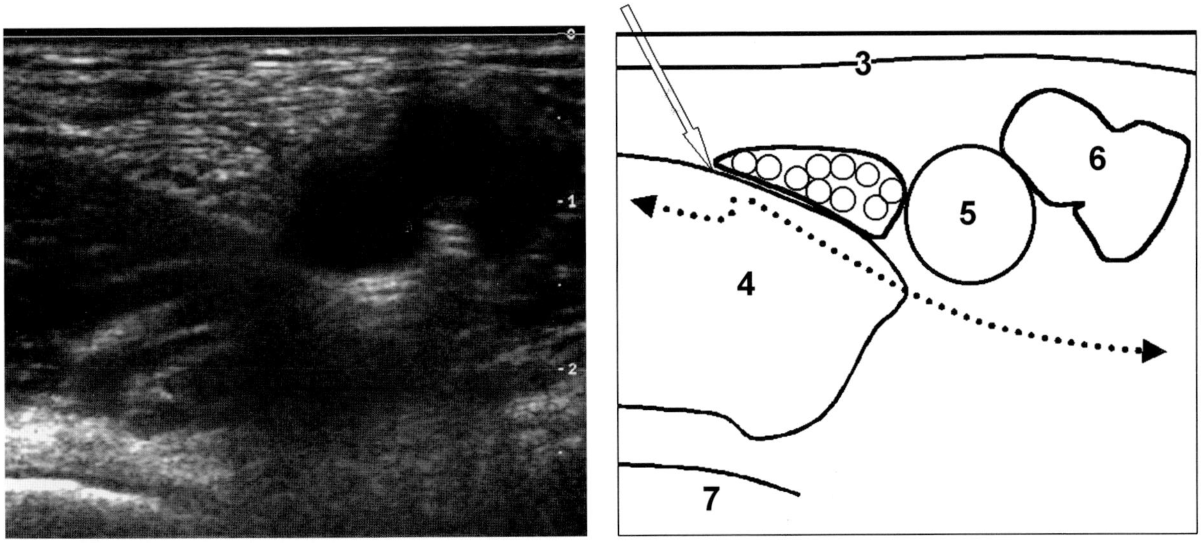

a b

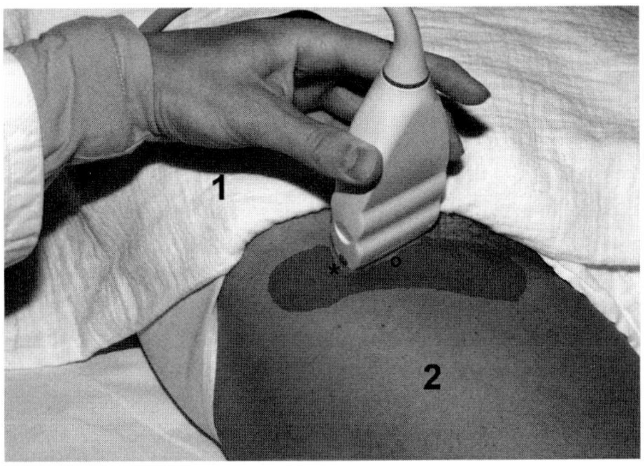

c

Fig. 6.9a–c. Sonographically guided three-in-one block. **a** Sonogram with (**b**) corresponding line drawing and recommended position of the needle (*arrow*). **c** Position of the transducer in the transverse plane with the site of needle insertion medial to the transducer (*asterisk*) or in the middle of the transducer (*circle*) (*1* anterior superior iliac spine, *2* quadriceps femoris muscle). Just distal to the inguinal ligament (*3*) the femoral nerve is aimed at between the iliopsoas muscle (*4*) and the femoral artery (*5*) (*6* great saphenous vein joining femoral vein, *7* head of femur). The *dotted arrows* indicate the supposed spreading of anesthetic to reach the lateral femoral cutaneous and obturator nerves (gray area in **c**)

is reached indirectly by lateral spread, and the anterior branch of the obturator nerve by medial spread of the local anesthetic during injection. The posterior branch of the obturator nerve is never reached by local anesthetic in guided or nonguided applications (Marhofer et al. 2000).

6.2.2.3
Pudendal Nerve Block

Instead of nonguided techniques or computed tomographic guidance (Thoumas et al. 1999), sonographic guidance can also be used to depict the site of injection for the pudendal nerve block (Kovacs et al. 2001). In a prone position the ischial spine, the sacrospinous ligament and the internal pudendal artery, which accompanies the pudendal nerve on its course around the mentioned musculoskeletal structures, are easily delineated with sonography. The needle should then be advanced under sonographic control almost to the level of the sacrospinous ligament 5 mm medial to the artery or 8 mm medial to the tip of the ischial spine (Fig. 6.10). Direct visualization of the pudendal nerve is possible in 47.2% of patients only (Kovacs et al. 2001). This is due to fatty connective tissue wrapping the nerve and impairing its sonographic detection (Gruber et al. 2001). Sonographic visualization of the region where the nerve is situated, however, allows the needle to be led into the common bed of connective tissue around the nerve and may allow a highly successful pudendal nerve block.

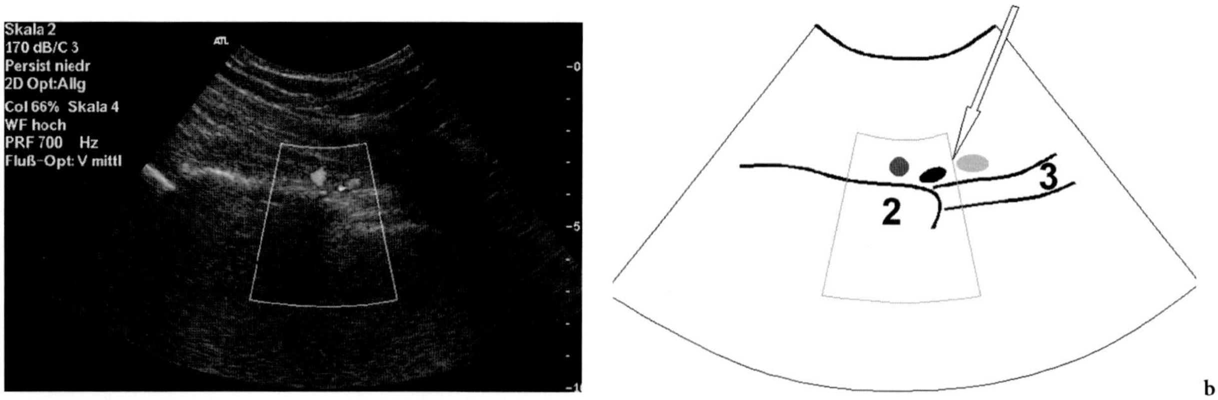

a b

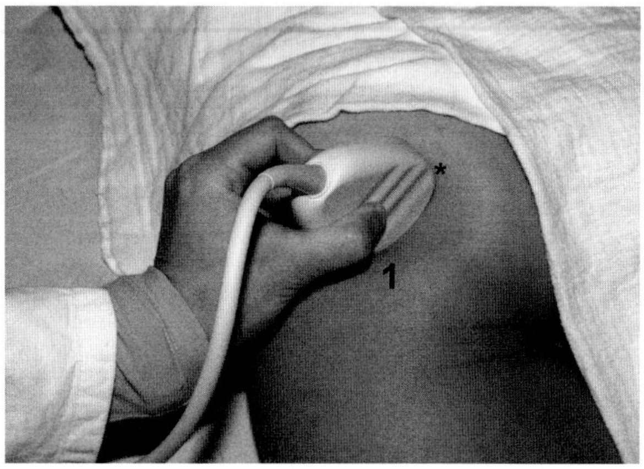

c

Fig. 6.10a–c. Sonographically guided pudendal nerve block. **a** Sonogram with (**b**) corresponding line drawing and recommended position of the needle (*arrow*). **c** Position of the transducer in an almost transverse plane with the site of needle insertion medial to the transducer (*asterisk*). The needle should be advanced through the gluteus maximus muscle (*1*) close to the ischial spine and the sacrospinous ligament. Using color-coded Doppler sonography the internal pudendal artery (*medium gray*) and vein (*black*) can be identified as a guide to the pudendal nerve (*light gray*)

References

Aida S, Takahashi H, Shimoji K (1996) Renal subcapsular hematoma after lumbar plexus block. Anesthesiology 84: 452–455

Bedder MD, Kozody R, Cronig DB (1988) Comparison of bupivacaine and alkalinised bupivacaine in brachial plexus anesthesia. Anesth Analg 67:48–52

Bridenbaugh LD (1988) The upper extremity: somatic blockade. In: Cousins MJ, Bridenbaugh PO (eds) Neural blockade in clinical anesthesia and management of pain. Lippincott, Philadelphia, pp 387–416

Dellon AL, Mackinnon SE (1986) Treatment of the painful neuroma by neuroma resection and muscle implantation. Plast Reconstr Surg 77:427–436

Dellon AL, Mackinnon SE, Pestronk A (1984) Implantation of sensory nerve into muscle: preliminary clinical and experimental observations on neuroma formation. Ann Plast Surg 12:30–40

Dockery GL (1999) The treatment of intermetatarsal neuromas with 4% alcohol sclerosing injections. J Foot Ankle Surg 38:403–408

Goldberg ME, Gregg C, Larijani GE, et al (1987) Comparison of three methods of axillary approach to brachial plexus blockade for upper extremity surgery. Anesthesiology 66: 814–816

Graf BM, Martin E (2001) Peripheral neuronal blockade. A review of new developments of an old technique (in German). fibsthetist 50:312–322

Gruber H, Kovacs P, Piegger J, et al (2001) New, simple, ultrasound-guided infiltration of the pudendal nerve: topographic basics. Dis Colon Rectum 44:1376–1380

Hanania M, Kitain E (1998) Perisciatic injection of steroid for the treatment of sciatica due to piriformis syndrome. Reg Anesth Pain Med 23:223–228

Jandrasits O, Likar R, Marhofer P, et al (1998) The use of ultrasonography for regional anesthetic techniques: upper extremity blockades. Acta Anaesthesiol Scand 42:48–51

Kapral S, Krafft P, Eibenberger K, et al (1994) Ultrasound-guided supraclavicular approach for regional anesthesia of the brachial plexus. Anesth Analg 78:507–513

Kirchmair L, Entner T, Wissel J, et al (2001) A study of the paravertebral anatomy for ultrasound-guided posterior lumbar plexus block. Anesth Analg 93:477–481

Kirchmair L, Entner T, Kapral S, et al (2002) Ultrasound guidance for the psoas compartment block: an imaging study. Anesth Analg 94:706–710

Kovacs P, Gruber H, Piegger J, et al (2001) New, simple, ultrasound-guided infiltration of the pudendal nerve: ultrasonographic technique. Dis Colon Rectum 44:1381–1385

Kovacs P, Gruber H, Peer S, et al (2003) Ultrasonographic guided phenol instillation in painful stump neuroma: inital ecperience. J Ultrasound Med (in press)

Lu L, Atchabahian A, Mackinnon SE, et al (1998) Nerve injection injury with botulinum toxin. Plast Reconstr Surg 101: 1875–1880

Marhofer P, Schrögendorfer K, Koinig H, et al (1997) Ultrasonographic guidance improves sensory block and onset time of three-in-one blocks. Anesth Analg 85:854–857

Marhofer P, Schrögendorfer K, Wallner T, et al (1998) Ultrasonographic guidance reduces the amount of local anesthetic for 3-in-1 blocks. Reg Anesth Pain Med 23:584–588

Marhofer P, Nasel C, Sitzwohl C, et al (2000) Magnetic resonance imaging of the distribution of local anesthetic during the three-in-one block. Anesth Analg 90:119–124

Masala S, Fanucci E, Ranconi P, et al (2001) Treatment of intermetatarsal neuromas with alcohol injection under US guidance (in Italian). Radiol Med (Torino) 102:370–373

Mooney V, Frykman G, McLamb J (1969) Current status of intraneural phenol injections. Clin Orthop 63:122–129

Moore D (1954) Regional block. Thomas, Springfield, p 60

Moorthy SS, Schmidt SI, Dierdorf SF, et al (1991) A supraclavicular lateral approach for brachial plexus regional anesthesia. Anesth Analg 72:241–244

Myers RR, Katz J (1988) Neuropathy of neurolytic and semidestructive agents. In: Cousins MJ, Bridenbaugh PO (eds) Neural blockade in clinical anesthesia and management of pain. Lippincott, Philadelphia, pp 1031–1051

Ootaki C, Hayashi H, Amano M (2000) Ultrasound-guided infraclavicular brachial plexus block: an alternative technique to landmark-guided approaches. Reg Anesth Pain Med 25:600–604

Rasmussen MR, Kitaoka HB, Patzer GL (1996) Nonoperative treatment of plantar interdigital neuroma with a single corticosteroid injection. Clin Orthop 326:188–193

Retzl G, Kapral S, Greher M, et al (2001) Ultrasonographic findings of the axillary part of the brachial plexus. Anesth Analg 92:1271–1275

Thomas AJ, Bull MJ, Howard AC, et al (1999) Perioperative ultrasound guided needle localisation of amputation stump neuroma. Injury 30:689–691

Thoumas D, Leroi AM, Mauillon J, et al (1999) Pudendal neuralgia: CT-guided pudendal nerve block technique. Abdom Imaging 24:309–312

Ting PL, Sivagnanaratnam V (1989) Ultrasonographic study of the spread of local anaesthetic during axillary brachial plexus block. Br J Anaesth 63:326–329

Tsukazaki T, Ito N, Maeda H, et al (1993) Effect of phenol block on peripheral nerve: morphometric and histochemical study in rats (abstract, in Japanese). Nippon Seikeigeka Gakkai Zasshi 67:473–479

Tuominen M, Haasio J, Hekali R, et al (1989) Continuous interscalene brachial plexus block: clinical efficacy, technical problems and bupivacaine plasma concentrations. Acta Anaesthesiol Scand 33:84–88

Westerlund T, Vuorinen V, Röyttä M (2001) Same axonal regeneration rate after different endoneural response to intraneural glycerol and phenol injection. Acta Neuropathol (Berl) 102:41:54

Winnie AP (1993) Axillary perivascular technique of brachial plexus block. In: Winnie AP, Håkansson L (eds) Plexus anesthesia, vol 1, 3rd edn. Saunders, Philadelphia, pp 121–143

Winnie AP, Ramamurthy S, Durrani Z (1973) The inguinal paravascular technique of lumbar plexus anesthesia: the 3-in-1 block. Anesth Analg 52:989–996

Winnie AP, Radonjic R, Akkineni SR, et al (1979) Factors influencing distribution of local anaesthetic injected into the brachial plexus sheath. Anesth Analg 58: 225–234

Yang WT, Chui PT, Metreweli C (1998) Anatomy of the normal brachial plexus revealed by sonography and the role of Sonographic guidance in anesthesia of the brachial plexus. AJR Am J Roentgenol 171:1631–1636

7 Clinical Considerations: The Surgeon's Perspective

H. Piza-Katzer

CONTENTS

7.1 Historical Introduction *107*
7.2 Anatomy of the Peripheral Nerve *108*
7.2.1 Nerve Fiber *108*
7.2.2 Fascicle *108*
7.2.3 Nerve Trunk *108*
7.2.4 Vascular Supply *108*
7.3 Nerve Injury, Degeneration and Regeneration *109*
7.4 Classification of Nerve Injuries *109*
7.4.1 Classification of Nerve Injuries According to Functional Loss and Severity *109*
7.4.2 Classification of Nerve Injuries According to Their Etiology *110*
7.5 Surgical Nerve Repair and Reconstruction: Techniques *112*
7.5.1 Nerve-in-continuity *112*
7.5.2 Nerve Injury with Loss of Continuity *115*
7.6 Timing of Nerve Repair *116*
7.7 Prognosis *118*
7.8 Future Directions in Peripheral Nerve Surgery *118*
7.9 Summary and Conclusion *119*
References *120*

7.1 Historical Introduction

The edifice of knowledge is built gradually over centuries of human history. We stand on the shoulders of those who went before us, profiting from their wisdom and learning from their mistakes. In this sense, a brief excursion into the history of peripheral nerves should contribute not only to the satisfaction of our sense of curiosity, but also serve as a homage to those who were at the frontiers of knowledge and opened up new territories for succeeding generations.

According to history, the world's first meticulous anatomist was the Greek physician Herophilus who lived in Alexandria around 300 BC. He practiced in Alexandria, where human dissections were permitted, and he even performed some in public. He also made careful comparisons between animal and human morphology. The results of the careful dissections of this physician – considered as the father of scientific anatomy – are recorded in his work *On Dissections,* and the world owes its first insight into the anatomy of peripheral nerves to his careful observations. He not only distinguished nerves from tendons, but also traced nerves to the spinal cord, and differentiated between the sensory and motor components of nerves.

Five centuries later, these initial findings were enormously extended by Galen (Brock 1929), who provided a comprehensive description of the peripheral nervous system as a whole, describing in detail the digital nerves as well. In his works we hear, possibly for the first time in the history of medicine, reports of the practice of nerve repair. From these early reports to contemporary practice, the history of peripheral nerve repair is very confused, with conflicting beliefs and expectations about the success of surgical interventions. The introduction of staining methods, improvements in staining techniques and powerful microscopes have enabled an understanding of the finer structural features of the nerve fibers and the nerve cell. Observations of spontaneous recovery of nerve function after transection, a gradually increasing knowledge of the processes involved in nerve regeneration, and advances in microsurgical techniques have all contributed to establishing faith in the significance and success of surgical repair of peripheral nerve lesions. It has been a long way to reach this point and there is still a long way to go.

H. Piza-Katzer, MD
Professor and Chairman, Department of Plastic and Reconstructive Surgery and Ludwig Boltzmann Institute for Quality Control in Plastic and Reconstructive Surgery, University Hospital Innsbruck, Anichstrasse 35, 6020 Innsbruck, Austria

7.2 Anatomy of the Peripheral Nerve

It goes without saying that operative repair and reconstruction of damaged nerves presupposes a very clear knowledge of the gross anatomy of the peripheral nerve as well as its complex internal features (Mumenthaler et al. 1998). The use of clearly defined terms is a prerequisite for understanding and precisely describing the pathophysiological sequelae and the morphological consequences of nerve injury.

7.2.1 Nerve Fiber

The basic structural unit of the peripheral nerve at the microscopic level is the nerve fiber which is responsible for conducting impulses to and from the peripheral organs. The nerve fiber has a complex structure. It consists of the axon, which is the central core, which is enveloped in a complex covering of a single layer of linked Schwann cells with and without a myelin component, the basement membrane external to this covering and a sheath of endoneurial connective tissue of collagen fibers which forms its outermost layer. This layer represents the supporting framework for the nerve fibers and capillaries inside the fascicle.

Nerve fibers are either myelinated or unmyelinated. The axon of a myelinated nerve fiber is individually enveloped by a single Schwann cell, the membrane of which forms a multilaminated myelin sheath. The sheath of an unmyelinated axon consists of a single layer of Schwann cells. The cytoplasm of a Schwann cell surrounds more than one axon so that the endoneural tube usually contains several axons, in contrast to that of a myelinated fiber, which contains only one axon.

7.2.2 Fascicle

Nerve fibers are bundled together to form a fascicle which is a macroscopic unit of the peripheral nervous system. The endoneurial space refers to tissue spaces within the nerve fascicle. Each fascicle is surrounded by the perineurium, a sheath of connective tissue formed by several layers of perineurial cells. The perineurium has an important barrier function, protecting the fascicle from interfascicular tissue fluids and from infection, and is responsible for maintaining a higher tissue pressure within the fascicle and also the elasticity and tensile strength of the nerve fibers.

7.2.3 Nerve Trunk

Many fascicles are bundled together by the epineurium to form a nerve, but the number of fascicles in a nerve can vary. There are monofascicular nerves composed of a single fasciculus, and polyfascicular nerves composed of a few large fasciculi or entirely of small fasciculi of the same size or a combination of large and small fasciculi. There are also fascicular groups outlined by spatial closeness, by encircling condensation of the epineurium around them or by an arbitrary selection. In monofascicular nerves, the greater part of the tissue in the nerve trunk is fascicular in nature; in polyfascicular nerves the ratio of fascicular to non-fascicular decreases according to the number of fascicles present – the larger the number of fascicles, the greater the amount of non-fascicular tissue. All these anatomical details play a role in determining the severity of injury (e.g. monofascicular nerves are more vulnerable to severe injuries than polyfascicular ones), and in the choice of the appropriate method of surgical repair of nerve lesions.

Nerve fibers branch within the tissue they innervate and also within the nerve trunk. It is clear that the number of fibers is greater distally than proximally. There are three different types of nerve fibers – motor, sensory and sympathetic. Sensory and motor nerves contain both myelinated and unmyelinated nerve fibers. The postganglionic sympathetic nerves contain unmyelinated fibers and innervate the skin, blood vessels and hair follicles.

7.2.4 Vascular Supply

Extensively interconnected microvascular systems ensure that the peripheral nerves are adequately vascularized. Intraneural microvessels extend longitudinally within the epineurium, with this system being reinforced by extrinsic segmental regional blood vessels. There are vascular plexus within the perineurium and within the fascicles, microvascular networks of capillaries, arterioles and venules, ensuring the supply and blood nutrients to the nerve structures. Intimate knowledge of the intraneural microvascular system is a precondition for microsurgical procedures on nerves such as mobilization, transposition, stretching and resection, all of which involve manipulation of the blood vessels, which, if improperly performed, will result in loss of blood supply to the nerve and all its associated adverse consequences.

7.3 Nerve Injury, Degeneration and Regeneration

Traumatic injury to a nerve might consist only of focal demyelination demonstrated by local conduction block. Regeneration in this case represents local myelin repair, resulting in restoration of excitability and conduction of nerve fibers.

Trauma that results in transection of the nerve fibers sets in motion several pathophysiological processes. There is focal demyelination at the site of injury, wallerian degeneration distally and proximally (WALLER 1850) and, depending on the site of injury, cell body death (KRISTENSSON 1981). The more proximal the injury, the greater is the danger of cell body death. All these occur because the axons, which carry information to and from the nerve cell body, depend on the nerve cell for their survival and function and the nerve cell reacts to signals from the periphery. When axons undergo damage, their transport functions – anterograde and retrograde – fail, causing structural and functional changes also in the nerve cell body (GELBERMANN 1991) including, under certain conditions, the death of the neuron.

Under these conditions, the process of regeneration consists of the surviving axons sprouting regenerating units proximally under the influence of neurotrophic factors (VARON and ADLER 1989), and their establishing contact with the corresponding part of the distal nerve through the transected part, now filled with proliferating fibroblasts. When that happens, functional recovery (sensory, motor, sympathetic) may occur to a greater or lesser extent. If, however, the gap between the transected ends is large, the axon sprouts may fail to reach the distal stump, getting lost in the surrounding proliferating connective tissue, or they may be misdirected. In the former case, painful neuromas may develop and the peripheral target structures may suffer irreversible damage. In the latter case, incorrect reinnervation of targets will occur, resulting in more or less serious functional consequences.

7.4 Classification of Nerve Injuries

7.4.1 Classification of Nerve Injuries According to Functional Loss and Severity

Sir Herbert SEDDON (1943) distinguished between three types of nerve injuries as follows:

1. *Neurapraxia* represents first-degree injury and stands for a nerve lesion in which there is a temporary local conduction block without any loss of continuity of axons or nerve trunk. Depending on the severity of injury, there may be histopathological changes consisting of focal demyelination, although this is not always present. When the cause of the local conduction block is lifted, recovery occurs, but this may not be very rapid (within minutes or days), but might be progressive and gradual, lasting over 12 weeks if a greater degree of injury has caused morphological alterations in the form of segmental demyelination. However, recovery is always complete, since there is no need for axonal regeneration. Tourniquet palsy and radial nerve paralysis resulting from the compression of the nerve in an alcoholic who falls asleep with his arm resting on the back of a chair or other hard object are typical examples of this kind of injury. The diagnosis of neurapraxia can be made on the basis of conduction block at the site of the lesion and response to electric stimulation of the nerve segment distal to it.
2. *Axonotmesis* is second-degree injury in which there is loss of continuity of axons, but the nerve trunk sheath is unbroken. Such an injury is followed by disintegration of the axon and its myelin sheath, so-called Wallerian degeneration, distal to the site of injury and to some extent proximally as well. The endoneurium and the perineurium are intact. Axon division can result from chronic compression syndromes such as carpal tunnel syndrome or compression injury to the ulnar nerve. Such an injury has also a good prognosis with complete spontaneous recovery, since the regenerating axons do not have to cross through scar tissue, and misdirection of axon sprouts also does not occur.
   In contrast to neurapraxia where there is no advancing Tinel's sign (because there is no axonal degeneration and regeneration), after axonotmesis, one can observe an advancing Hoffmann-Tinel sign, with recovery occurring at the rate of 1 mm/day in a 20-year-old individual and correspondingly more slowly in older subjects with nerve injuries.
3. *Neurotmesis* stands for complete transection of a nerve. In view of the longitudinal elasticity of nerve sheaths, such an injury is followed by complete dehiscence of the severed ends of the nerve trunk. Neurotmesis is observed in open wounds and may or may not be associated with nerve deficit. Such injuries need to be surgically repaired by different methods, depending on the nature of the injury, and complete recovery of function may not be achieved.

Sunderland classified nerve injuries into five types (Sunderland 1951), according to the extent of damage that has occurred. Neurapraxia is defined as in the classification of Seddon and constitutes *first-degree injury*. Sunderland elaborates Seddon's classification by distinguishing under axonotmesis between axon severance or damage alone (*second-degree injury),* axon severance or damage together with damage to endoneurial sheaths, but with intact perineurium that enables maintenance of fascicular continuity (e.g. after acute blunt injuries with extensive endoneural bleeding and scar formation) – *third-degree injury* – and axonal severance with damage to the endoneurium and the perineurium as well (e.g. after severe traction or stretch injury with massive scarring, after severe blunt injuries or incomplete severance of the nerve trunk) -*fourth-degree injury*. Neurotmesis is the most severe form of injury (*fifth-degree injury*) where the entire nerve trunk is transected and nerve continuity is completely lost.

Spontaneous and complete regeneration can occur after first- and second-degree injuries. After third-degree injury, spontaneous recovery can occur, but it will be incomplete, since the regenerating nerve fibers – the axon sprouts – although restricted in their growth within the fascicle, may yet grow towards different distal paths because of mismatching of nerve fibers. Furthermore, because of the presence of scar tissue, not all axon sprouts will be able to make contact with the distal receptors and end organs. To this must be added that the more proximal the injury is the poorer the prognosis for the following reason. In the proximal regions, fascicles are mixed, with motor and sensory fibers lying adjacent to each other. Mismatch of regenerating fibers present a greater threat to recovery. At a more distal part, a third-degree injury is likely to cause less chaotic recovery, since at this level, the fascicles contain either motor or sensory fibers alone. Misdirected regeneration is not a problem here, although incomplete regeneration is still a possibility.

After a fourth-degree injury where the perineurium is also damaged, spontaneous recovery is not to be expected. Such damage to the nerve is the result of very severe stretch or traction injuries or it can occur after nerve injections. Clinical and electrodiagnostic tests will provide evidence of recovery. First-, second- and third-degree injuries will demonstrate progression of recovery within the first 3 months after they have been sustained, but if by 3 months there is no evidence of recovery, the injury will have to be considered as a fourth-degree injury and surgical intervention must be considered and initiated.

Fifth-degree injuries involving complete severance of a nerve can only be managed surgically.

Mackinnon and Dellon add a *sixth-degree injury* (Mackinnon and Dellon 1988), within one and the same nerve, in which all the five or varying combinations of Sunderland's five types of injuries may be present, presenting the so-called *neuroma-in-continuity*. Various fascicles of a nerve show varying degrees of injuries (I, II, III, IV, V) and some may even have normal function. This type of injury presents a surgical dilemma, since the surgeon must assess the patient clinically and determine the degrees of function loss caused by injuries to different fascicles. During surgical management, the surgeon must be careful not to manipulate the intact fascicles and those with first-, second- or third-degree injury, since spontaneous recovery might occur in these fascicles, and this is far superior to that which can be achieved by end-to-end coaptation or surgical grafting techniques.

Nerve injuries are followed by temporary or long-lasting loss of sensory and motor function and in some cases by pain. The type of nerve injury will determine both the method of repair to be employed and the prognosis for recovery of motor and sensory functions and alleviation of pain symptoms after surgical repair.

7.4.2 Classification of Nerve Injuries According to Their Etiology

A nerve injury is defined as any damage caused to a nerve by a physical force applied externally or generated by a disturbed internal anatomical situation. Neuropathy refers to nerve lesions caused not by physical injury but by underlying systemic diseases, metabolic and toxic disturbances, and primary vascular disease. The primary causes of nerve injuries are physical trauma, ischaemia, action of sclerosing and toxic agents, cooling, freezing and ionizing radiation and a combination of these causes. These injuries can also be the result of medical and surgical interventions (Piza-Katzer et al. 1994, 1995).

7.4.2.1 Physical Trauma

7.4.2.1.1 Compression

Compression trauma can occur with closed or open wounds. There are two kinds of compression injury that should be distinguished: acute and chronic. *Acute* compression can be caused by exogenous or endogenous forces. Examples of exogenous forces are a blow from a blunt object, tight bandages, tourniquet, splints and plaster casts. Dislocated bone, a fragment of broken bone, a clamped nerve during surgery or unrelieved pressure on a nerve, for example, during anesthesia or under coma, severely compress a nerve by forcing it against an unyielding surface such as a bone. The famous "Saturday night paralysis" is the result of an acute compression. During pregnancy and delivery, a nerve in the mother may be compressed. The severity of the injury can vary between first- and third-degree and when the offending forces are removed, recovery should occur spontaneously and completely at the latest by 6 months after injury. Motor function failure is the first to occur and the last to recover. Endogenous forces responsible for acute nerve compression are hemorrhage into a confined compartment containing a nerve such as the carpal tunnel or the psoas compartment.

Chronic compression develops slowly and can be progressive or intermittent. There are irregular remissions and exacerbations in the signs and symptoms associated with these lesions. The effect on the nerve fibers is produced by physical trauma, impaired blood supply (caused, for example, by a hematoma, and enlarging tumor or inflamed tissue) and resulting fibrosis that constricts the fasciculi and the nerve trunk. The severity of the injury can progress from first-degree to even fourth-degree damage unless the nerve is decompressed.

It is a matter of controversy whether the primary pathology in chronic nerve compression is the result of physical deformation of the nerve fibers or vascular complications caused by compression. However, regardless of the cause of the pathology, the injured nerve fibers suffer the same fate, namely progressive segmental demyelination, axon thinning and destruction of the axon with Wallerian degeneration. Some classical examples of nerve compression injuries in the upper extremity are:

1. radial nerve entrapment at the elbow
2. ulnar nerve compression at the elbow
3. median nerve compression in the forearm
4. median nerve compression in the carpal tunnel
5. ulnar nerve compression at he wrist
6. radial sensory nerve compression in the forearm

and in the lower extremity are:

1. femoral nerve
2. common peroneal nerve entrapment
3. deep peroneal nerve entrapment
4. superficial peroneal nerve entrapment
5. sural nerve entrapment
6. tarsal tunnel syndrome
7. plantar nerve compression

Two other most common injuries that a surgeon has to deal with are those affecting the facial and the accessory nerve.

7.4.2.1.2 Friction and Nerve Entrapment Lesions

Entrapment lesions are the most common of the mechanically caused nerve injuries. They develop in anatomical regions where a nerve runs through a confined space, a constricted opening or over or around a fibrous band where it is susceptible to mechanical irritation. In entrapment lesions, a nerve is fixed in some confined position because of adhesions. In compartment compression, the nerve is not fixed to any tissue, but suffers injury because of compression. Thus carpal and tarsal tunnel syndromes are compartment compression lesions and not entrapment lesions. Entrapment may subsequently develop as a result of hemorrhage within the tunnel, mechanical irritation leading to friction damage, inflammatory reaction and fibrosis. The key pathogenetic factor in entrapment nerve lesions is local inflammatory reactions to repeated mechanical irritations.

Although there is a difference between compression and entrapment injuries, they are combined by convention under the heading of compression lesions.

7.4.2.1.3 Traction

Traction injury can be *acute* or *chronic*. In the former, an abruptly applied force causes destructive structural changes in a nerve and results in immediate loss of function. In the latter, a nerve is stretched gradually and symptoms appear only after considerable deformation has taken place. Adhesions, dislocation of bones, fractures, injuries that forcibly displace body parts so as to stretch the nerves passing between them, high velocity missile injuries, nerves repaired end-to-end under tension, and premature postoperative limb extension in the course of mobilization are some of the basic causes of traction injury.

Nerves composed of a single or a few fascicles with little supporting epineurial tissue are at greater risk of sustaining traction injuries. When a nerve has a short free-running course and is fixed at one or both ends, such as, for example, the suprascapular nerve, the elastic limit of the nerve is rapidly exceeded when it is stretched and it is thus more vulnerable to traction injury. In contrast, in a nerve such as the medial division of the sciatic nerve, a considerable length of which is free-running, traction forces are fully spent in taking up the slack in the nerve and the fasciculi so that the nerve fibers escape injury. Proximity to a joint also predisposes a nerve to traction injury. The axillary nerve, the median and ulnar nerves at the elbow joint and the common peroneal nerve at the knee joint are particularly vulnerable to traction injuries after joint dislocation.

7.4.2.1.4 Ischaemic Lesions

Maintenance of the structural and functional integrity of the nerve requires adequate local blood supply. When the blood supply is impaired, nerve conduction is lost first before structural damage takes place. With increasing ischaemia, conduction block, Wallerian degeneration, and necrosis of the nerve take place, and finally the nerve is transformed into a fibrotic cord. In view of considerable overlap in the distribution of blood vessels and extensive anastomoses between their branches, there is a margin of safety and the collateral circulatory mechanisms protect blood supply to the nerves from interruption caused by the failure of a few arteries. However, extensive occlusions that involve intraneural ramifications of vessels will affect the collateral circulation, which, when prolonged, can cause ischaemic nerve damage. Ischaemia may be the result of compression or stretch or due to damage to the arteries supplying the nerve (for example, as a result of arteriolar spasm, arterial embolism, laceration, severance, ligation, aneurysms, damage during mobilization of an injured nerve preparatory to transposition and nerve repair).The severity of the consequences of ischaemia – disturbances in motor and sensory functions – will depend on the duration of the ischaemia and whether collateral circulation is available.

7.4.2.1.5 Complete Transection

Injuries resulting in loss of continuity of the nerve trunk can present in basically three different forms: (1) clean severance; (2) severance with lacerated, crushed and contused nerve ends; and (3) trauma causing destruction of a nerve segment, so that there is a nerve defect that will have to be bridged. In each of these situations, the methods of nerve repair employed are distinctly different.

7.5 Surgical Nerve Repair and Reconstruction: Techniques

7.5.1 Nerve-in-continuity

7.5.1.1 Neurolysis

This is the method of surgical repair of nerves when neural fibrosis has developed as a result of physical, chemical, or ischaemic insult to a nerve. Scar tissue can cause compression, adhesion, and thus loss of longitudinal mobility. When expected spontaneous regeneration does not take place within the normal period of time (8–12 weeks) and when in addition the patient complains of pain, an exploration of the site of injury may show fibrosis and adhesions which may be responsible for delayed regeneration.

By means of external neurolysis a nerve is freed segment by segment from its bed by removing adhesions that attach it to surrounding structures and by resecting constrictive scar tissue from around the nerve (Fig. 7.1). By resecting fibrotic tissues, impairment to the blood supply can be eliminated. It is important that during neurolysis, great care is taken not to injure blood vessels in the region. In epineuriotomy, the fibrotic superficial epineurium is opened under the microscope with a longitudinal incision in order to decompress the fasciculi contained within it. Epifascicular epineuriectomy consists of totally or partially resecting the thickened fibrotic tissue surrounding the nerve. This is done when decompression is not achieved by epineuriotomy alone. This can happen if fibrotic tissue has reached the spaces between the fascicles. The aim here again is to free the nerve from compression. For surgery, blunt instruments are used except where fibrotic tissue reaches deeper layers, when the scalpel will have to be used.

Interfascicular epineuriectomy will be needed in cases where deep layers and larger areas of the interfascicular epineurium are fibrotic. The surgical procedure should be stopped as soon as decompression is achieved.

Internal neurolysis is controversial. It is claimed that removal of epineural scar tissue will damage the blood vessels that run on the surface of the superficial and in the deeper interfascicular epineurium and compromise the blood supply to the nerve, causing ischaemia, that fine fascicular intercommunications will be destroyed, and that additional scar tissue that develops during the process of healing will again lead

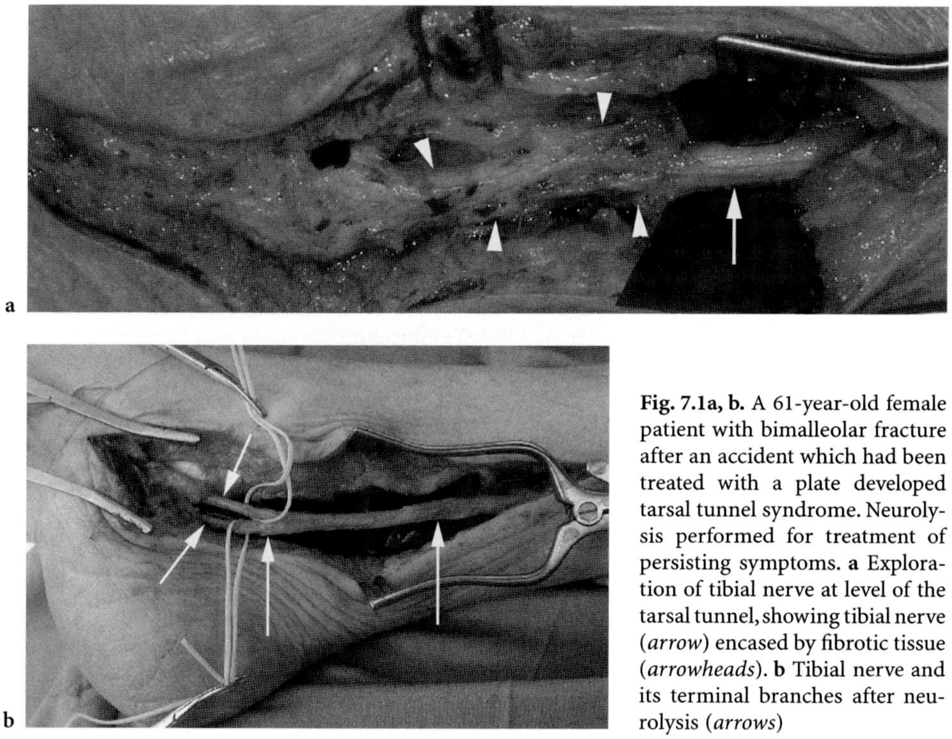

Fig. 7.1a, b. A 61-year-old female patient with bimalleolar fracture after an accident which had been treated with a plate developed tarsal tunnel syndrome. Neurolysis performed for treatment of persisting symptoms. **a** Exploration of tibial nerve at level of the tarsal tunnel, showing tibial nerve (*arrow*) encased by fibrotic tissue (*arrowheads*). **b** Tibial nerve and its terminal branches after neurolysis (*arrows*)

to troublesome nerve compression (Rydevik et al. 1976; Frykman et al. 1981; Lundborg 1988). Millesi states that by taking adequate care to maintain at least a part of the longitudinal blood supply, the problem of ischaemia can be avoided; furthermore, if surgery is performed in an atraumatic way with microsurgical techniques and if the causes of compression are eliminated (e.g. by completely releasing the carpal tunnel), development of fibrotic tissue can be eliminated (Millesi 1992). However, internal neurolysis continues to be a procedure that is rarely performed except where there is no alternative (Fig. 7.2).

Damage to a nerve caused by the development of fibrosis subsequent to compression and traction can only be handled surgically by an appropriate form of neurolysis (Millesi 1981).

7.5.1.2
Mobilization

Nerves may need to be extensively mobilized so that they can be transposed to a new bed or for joining nerve ends with a wide gap between them in the process of tensionless coaptation. Mobilization carries several risks such as destruction of the complex fascicular plexus formations, which are often variable in individuals and unintentional severance of nutrient vessels. This is particularly the case if surgery is performed under tourniquet control when an artery may be severed and may retract without being noticed. When the tourniquet is released, bleeding might occur. An attempt to secure the severed ends of the vessel can cause fascicular damage and bleeding from such arteries can cause scar tissue leading to the formation of fibrosis and result in associated damage and regeneration block. All mobilization requires stripping of branches and sacrifice of some nutrient blood vessels. How much sacrifice is needed for mobilization and how much is permissible without causing additional lesions are issues that an experienced surgeon will have to decide case by case (Sunderland 1991).

7.5.1.3
Transposition

This is performed in cases where an injured nerve needs a new bed for regeneration after extensive injury to the original bed, to shorten the course of a nerve to enable joining the ends of a transected nerve or to protect a repaired nerve from undue tension. An instance of the value of this procedure for dealing with a lesion in a nerve in continuity is provided by transposition of the ulnar nerve anterior to the medial humeral epicondyle for dealing with traumatic neuritis caused by repeated tension behind

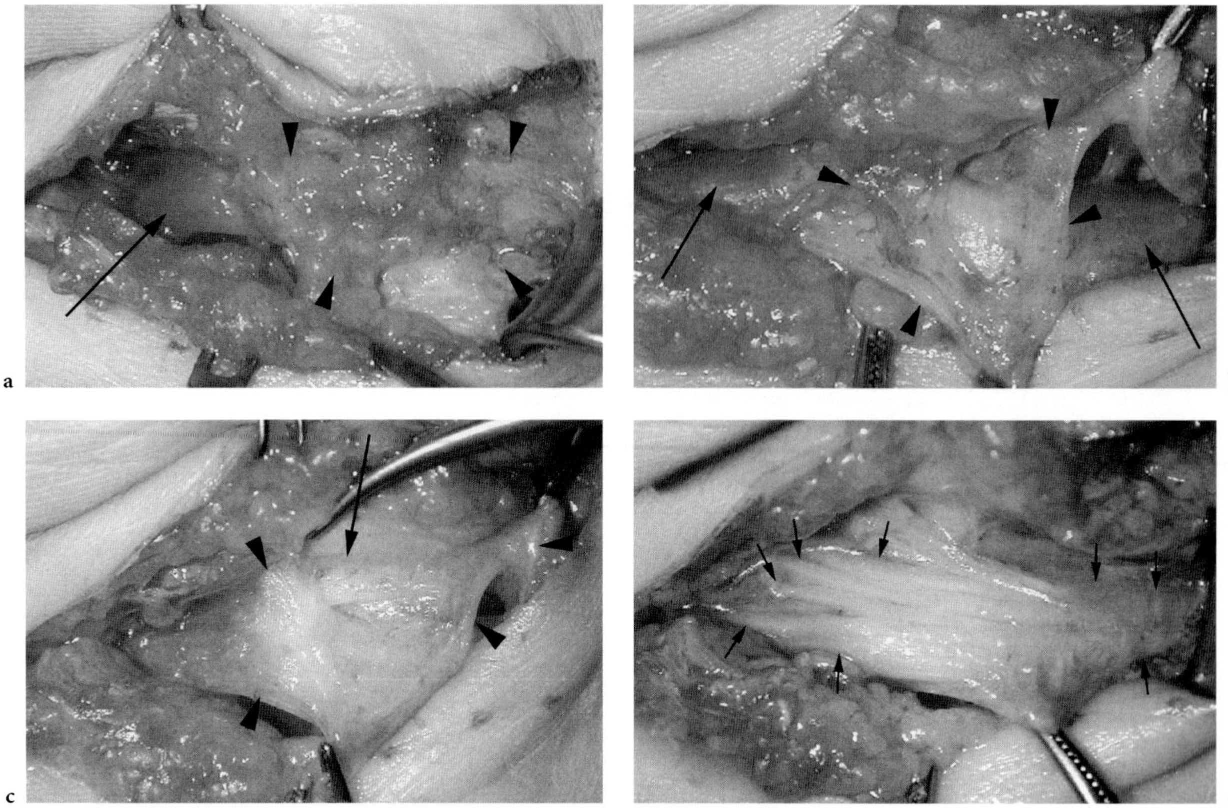

Fig. 7.2a–d. A 59-year-old female patient with worsening clinical symptoms and electrophysiological test results after surgery for carpal tunnel syndrome. **a** During surgical revision tight scar tissue encasing the median nerve was detected. **b**, **c** Gradual resection of scar tissue and internal neurolysis (**d**) was performed (*arrowheads* scar tissue, *long arrow* median nerve, **d** *short arrows* median nerve fascicles)

the epicondyle during elbow movement. In bringing together severed ends of nerves, this procedure has also been observed to be associated with improvement and recovery.

7.5.1.4 Neuromas

Painful neuromas can develop on an injured nerve in continuity, at the suture site of a repaired nerve, at the proximal end of a nerve that cannot be repaired and at the proximal end of a severed nerve in an amputated stump. If the pain cannot be handled with conservative measures such as flooding the neuroma and the surrounding tissue with a local anesthetic and there is failed recovery in the injured nerve, surgical intervention must be considered. However, timing of resection is crucial, since nerve regeneration may occur even in the presence of a neuroma if the nerve is in continuity. Premature resection might result in further suture site neuromas that may be even more troublesome than the original one. Thus, adequate time must be allowed – even as long as several months – to see if spontaneous regeneration takes place. In any case, the aim of surgery is to remove the neuroma from an area where it is subject to pressure and to free it from adhesions that worsen the condition. In severed nerves, neuromas represent a circumscribed mass of axon terminals which have no potential to reach the distal nerve end – they can be called wasted axon regeneration. One way, then, to deal with neuromas would be dysregulate or prevent such regeneration. However, all the methods currently available such as fascicle ligation (Battista et al. 1981) or cross-uniting the stumps of severed nerves in order to confine regenerating axons to the anastomotic loop (Wood and Mudge 1987), implanting the nerve end directly into a muscle after cutting it short (Sunderland 1991) are all only about 80% successful (Tupper 1986). This is because axons have an unlimited capacity to regenerate and can even force their way through dense fibrous tissue. Sealing the severed fasciculi so as to prevent axons from escaping into the surrounding connective tissue would appear to be the best method for preventing the formation of painful neuromas; an effective sealant, however, is not yet available

7.5.2 Nerve Injury with Loss of Continuity

7.5.2.1 Coaptation

Depending on the type of nerve continuity loss, different methods of repair will have to employed. If there is clean severance, and the nerve ends can be brought together without tension, primary repair with end-to-end coaptation can be performed using epineural suture. With this method, nerve trunk continuity is restored and if correct axial alignment of the nerve ends is established, fascicular continuity can be achieved.

7.5.2.2 Group Fascicular Repair

This is resorted to when it is obvious that epineural repair would result in major loss of regenerating axons at the suture line. For instance, if epineural repair will unavoidably result in opposing fascicular tissue at one end of the nerve to interfascicular tissue at the other end, there will be serious loss of regenerating axons that get lost in the interfascicular tissue. Or again, if there is great danger of mismatching of sensory and motor fibers, then group fascicular repair must be considered. Thus, the primary aim of such repair is to obtain the best possible fascicular apposition. However, it should be remembered that it is a long and complicated method and is not recommended for all occasions. This procedure calls for microsurgical skills and, as it involves preparation of the fasciculi, there is increased danger of trauma to the blood vessels and epineural tissue, with the associated dangers of scar formation.

7.5.2.3 Sutureless Repair

To obtain a tension-free suture and avoid possible reaction to suture materials, certain methods have been tried for maintaining coaptation of the nerve ends such as welding with fibrin glue, by laser, by using various adhesives such as fibrin, Micropore surgical tape or tissue adhesives, or by performing a tubular or cuff union. The last of these is intended to restrict axons from getting lost in neighboring tissue and to protect the site of repair from adhesions caused by formation of scar tissue. Biological sleeves of arteries and veins have also been investigated to achieve nerve repair without using sutures. All these methods have their advantages and disadvantages. The point to keep in mind is that union of nerve ends must be achieved as far as possible in a tension-free manner so that postoperative stretching does not result in failure of the suture line (Millesi and Meissl 1981), and the nerve tissue must be handled very delicately to avoid additional trauma.

7.5.2.4 Nerve Graft

Where no coaptation can be achieved without tension because there is a nerve defect that can only be dealt with by a bridge, nerve grafting becomes the method of choice. It is thanks to Millesi's pioneering work that the technique of nerve grafting has acquired respectability (Millesi 1986). If all methods of gaining length, such as mobilization, transposition and gentle stretching, fail in approximating the nerve ends so that an end-to-end coaptation cannot be performed without tension, then grafting is the alternative (Miyamoto and Tsuge 1981). However, nerve grafts involve sacrifice of functional nerves. A surgeon must carefully consider whether a nerve defect represents a serious handicap (for instance, loss of median nerve), or is a disability with which a patient can live, especially considering that re-educational training and reconstructive surgery can help a patient adjust to certain functional loss (e.g. irreparable radial, ulnar and lateral popliteal nerve lesions).

As Sunderland emphasizes again and again, the function of nerve repair is not just to establish nerve continuity but to restore lost functions (Sunderland 1991). If there are no reasonable prospects for achieving the latter, for example because prolonged denervation of muscles has led to their atrophy, then the surgeon has the responsibility to weigh the sacrifice of a functional nerve to be used in autograft against failure of the graft to restore function.

The nerve that is generally harvested for graft purposes is the sural nerve, its advantages being its length, its thickness that permits splitting so that double the length of the nerve is available for grafting and low donor site morbidity.

There are different kinds of nerve grafts – full thickness, cable, group fascicular and free neurovascular. Once again, depending on the site of defect, one or the other method of nerve grafting will have to employed (Fig. 7.3).

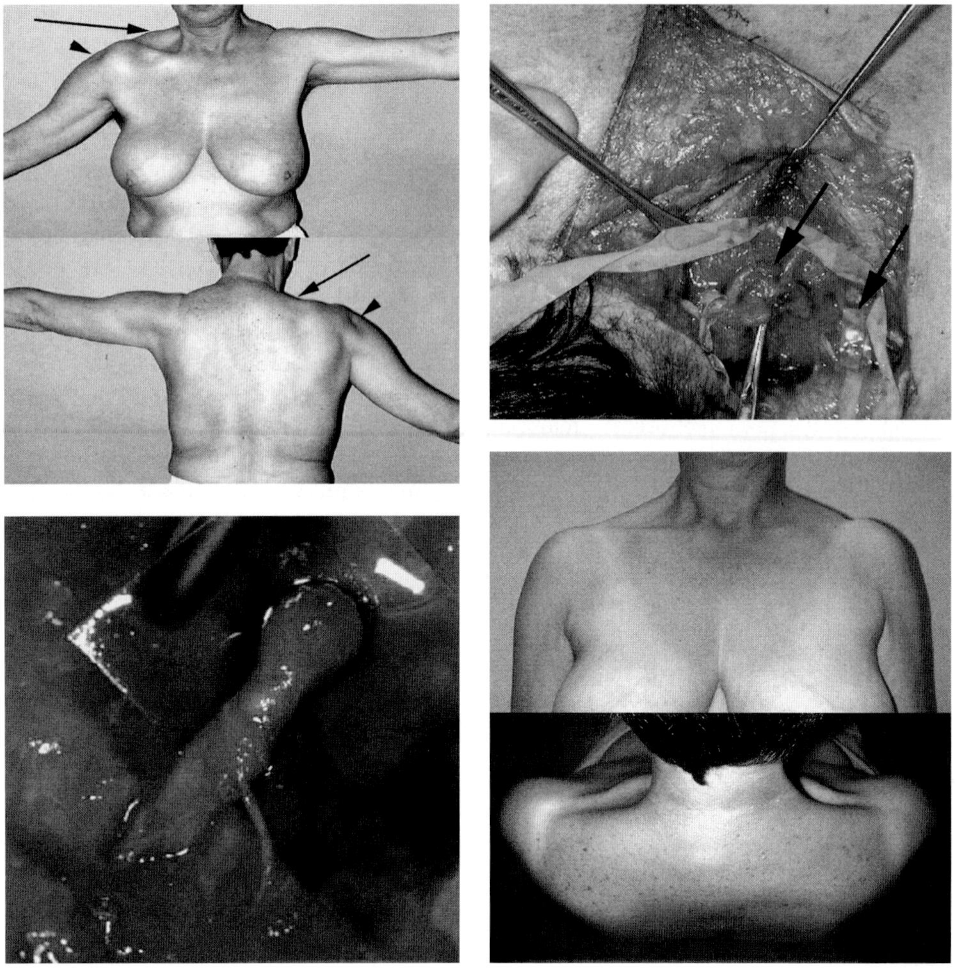

Fig. 7.3. a Condition 5 months after lymph node biopsy (neck, right) in a 48-year-old patient showing atrophy of the trapezius muscle (*arrows*) and inactivity atrophy of the deltoid muscle (*arrowheads*) with reduced ability to elevate the right arm. Sonography revealed dissection at accessory nerve. **b, c** Surgical revision with exposure of the transected accessory nerve (**b** *arrows*), complete resection of the distal and proximal neuroma (**c**), and interposition of graft 2×2.5 cm. **d** Result 2 years after reconstruction – note complete restitution in the area of the trapezius and deltoideus muscle

7.6 Timing of Nerve Repair

Restoration of function depends, among other factors, on the timing of the nerve repair. The question therefore is when are conservative methods to be employed and when is surgical intervention indicated. How long should one wait to see if spontaneous regeneration takes place and when does such waiting result in irreparable damage? When is surgical intervention to be considered as being too soon and when is it too late?

Here we must distinguish between open and closed wounds. Open wounds can be clean and simple penetrating injuries and lacerations with minimal tissue damage, or complex injuries involving extensive tissue damage, fractures and dislocations with joint involvement, and rupture of blood vessels. However, the severity of the wound is not a reliable guide to the nature of nerve injury. This is because the tensile strength and mobility of nerves may protect them from injury or, when injury is sustained, may help preserve continuity of the nerves, and spontaneous regeneration may occur. On the other hand, a small penetrating wound from a sharp object might result in nerve transection. In any case, an immediate exploration of the wound should be performed.

When a nerve has been cleanly severed, and there is loss of nerve continuity without loss of nerve tissue, and when the patient presents within a few hours of injury, immediate primary repair is advisable for reestablishing continuity. The advantages of primary repair are:

1. Only one surgical intervention is required, obviating the need for further surgery.
2. No fibrotic changes have occurred and no scar tissue has developed through which regenerating axon sprouts have to push.
3. One need only deal with the elastic retraction of the nerve stumps.
4. There is no need for preparatory trimming of the nerve ends.
5. There is no need for mobilization to achieve end-to-end coaptation.
6. Union of the nerve can be achieved without tension.
7. It is easier to align the opposing ends, since there is no disturbance of the fascicular relations.
8. The longitudinal mobility of the nerve is still intact.
9. There is clear visualization of the anatomic region since the neighboring structures are free from scar tissue.
10. Wound infection can be prevented by appropriate antibiotic therapy.

Although primary repair has the best prognosis under the wound conditions described above, it must be pointed out that unless skilled and experienced surgeons are available for performing primary repair, it is better to perform early secondary repair even when the conditions of the wound would justify primary repair. A good secondary repair is better than a primary repair inefficiently executed. An inexperienced casualty surgeon can do more harm than good in attempting primary repair of a severed nerve.

In cases of blunt injuries or those caused by high velocity missiles involving massive tissue damage, or in bleeding and contaminated wounds with danger of infection, primary nerve repair should not be attempted for the following reasons.

First, the nerve ends are ragged and contused and are sites of inflammation. It is not easy to determine the longitudinal extent and severity of the injury and to decide how far the severed ends of the nerve should be resected in order to perform coaptation. It may take 3 to 4 weeks before the extent of nerve damage can be ascertained (Zachary et al. 1987). Second, in the process of nerve end preparation for coaptation by mobilization and transposition of the nerve in order to gain sufficient length for union without excessive tension (especially when the nerve stumps have retracted and can only be found by additional resection), there is the danger of introducing infection in areas not damaged by the trauma itself. Third, the scarring associated with healing of lesions in the neighboring structures such as the nerve bed can negatively affect healing at the suture site of the coapted nerve. In addition, the patient is most likely in a state of shock and should not be subjected to long surgical interventions. Furthermore, in most trauma surgery units, often a skilled surgeon with specialist knowledge of the microsurgical techniques of nerve repair may not be available and, quite simply, the necessary operative conditions for optimal nerve surgery are often not present.

For these reasons, primary repair must be delayed. For how long will depend on the condition of the wound, but the negative consequences of this delay can probably be reduced by a so-called delayed primary repair for establishing nerve continuity (Millesi 1992). Delayed primary repair means wound closure on the day of injury and then a few days later, under optimal institutional and personnel conditions, reopening the wound which has not yet healed in order to perform nerve repair. If the wound does not permit such an early repair, then it is generally thought that the most favorable time for repair is 3–5 weeks after injury. The timing is dependent on the clinical conditions.

Closed injuries require a different timing of repair. If after a closed nerve injury, a patient demonstrates nerve function deficit, there is no occasion to perform primary surgery. The patient is monitored over a period of 3 months. If at the end of this period, there are some clinical signs of recovery or some electrical evidence of regeneration, then it would be worth waiting for complete recovery to take place, monitoring the patient carefully. Of course, it will have to be kept in mind that, depending on the level of injury, complete return of function may take several months. If, however, after a 3-month waiting period, no signs of recovery are present, the nerve needs to be surgically explored, and depending on the results of intraoperative evaluation, different methods of nerve repair such as neurolysis or nerve graft will have to employed.

The maximum tolerated interval between injury and recovery of function depends on whether the loss involved is motor or sensory. It has been suggested that the maximum time interval that can be tolerated between the time of injury and the reestablishment of neuromuscular connection is between 1 year and 18 months. This can vary depending on the muscles involved. The smaller intrinsic muscles in the hand must be innervated even sooner than that in order to reinstate motor function. In any case, the time interval between injury and repair should not exceed 4–5 months. The time limits for return of sensory function are different from those for return of motor function; sensation can return many years after repair of injury to the nerve (Mackinnon and Dellon 1998). Thus, in treating closed nerve injuries, the principle is fundamentally conservative, with the expectation of return of function, and the patient is frequently followed-up with clinical examination and electrodiagnostic tests.

The situation is different when the closed nerve injury is in an area which has a known predilection for compression of nerves. In such cases, it is recommended that surgery be performed immediately in order to decompress the nerve. Unless this done, recovery of the injured nerve will be delayed because of the added insult of compression effects. For example, in a patient presenting with traumatic injury to the hand or forearm associated with deficits in sensory and motor functions, one should suspect an acute carpal tunnel syndrome and immediate decompression of the nerve involved should be performed. Similarly, a patient who demonstrates signs of complete peroneal nerve paralysis after undergoing a crush injury to the leg should also be considered as a candidate for decompression surgery. The pathological conditions involved and the anatomic sites of injury in these two cases are very similar and consequently should be treated in similar ways. The nerve involved should be decompressed at the site of compression.

7.7 Prognosis

The success of nerve repair depends on a large number of factors that have to do with the kind of nerve injured (monofascicular, polyfascicular), the level of injury, the kind and severity of injury, factors operating at and below the site of repair (e.g. how easily regenerating axons can pass through the site of repair to the distal end), the time between injury and repair, the skill of the surgeon carrying out the microsurgical procedures and the techniques employed, to name just a few. One extremely critical factor is that of timing. Here the motto is, the sooner the repair is carried out, the sooner the endoneurial tubes are reoccupied by regenerating axons, and the better is the chance that functional deficits will be overcome. The longer a nerve injury is left untreated, the greater are the chances of endoneurial tube atrophy, fascicular shrinkage and intrafascicular fibrosis, and end-organ atrophy because of denervation, and consequently the poorer the chance of recovery of function.

Generally, the more proximal the lesion, the poorer is the prognosis. Pure nerves have a better chance of recovery than mixed motor and sensory nerves. End-to-end repairs are better than nerve grafts and shorter grafts do better than long grafts. Age is also a relevant factor. Better recovery can be achieved in younger than in older patients, and the very young have a decided advantage.

Postoperative procedures also contribute significantly to recovery. Training and practice do contribute to improvement of motor performance and the sharpening of sensory perceptions. Even if nerve repair is followed by residual sensory and motor deficits because of incomplete or defective axonal regeneration, it should be kept in mind that with training (for example, with sensory reeducation consisting of desensitization, early phase discrimination and localization and late phase discrimination and tactile gnosis), a patient can be helped to learn to deal with new and altered patterns of innervation. The role of cortical plasticity in regaining function after nerve injury should not be underestimated.

Furthermore, the condition of the patient is important. Factors such as whether the patient is a smoker, an alcoholic, or has underlying systemic diseases will affect the final results of nerve repair.

7.8 Future Directions in Peripheral Nerve Surgery

Problems preventing successful nerve repair associated with difficulties in proper axial alignment and fascicular approximation need to be resolved. "The most important single technical factor in peripheral nerve repair is the coaptation of fascicular tissue" (Millesi 1985). This is as true today as when these words were written in 1985. Problems at the suture line are also caused by scar tissue, but no effective methods to reduce fibroblast activity are yet available. Atraumatic surgical techniques currently offer the only method to keep scarring to a minimum. Several in vitro experiments have shown that survival of nerve cells and axon growth depend on certain biomolecules such as nerve growth factor, fibroblast growth factor (Morrison et al. 1986) and somatomedin C, which are produced by peripheral target cells and transmitted via retrograde axonal transport along the axon to the nerve cell body and exert a trophic influence on them (Hansson et al. 1986). This function of the target cells is disrupted after nerve transection that separates end-organs from the nerve cell, and is taken over by the non-neuronal cells in the distal and proximal stumps.

Promotion and acceleration of nerve regeneration and selective reinnervation after injury might be achieved by altering the microenvironment with the help of various neurotrophic factors administered in the region between the nerve stumps. This is one exciting avenue that might lead to advances in clinical nerve regeneration. Nerve grafts involve sacrifice of functional nerves to achieve repair. Investigations into alternatives to conventional grafts, therefore, are highly interesting. One such method that is being studied is that of nerve guides seeded with adult Schwann cells that provide the necessary and continuing trophic factors for regeneration (Ansselin et al. 1997). Gene therapy holds out the promise of delivering a gene together with its necessary regulatory elements (the gene construct) to the cell surface, using a vector to mediate the transfer across the cell membrane and in some cases into the nuclei. This might prove to be useful in stimulating the growth of adult nerve cells, a process that might be important in situations where nerve cell destruction has occurred following axonal injury. Thus, despite the remarkable advances in peripheral nerve repair made in the past five decades, there are still several problems that need to be addressed. The future of nerve repair is challenging, adventurous and also promising.

7.9 Summary and Conclusion

Decision making in the clinical management of nerve injury and repair is a complex and difficult task. A patient presenting with nerve injury must be carefully investigated with appropriate methods in order to determine the exact site, accompanying tissue involvement, the nerve affected, cause (compression, traction, ischaemia or a combination of causes), severity (five grades), time elapsed since injury, prior interventions, underlying systemic diseases if any, and consequences in terms of functional disturbance (sensory, motor, pain) of the injury. All these factors will play a role in recovery of function and will determine the surgeon's approach to the case. When and how a transected nerve should be repaired, whether coaptation will do the job adequately or whether nerve grafts must be used are decisions a surgeon has to make based on the particular case at hand.

Where pain is a major symptom, the cause must be looked for and eliminated. Factors at the site of a nerve lesion that cause pain and threaten injury to nerve fibers, such as compression because of inflamed tissue, hematoma or tumor, traction because of adhesion or ischaemia because of compression, will have to be dealt with in an appropriate way. A compartment entrapment syndrome will have to be dealt with by decompression of the nerve by surgically releasing the compartment it is trapped in, and adhesions and fibrosis should be dealt with by the appropriate form of neurolysis.

Complex nerve lesions where different fascicles have suffered injuries of different grades of severity present a great challenge to even the most experienced and skilled surgeon. If clinical and electrodiagnostic methods of investigation of the nature and severity of a nerve injury suggest the possibility of spontaneous regeneration of the nerve and recovery of motor and sensory functions (more distal than proximal, first to third degree of severity, less than 3 months after injury), the reasonable approach will be one of expectation and conservative management, accompanied by careful and frequent monitoring. Where there is no evidence of recovery after a period of 3 months following injury, the need for surgical intervention must be considered. What form this should take will depend on the causes that are arresting or preventing recovery and regeneration. Since every such intervention represents additional trauma and causes scar tissue, surgery should be an option only when no spontaneous regeneration can be expected. On the other hand, if recovery and regeneration are being interfered with because of the presence of scar tissue that hinders axons from reaching their distal end-organs or receptors, appropriate surgical measures must be instituted in order to resect this tissue. Furthermore, the longer the period of denervation of end organs and distal receptors, the less complete will be the recovery, and in some cases, all chances of recovery may be lost.

The surgeon has the responsibility to make careful investigation, interpret the results, decide if surgical management is necessary and if so, the most appropriate timing for it, and meticulously carry out nerve repair using the most suitable method under optimal institutional and personnel conditions. Finally, surgical nerve repair is an extremely demanding and skilful task – it should be undertaken only by a surgeon with a deep knowledge of the complex and often variable anatomy of the peripheral nervous system, special training in microsurgical techniques and extensive experience.

References

Ansselin AD, Fink T, Davey DF (1997) Peripheral nerve regeneration through nerve guides seeded with adult Schwann cells. Neuropathol Appl Neurobiol 23:387–398

Brock AJ (1929) Greek medicine. Dent, New York

Battista AF, Cravioto HM, Budzilovich GN (1981) Painful neuroma: changes produced in peripheral nerve after fascicle ligation. Neurosurgery 9:589

Frykman GK, Adams J, Bowen WW (1981) Neurolysis. Orthop Clin North Am 12:325

Gelbermann RH (1991) Operative nerve repair and reconstruction, vol 1. Lippincott, Philadelphia

Hansson HA, Dahlin LB, Danielsen N, et al (1986) Evidence indicating trophic importance of IGF-1 in regenerating peripheral nerves. Acta Physiol Scand 126:609–614

Kristensson K (1981) Retrograde signalling of nerve cell body response to trauma. In: Gorio A, Millesi H, Mingrino S (eds) Posttraumatic peripheral nerve regeneration. Raven, New York, pp 27–34

Lundborg G (1988) Nerve injury and repair. Churchill Livingstone, Edinburgh, p 105

Mackinnon SE, Dellon AL (1988) Surgery of the peripheral nerve. Thieme Medical, New York

Millesi H (1981) Reappraisal of nerve repair. Surg Clin North Am 61:321

Millesi H (1985) Peripheral nerve repair: terminology, questions and facts. J Reconstr Microsurg 2:21–31

Millesi H (1986) The nerve gap. Hand Clin 2:651–663

Millesi H (1992) Chirurgie der peripheren Nerven. Urban and Schwarzenberg, Munich

Millesi H, Meissl G (1981) Consequences of tension at the suture line. In: Gorio A, Millesi H, Mingrino S (eds) Posttraumatic peripheral nerve regeneration. Raven, New York, p 277

Miyamoto Y, Tsuge K (1981) Grafting vs end-to-end coaptation of nerves. In: Gorio A, Millesi H, Mingrino S (eds) Posttraumatic peripheral nerve regeneration. Raven, New York, p 351

Morrison RS, Sharma A, de Vellis J, et al (1986) Basic fibroblast growth factor supports the survival of cerebral cortical neurons in primary culture. Proc Natl Acad Sci U S A 83: 7537–7541

Mumenthaler M, Schliack H, Stöhr M (1998) Läsionen peripherer Nerven und radikuläre Syndrome. Thieme, Stuttgart

Piza-Katzer H, Herczeg E, Balogh B, et al (1994) Intra- und postoperative Nervenläsionen und ihre Behandlung. Nervenarzt 65:375–380

Piza-Katzer H, Balogh B, Herczeg E, et al (1995) Iatrogene Nervenläsionen und ihre mikrochirurgische Behandlung. Chirurg 66:1146–1153

Rydevik B, Lundborg G, Nordborg C (1976) Intraneural tissue reactions induced by internal neurolysis. An experimental study on the blood nerve barrier, connective tissues and nerve fibres of rabbit tibial nerve. Scand J Plast Reconstr Surg 10:3

Seddon HJ (1943) Three types of nerve injury. Brain 66:237

Sunderland S (1951) A classification of peripheral nerve injuries producing loss of function. Brain 74:491

Sunderland S (1991) Nerve injuries and their repair: a critical appraisal. Churchill Livingstone, New York

Tupper JW (1986) Discussion of paper by Dellon AL and Mackinnon SE 1986. J Plast Reconstr Surg 77:437

Varon S, Adler R (1989) Nerve growth factors and control of nerve growth. Curr Top Dev Biol 16:207–252

Waller AV (1850) Experiments on the glossopharyngeal and hypoglossal nerves of the frog and observations produced thereby in the structure of their primitive fibres. Philos Trans R Soc Lond 140:423

Wood VE, Mudge MK (1987) Treatment of neuromas about a major amputation stump. J Hand Surg [Am] 12:302

Zachary LS, Dellon AL, Seiler WA (1987) Relationship of intraneural damage in the rat sciatic nerve to the method of injury. Microsurgery 8:182–185

8 An Introduction to Electrodiagnostic Testing

S. Kiechl

CONTENTS

8.1 Basic Principles *121*
8.1.1 Nerve Conduction Studies *121*
8.1.2 Late Responses – the F-wave *124*
8.1.3 Needle Electromyography *125*
8.2 Significance of Electrodiagnostic Testing in the Management of Peripheral Nerve Lesions *127*
8.2.1 Diagnosis of Peripheral Nerve Lesions *128*
8.2.2 Severity of Peripheral Nerve Lesions *128*
8.2.3 Localization of Peripheral Nerve Lesions *130*
8.2.4 Etiology of Peripheral Nerve Lesions *131*
8.2.5 Detection of Innervation Anomalies *131*
8.2.6 Follow-up of Peripheral Nerve Lesions *132*
8.2.7 Diagnostic Work-up in Patients with Peripheral Nerve Lesions *133*
References 134

8.1 Basic Principles

Standard electrodiagnostic (EDX) examination consists of nerve conduction studies, recording of late responses and needle electromyography (EMG) (Guidelines in Electrodiagnostic Medicine 1999). On performing EDX testing a few contraindications have to be considered (Table 8.1).

8.1.1 Nerve Conduction Studies

The study of nerve conduction entails depolarizing the nerve fibers with an electric stimulus and subsequent recording the evoked motor or sensory responses by means of various types of surface electrodes (Fig. 8.1). Exceptionally, if responses are very small and the initial deflection cannot be reliably assessed, recording with needle electrodes from atrophic muscles or sensory nerves may be more appropriate. The stimulus is applied percutaneously with the cathode held distally and the ground is best placed between the stimulation and recording site.

Table 8.1. Contraindications to EDX testing

Electromyography

- Any kind of coagulation disorder rendering patients at risk of muscle hemorrhage such as hemophilia, oral anticoagulation (INR >1.7) or dose-adjusted intravenous heparin therapy.
- Wounds or infected skin covering the muscles of interest

Nerve conduction studies

- Pacemakers: proximal stimulation at Erb's point (brachial plexus) or axilla ipsilateral to a pacemaker may cause dysfunction of the technical device

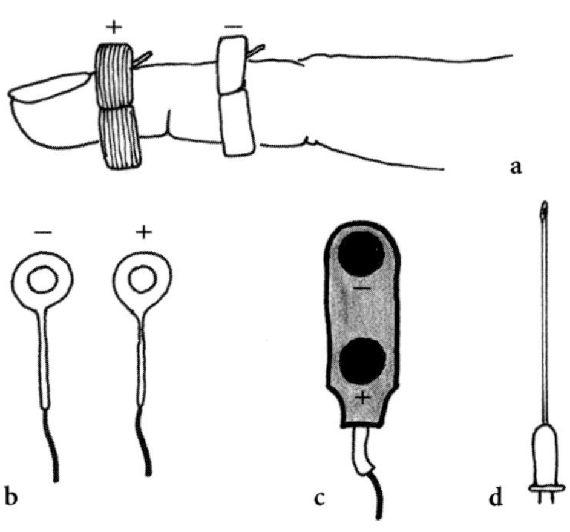

Fig. 8.1. a Ring electrodes for antidromic sensory nerve conduction studies. **b** Disk electrodes for motor and orthodromic sensory nerve conduction studies and F-wave recording. **c** Stimulator and (**d**) concentric needle electrode for standard EMG

S. Kiechl, MD
Professor, Department of Neurology, Section for Electrodiagnosis (EMG/NLG), University Hospital Innsbruck, Anichstrasse 35, 6020 Innsbruck, Austria

8.1.1.1 Motor Nerve Conduction Studies

According to the tendon montage the active recording electrode is fixed on the center of the muscle belly usually resembling the end-plate region and the reference electrode is placed over the insertion of the tendon (Fig. 8.2).

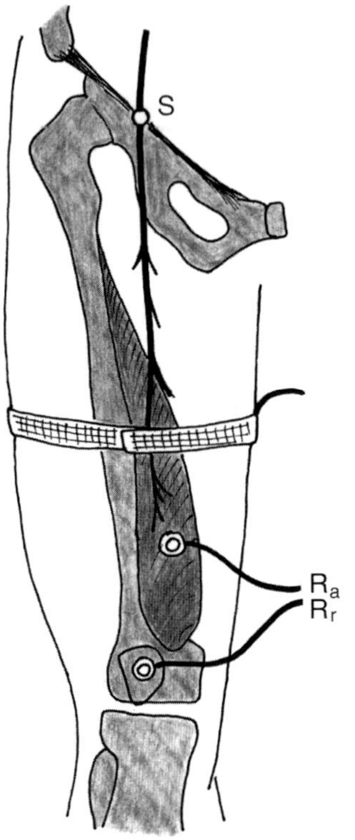

Fig. 8.2. Belly-tendon method of electrode placing in femoral nerve studies. The active recording electrode (R_a) is fixed on the center of the muscle belly resembling the end-plate region and the reference electrode (R_r) is placed over the insertion of the tendon

If properly performed, this technique produces a biphasic motor potential with an initial negativity and steep upward deflection from baseline. The M-response results from summation of the muscle fiber action potentials and is termed *compound muscle action potential* (CMAP) if virtually all nerve and muscle fibers depolarize (Fig. 8.3a). To ensure sufficient stimulation of the nerve, the current applied is slowly increased until the generated motor response no longer increases, and a final recording is performed with an electric stimulus 20% above this level (i.e. *supramaximal stimulation*). Standard machine settings are a gain of 5 mV per division (*y*-axis of the screen – amplitude), sweep duration of 2–5 ms per division (*x*-axis of the screen) and a duration of the electrical impulse of 200 ms. Routinely, the following parameters of the M-response are assessed.

Latency. The latency is the time elapsing between onset of the stimulus and the initial negative deflection from baseline (in milliseconds, this is the onset latency; Fig. 8.3a). It includes the time required for initiation of the action potential (about 0.1 ms), the orthodromic propagation of the action potential to the motor end plate, the time delay across the neuromuscular junction and the slow depolarization of given muscle fibers (3–5 m/s). Reporting of the distal motor latency is very convenient, whereas latencies from proximal stimulation are incorporated in the calculation of conduction velocities (CVs).

Conduction Velocities. Motor CVs (in meters per second) are simply computed by dividing the distance between two stimulation points (tape measurement of surface distance in a standardized limb position, in millimeters) by the nerve conduction time (proximal minus distal motor latency, in millisecond). CVs assessed in this way reflect the fast-

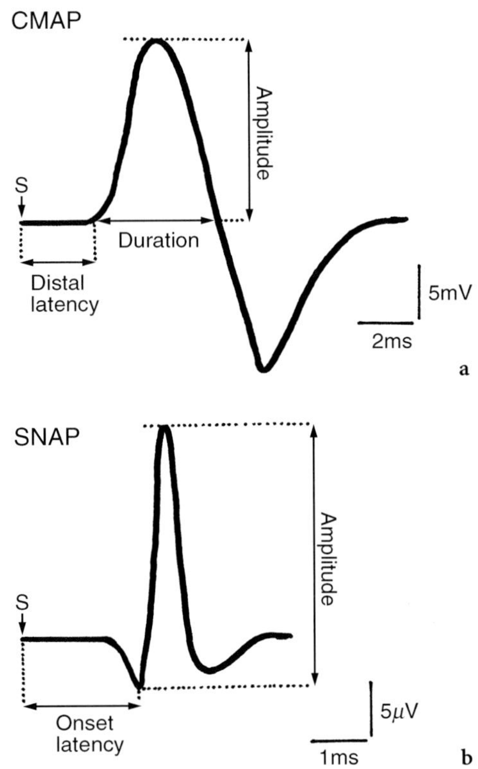

Fig. 8.3. a Compound muscle action potential (*CMAP*). CMAP represents the summation of all the underlying muscle fiber action potentials and is biphasic with an initial negative deflection. The latency, amplitude and potential duration are routinely assessed. **b** Sensory nerve action potential (SNAP). SNAP represents the summation of all the underlying sensory fiber action potentials and is bi- or triphasic. The onset latency and amplitude are routinely assessed

est conducting axons, which determine the initial deflection of the CMAPs. Focal slowing of CVs commonly occurs in entrapment syndromes, whereas diffuse slowing is typical of generalized disorders of the peripheral nervous system. Accordingly, nerve conduction studies find application for pinpointing focal (compressive) nerve lesions and for classifying polyneuropathies as primarily axonal or demyelinating. It has to be considered that mild slowing is not specific for demyelination but may also arise from selective loss of large, fast conducting fibers prone to pressure damage.

Amplitude. CMAP amplitudes are measured as base-to-peak amplitudes (initial negative component of the potential; Fig. 8.3a) or, less commonly, as peak-to-peak amplitudes. Amplitudes mirror the number and synchrony of depolarizing muscle fibers. Low CMAP amplitudes upon distal stimulation are either a consequence of motor axon loss or distally located conduction blocks.

Duration. CMAP duration is measured from the initial deflection from baseline to the first baseline crossing and serves as a measure of synchrony (Fig. 8.3a).

8.1.1.2 Sensory Nerve Conduction Studies

Sensory nerve conduction studies are technically more demanding because sensory nerve action potentials (SNAPs) are small, being in the range of 1 to 50 μV (Fig. 8.3b). The SNAP is a compound potential representing the summation of the individual nerve action potentials of all sensory axons. It is recorded directly from the nerve with two ring or disk electrodes placed in a line over the nerve (interelectrode distance 3–4 cm) and the gain set to 5 to 20 μV per division. Signal averaging is often necessary to suppress background noise and other artifacts. Other technical requirements resemble those described for motor nerve conduction studies except for a usually much lower stimulation threshold.

SNAPs are bi- or triphasic and are characterized by the following parameters.

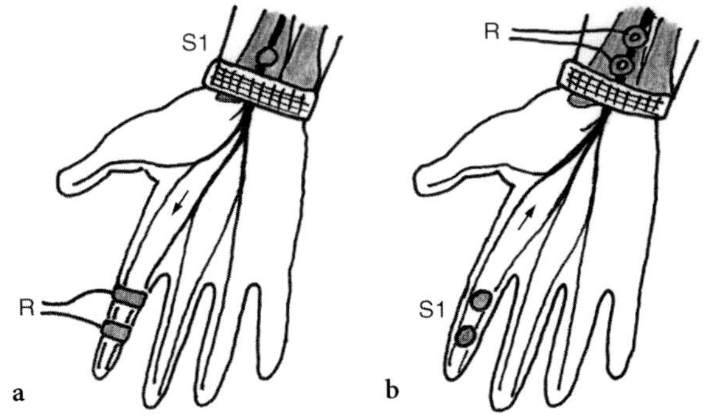

Fig. 8.4. **a** Antidromic (stimulation towards the sensory receptors) and (**b**) orthodromic (stimulation away from the sensory receptors) sensory studies. The amplitudes of the SNAPs are generally higher in the antidromic potentials (*S1* site of stimulation, *R* site of potential recording)

SNAP Amplitude. In most laboratories peak-to-peak amplitudes (Fig. 8.3b) are assessed. Low SNAP amplitudes may result from technical factors (edema, incorrect placement, etc), axon loss or asynchrony of conduction velocities in demyelinating disorders. Due to the phenomena of temporal dispersion and phase cancellation, SNAPs elicited by proximal stimulation are much lower in amplitude while the duration of the potential (distance between onset and first baseline crossing) is increased.

SNAP Latency. So called *onset latencies* are routinely used and represent the time interval from stimulus to the initial negative deflection of biphasic potentials or the initial positive peak of triphasic potentials (Fig. 8.3b). Unlike motor conduction studies, distal conduction velocities can be calculated with only one stimulation by dividing the distance between the active recording electrode and stimulation point by the onset latency. Assessment of proximal conduction velocities matches the procedure described for motor nerves. As a rule, sensory nerve conduction studies are more sensitive than motor studies in detecting focal and generalized neuropathies.

Stimulation and Recording Procedures. Both antidromic (stimulation towards the sensory receptors) and orthodromic (stimulation away from the sensory receptors) sensory studies are available (Fig. 8.4). Whereas conduction velocities are the same with either method, amplitudes are generally higher in the antidromic potentials because recording electrodes are closer to the nerve. Because of this advantage and the ease of application, preference is usually given to the antidromic technique unless SNAPs are superimposed by a volume-conducted motor potential and the onset of the potential cannot be identified.

8.1.1.3
Reliability and External Influences

Fast saltatory conduction of peripheral nerves depends on a mature nerve architecture. Accordingly, motor and sensory conduction velocities markedly increase in the first years of life parallel to advancing myelination, and decrease after age 60 years due to slow axon and myelin degeneration at higher ages. Apart from age, nerve conduction is influenced by the skin temperature (0.7–2.4 m/s change for each degree centigrade) (Liveson and Ma 1992). In many laboratories temperature is measured and corrected for by heating or computational adjustment. Reproducibility studies have yielded measurement errors ranging from some 5% (about 3 m/s) (intraobserver reliability) up to 10% (about 6 m/s) if weeks elapse between examinations and the examiner changes (long-term interobserver reliability) (Gassel 1964; Honet et al. 1968). This inaccuracy is inherently related to the complex methodological requirements of EDX studies and should be born in mind when interpreting alterations in nerve conduction over time.

8.1.2
Late Responses – the F-wave

Nerve conduction studies are appropriate for assessing peripheral nerves up to Erb's point (upper extremities) and the gluteal fold/inguinal ligament (lower extremities) but are not applicable to the very proximal nerve segments (plexus) and nerve roots. Recording of late responses, especially the F-wave, permits this gap to be closed (Eisen et al. 1977). After routine (supramaximal) motor nerve stimulation the action potential conducts distally to the neuromuscular junction eliciting the CMAP or M-response and proximally towards anterior horn cells (via the motor nerve roots) where it triggers a backfiring of a small and variable subpopulation of these cells (Fig. 8.5). This action potential again spreads distally and causes a second low-amplitude response (1–5% of the CMAP). Strictly speaking, the F-wave is not a reflex since both the efferent and afferent loops are purely motor without an intervening synapse (Fig. 8.5).

The technical equipment and recording set-up is the same as in standard motor nerve conduction studies except for an increase in gain (100 to 200 μV) and sweep speed (5 to 10 ms). In clinical routine 10 to 20 responses are recorded, which typically vary in latency and amplitude owing to the continuously changing population of anterior horn cells involved in the generation of this potential (Fig. 8.6). The minimal F-wave latency reflecting conduction of the fastest motor fibers (normative values depend on body height) and the F-wave persistence (normal, 80–100%) are the best standardized and most reliable measures obtainable from F-wave studies (Fig. 8.6).

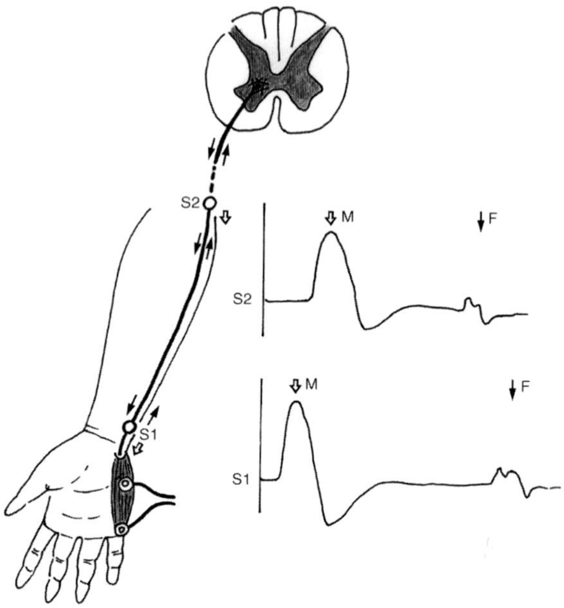

Fig. 8.5. F-response circuitry. The direct muscle response (*M*) occurs from orthodromic travel. The F-wave (*F*) is derived by antidromic travel to the anterior horn cells, back firing of some anterior horn cells, and orthodromic travel down to the muscle. With proximal stimulation (*S2*) the latency of the M-response increases but the F-wave latency decreases

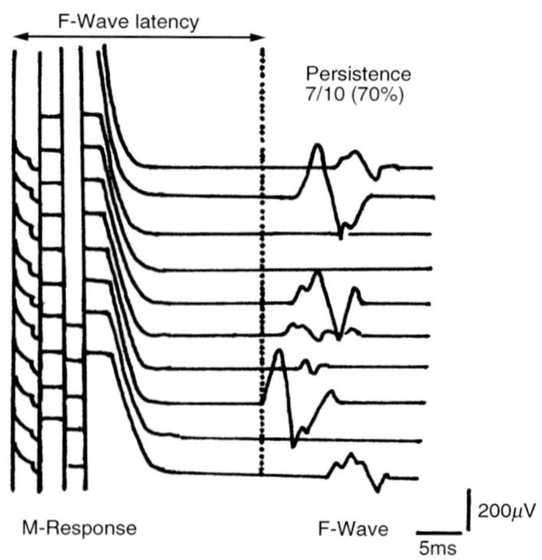

Fig. 8.6. F-wave measurements. The minimal F-wave *latency* is the shortest of the ten responses, representing the largest and fastest conducting fibers. The F-wave *persistence* is the number of responses obtained per number of stimulations (70% in this case)

If nerve conduction velocities are unremarkable, a prolonged F-wave latency and/or inconsistent response are strongly suggestive of a proximal nerve lesion, e.g. plexus palsy. Otherwise, F-waves can be adjusted for distal conduction abnormalities by calculation of corrected F-waves. On interpreting F-wave parameters several limitations have to be considered. F-wave responses are often unrecordable from nerves with severe axonal damage and difficult to obtain from muscles supplied by the nerve roots L2 to L4 and C5 to C7. In addition, the sensitivity of the test for assessing abnormalities confined to a single nerve root is low.

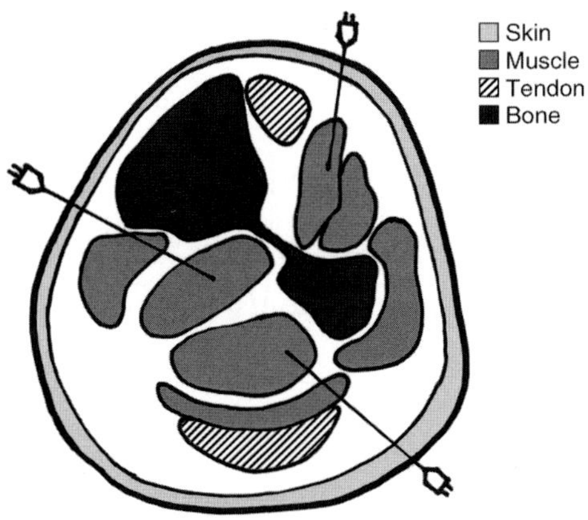

Fig. 8.7. Needle EMG. Correct placement of the needle is mandatory for a reliable examination as exemplified for the lower calf

8.1.3 Needle Electromyography

As with nerve conduction studies, needle EMG has to be individualized for each patient based on the clinical problem and results of the ongoing evaluation. The conduct of EMG especially the correct placing of the needle and sampling of muscles (Fig. 8.7), and interpretation of the recordings obtained, are a challenging part of the EDX examination.

Usually, concentric bipolar needle electrodes are used containing both the active (wire in the center of the needle) and reference electrode (shaft) (Fig. 8.1). The ground electrode is placed on the limb being investigated to suppress background noise. Insertion of the needle into the muscle may produce some discomfort. If performed skillfully, however, the examination is usually well tolerated even when numerous muscles are sampled.

The EMG examination is routinely composed of three stages – recording of rest activity, analysis of voluntary motor unit action potentials (MUAPs) and registration of the interference pattern during maximal muscle contraction. Electrical signals from the muscle are displayed on the screen and simultaneously presented acoustically over a loudspeaker.

8.1.3.1 Rest Activity

Normal muscle does not show any activity at rest (i.e. *spontaneous activity*) except for the end-plate region where end-plate noise (irregular monophasic negative potentials) and end-plate spikes (irregular biphasic potentials with an initial negative deflection) occur (Fig. 8.8a). Pathological spontaneous activity in terms of fibrillation potentials and positive waves manifests in denervated muscle during the 2nd to 3rd week. Both signals have the same significance but differ in configuration. Fibrillations (fib.) are brief triphasic spikes with an initial positive deflection (duration 1–5 ms, amplitude 10–20 μV) and a regular firing pattern, whereas positive waves (pw.) have a brief initial positive signal followed by a long negative phase (Fig. 8.8a). There are two common ways of quantifying the density of pathological spontaneous activity also referred to as *denervation activity*. Either it is graded on a scale ranging from 0 to 3 (0 no fib./pw., + persistent single fib./pw., ++ moderate numbers of fib./pw. in two or more areas, +++ many fib./pw. in all areas tested) or depicted as the number of recording sites in a muscle where fib./pw. emerge relative to the number of areas examined (e.g. seven of ten or "7/10").

8.1.3.2 Analysis of Voluntary MUAPs

A motor unit consists of all muscle fibers (usually five to several hundreds) supplied by a single motor neuron. Physiologically, the territories of motor units show a broad overlap and cover an area of 5–10 mm (Fig. 8.9a).

MUAPs recorded during needle EMG represent the compound action potential of all muscle fibers of a single motor unit, weighted towards the fibers nearest to the needle (Fig. 8.10). The morphology of MUAPs (duration, amplitude and phases) reflects the architecture of given motor units and thus permits a reliable differentiation of myopathic and neuropathic processes (Figs. 8.8b, 8.9d, e). By definition, the *MUAP duration* is measured from the initial deflection of the potential towards the final return to baseline (in mil-

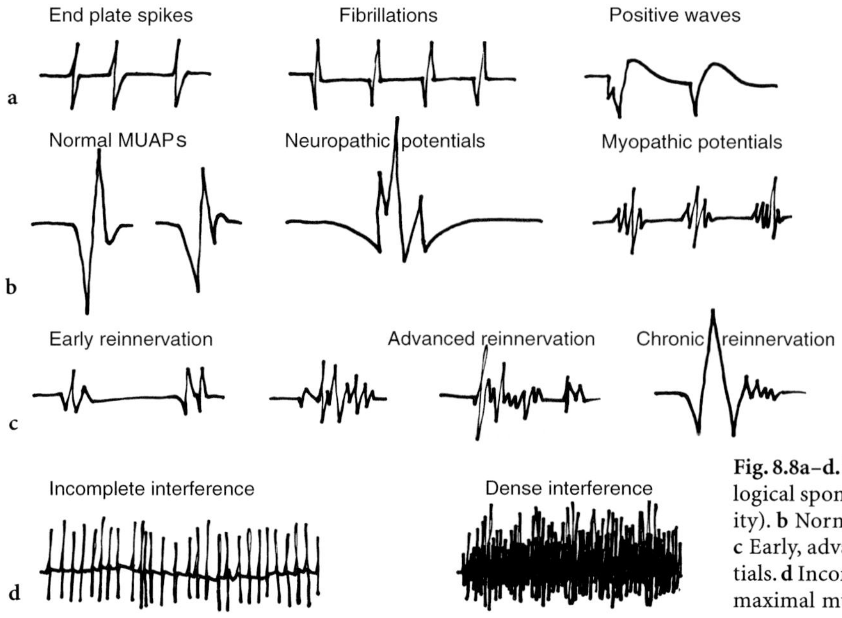

Fig. 8.8a–d. Needle EMG. **a** Physiological and pathological spontaneous activity (recording of rest activity). **b** Normal, neuropathic and myopathic MUAPs. **c** Early, advanced and chronic reinnervation potentials. **d** Incomplete and complete interference during maximal muscle contraction

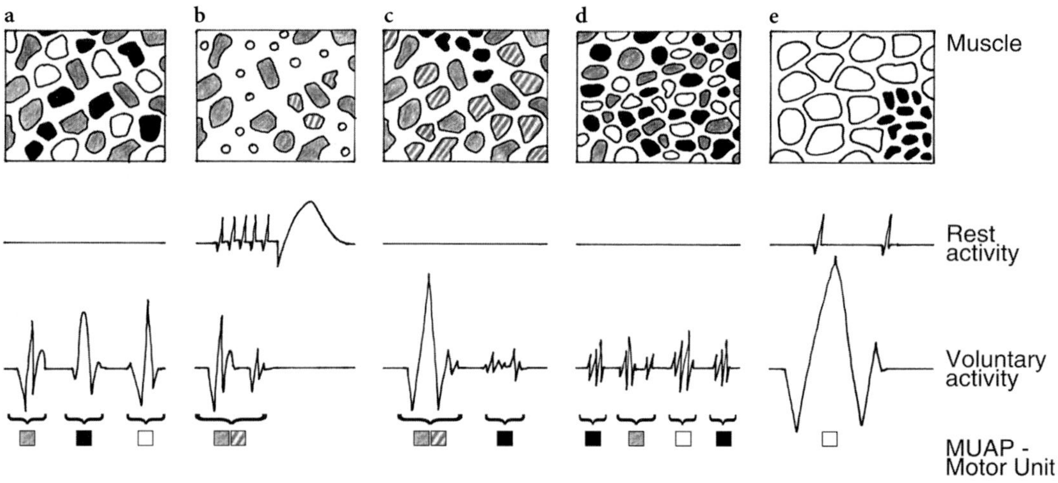

Fig. 8.9a–e. Architecture of motor units and corresponding EMG findings. **a** Normal muscle. The territories of three motor units (*black*, *gray* and *white*) show a broad overlap. The morphology of the corresponding three MUAPs is unremarkable. **b** Axonotmesis of two of the three motor axons. Muscle fibers supplied by these axons are denervated (spontaneous activity). The intact third (*gray*) axon shows collateral sprouting – one of two main mechanisms of regeneration – and has formed new end plates to three additional muscle fibers (*gray*, *white*). Accordingly the MUAP shows a late component. **c** Advanced stage of reinnervation. Meanwhile the gray motor axon has formed end plates to most denervated muscle fibers (*gray*, *white*). As a consequence, the size of the motor unit has substantially increased and a typical long-duration high-amplitude MUAP is recordable on EMG (neuropathic potential). In addition the black motor axon has again reached the muscle by true axonal sprouting from the lesion site, and formed the first end plates to a few muscle fibers (early reinnervation potential). **d** Myopathy. Short-duration low-amplitude MUAPs are the typical EMG finding and originate from a loss or atrophy of muscle fibers. **e** Severe chronic neurogenic damage with a grouped atrophy of muscle fibers and giant potentials on EMG. Such findings are typical of motor neuron diseases and chronic reinnervation processes

liseconds), the *MUAP amplitude* denotes the distance between the maximum positive and negative peaks (in millivolts) and *MUAP phases* are calculated by counting the number of baseline crossings (Fig. 8.10). As a standard, 10 to 20 distinct MUAPs are recorded from each muscle with the needle placed within or close to the motor unit (rise time <0.5 ms), and analyzed on a quantitative or qualitative basis. Because MUAP configuration varies substantially in various muscles and changes with advancing age, examinations will yield valid interpretations only if in the hands of an experienced electromyographer.

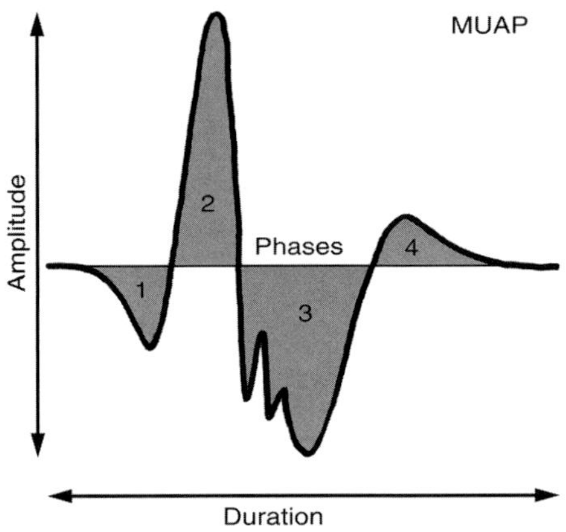

Fig. 8.10. Motor unit action potential (MUAP) measurements – *amplitude*, *duration* and *phases*

Long-duration high-amplitude MUAPs result from prominent enlargement of motor units, which is usually the consequence of axon loss and collateral sprouting of the remaining intact nerve fibers, and therefore characteristic of chronic neuropathic disorders (Figs. 8.8b, 8.9e). Short-duration low-amplitude MUAPs are the hallmark of myopathic disorders and originate from a loss or atrophy of muscle fibers and/or blockage of end plates (Figs. 8.8b, 8.9d). Polyphasia in turn (five or more baseline crossings of a MUAP) is a nonspecific abnormality occurring both in neurogenic diseases and myopathies (Fig. 8.10). It depends primarily on the synchrony of muscle fiber firing and secondarily on the architecture of the motor unit.

In early reinnervation processes thinly myelinated axonal sprouts form new neuromuscular junctions to denervated muscle fibers, which corresponds with the emergence of low-amplitude desynchronized MUAPs on EMG ("early reinnervation potentials") (Figs. 8.8c, 8.9b). Over time, MUAPs continuously grow in size, number of phases and duration ("advanced reinnervation potentials"), the myelin of sprouts matures and depolarization of muscle fibers synchronizes, thereby producing an increase in the amplitude along with a decrease in the number of phases and potential duration ("chronic reinnervation potential") (Figs. 8.8c, 8.9c, e).

8.1.3.3 Interference Pattern

During maximal contraction MUAPs normally overlap creating a "dense" or "complete" interference pattern with no single MUAPs being distinguishable given an appropriate sweep speed of 50–100 ms (Fig. 8.8d). An incomplete interference pattern is either due to poor central motor activation (central nervous system disorders) or, more frequently, due to reduced recruitment of MUAPs in the case of severe axon loss (neurogenic disorder) or manifestation of conduction blocks (Fig. 8.8d). A mild loss in the number of elicitable motor units is compensated for by a higher firing frequency of the remaining intact units. In myopathy an early (increased) recruitment of many motor units is seen if the muscle is activated with only a small force.

8.2 Significance of Electrodiagnostic Testing in the Management of Peripheral Nerve Lesions

In peripheral nerve lesions EDX studies are used for several purposes such as confirmation of the diagnosis, classification of nerve injury, localization of the lesion site, assessment of the underlying pathology, detection of nerve anastomosis and monitoring of regenerative processes (Katirji 2002). Relevancy, strengths and limitations of EDX testing, its potential impacts on case management and its significance in relation to other diagnostic procedures, especially the clinical evaluation (Table 8.2), are discussed in the following chapters. Commonly used terms in electrophysiology are summarized in Table 8.3.

Table 8.2. Significance of the clinical examination and of EDX studies in the evaluation and management of peripheral nerve lesions (+++ method of choice, ++ substantial contribution, + substantial contribution in selected patients, (+) usually not helpful; *NCS* nerve conduction studies, *EMG* electromyography)

	Clinical assessment	NCS/EMG
Establishment of the diagnosis	+++	+
Assessment of the severity of nerve damage	+	+++
Localization of nerve damage	++	++
Follow-up and prognosis	++	+++
Etiological classification	+	(+)
Detection of innervation anomalies	(+)	+++

8.2.1
Diagnosis of Peripheral Nerve Lesions

In most instances the correct diagnosis can be established based on the clinical pattern of motor and sensory deficits, localization and radiation of pain and eventually vegetative disturbances. A thorough review of the patient's medical history with emphasis on potential trigger events, demonstration of a Tinel's sign (Tinel 1915) at the site of suspected entrapment and results of provocation tests may serve to further substantiate the diagnosis. In some patients, however, diagnostic inaccuracies remain and EDX testing can substantially contribute to the classification of peripheral nerve lesions. Such pitfalls are often related to one of the following differential diagnoses:

- Plexus palsy versus polysegmental radiculopathies: differentiation can easily be achieved by the simple principle that SNAPs are diminished or absent in postganglionic damage (plexus) (Levin 2001; Ma et al. 1984) but normally preserved in preganglionic, i.e. root lesions (Fig. 8.11). Sometimes EMG of paravertebral muscles is required as a supplementary test.
- Peripheral versus central paresis: radial, ulnar and peroneal nerve palsy is sometimes mimicked by small cortical or subcortical brain lesions along the pyramidal tract. In cases of a peripheral origin, documentation of conduction abnormalities or axonal damage allows an accurate classification.
- Pure pain syndromes (e.g. nonparetic compression of the radial nerve under the arcade of Frohse (Rosenbaum 1999) or tarsal tunnel syndrome without sensorimotor deficits): EDX testing may yield evidence of subclinical nerve damage and thus lead to the correct diagnosis.

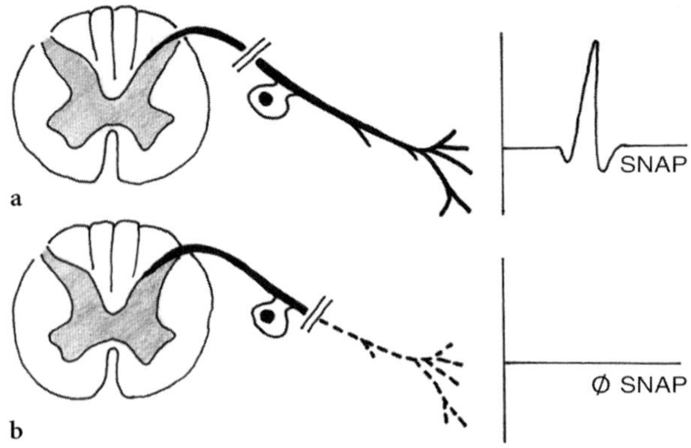

Fig. 8.11a, b. Sensory nerve conduction studies in (a) nerve root and (b) peripheral nerve lesions. The dorsal root ganglia are bipolar cells whose central processes form the sensory roots, and the distal processes continue as the peripheral sensory nerve fibers. In the case of a root lesions (a) the distal sensory nerve does not degenerate and normal SNAPs are elicitable because the lesion is proximal to the ganglia

8.2.2
Severity of Peripheral Nerve Lesions

The clinical impression alone is often insufficient for an early and adequate estimation of the severity of nerve damage – especially in the clinically relevant case of severe motor deficits. A reliable differentiation between neurapraxia and partial or total axonotmesis (Guitierrez and England 2002; Seddon 1943) is a domain of electrophysiology and crucial to all therapeutic decisions (Fig. 8.12). Both conditions may produce an identical amount of clinical weakness when the same number of motor fibers are involved. Whereas in neurapraxia impulses cannot pass across the lesion site due to a myelin disorder, in axonotmesis the nerve stump distal to the lesion undergoes degeneration and phagocytosis (Wallerian degeneration) (Lubinska 1977; Gutierrez and England 2001; Mumenthaler et al. 1998) (Fig. 8.13).

The electrophysiological hallmarks of neurapraxia are a synchronized or desynchronized slowing of nerve conduction (Fig. 8.12). In addition, conduction studies may identify typical conduction blocks or yield evidence of severe proximal conduction abnormalities. The latter phenomenon is characterized by a (near) normal motor response to electric nerve stimulation despite high-grade paresis, and absent or inconsistent F-wave responses. Conduction blocks are variably defined by a >30–50% loss in the amplitude of the CMAP without substantial increase in the potential duration (<20%) on sequential nerve stimulation (Oh et al. 1994) (Fig. 8.12). Acute axonal nerve damage (axonotmesis), in contrast, results in low-amplitude CMAPs regardless of whether the affected nerve is stimulated above or below the level of the lesion (Fig. 8.12). On needle EMG denervation activity emerges along with a drop-out of MUAPs on maximal effort (Figs. 8.8, 8.9b).

Prognosis of neurapraxia is generally favorable (Table 8.4), whereas in axonotmesis functional outcome relies on the efficacy of distal collateral sprouting of preserved nerve fibers and/or on adequate axonal sprouting from the lesion site (Fig. 8.9), both of which are influenced by factors such as the regeneration distance, intactness of the epi-/perineurium, mechanism of nerve damage, evidence of com-

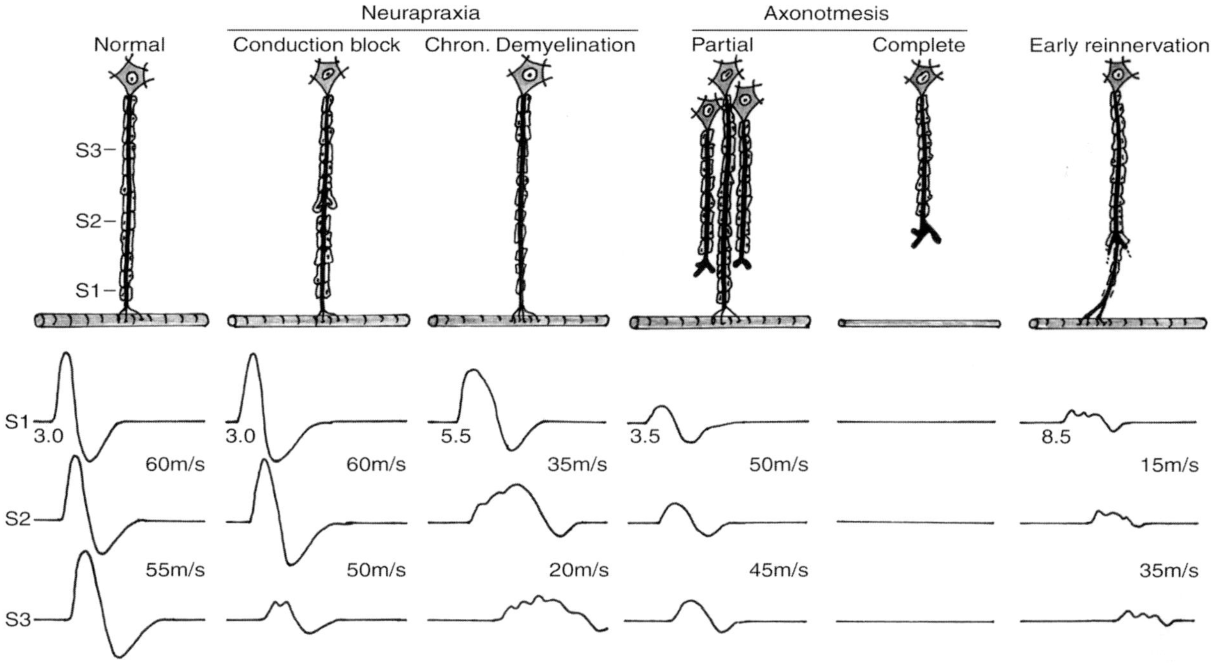

Fig. 8.12. Typical abnormalities of nerve conduction studies in neurapraxia (chronic demyelination and conduction blocks), partial and complete axonotmesis and reinnervation after axonotmesis

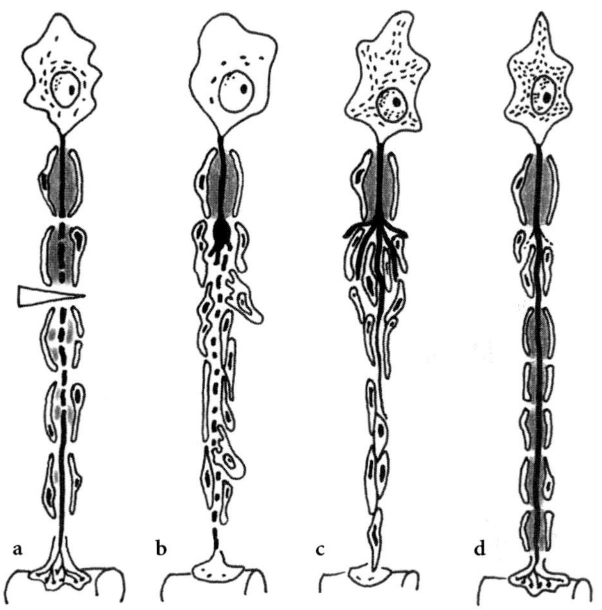

Fig. 8.13a–d. Wallerian degeneration. **a** Axonotmesis (*arrow* site of nerve transaction). **b** Within 4 to 7 days axonal enlargement and breakdown (fragmentation of axon and myelin) with subsequent phagocytosis of the entire axonal material distally to the site of injury emerges. **c** The degenerative process is followed by slow axonal regeneration (sprouting). **d** Late stage of reinnervation, which is favorable in this case (reproduced with modification from Mumenthaler et al. 1998, with permission)

pressive disorders, scarring and presence or absence of polyneuropathy.

As an important limitation, there is no way to distinguish between complete axonotmesis and neurotmesis by electrophysiological means. High-resolution nerve ultrasound or MRI are usually used for accurately assessing discontinuity of the damaged nerve.

An illustrative example showing how EDX studies assist in the therapeutic management is given below.

Illustrative case report

A 60-year-old woman noticed leg weakness immediately after abdominal hysterectomy. Clinical examination revealed severe weakness of knee extension and hip flexion (one-fifth on the Medical Research Council Scale), hypesthesia at the anteromedial thigh and absence of the patellar tendon reflex allowing the diagnosis of a femoral nerve lesion to be established. The patient was unable to walk without aid. Computed tomography of the pelvis was performed to rule out compression by a retroperitoneal hematoma.

Comment: iatrogenic injury of the femoral nerve during pelvic surgery most commonly arises from compression with the lateral retractor blade.

The first EDX testing was performed 3 weeks after surgical intervention. Remarkably, inguinal stimulation of the diseased femoral nerve elicited a near-normal motor response in spite of high-grade paresis (CMAP recorded from the vastus medialis head of the quadriceps muscle (Fig. 8.2) 8 mV versus 10.5 mV at the normal side), and EMG disclosed low-density denervation activity restricted to parts of the vastus lateralis muscle (fibrillation potentials 2/10).

Comment: this finding clearly indicates the presence of a proximal conduction block as the main mechanism of muscle weakness – and an overall good prognosis. Because conduction blocks frequently recover spontaneously over a period of up to 3 to 6 weeks early explorative surgery is usually not performed.

In this patient, however, the further clinical course was unfavorable without any improvement in muscle strength over the following 3 months. Results of control EDX studies remained virtually unchanged except for a disappearance of pathological spontaneous activity and beginning of reinnervation in the vastus lateralis muscle. MRI of the pelvis did not reveal any pathological finding. Ultrasonography, however, showed segmental thickening of the nerve 8 cm rostral to the inguinal ligament as indirect evidence of nerve compression.

Comment: if blockage of nerve conduction is maintained over several months the conditions is termed "persistent conduction block". Such abnormalities are either of immunological origin, which could be ruled out in our patient, or are caused by constrictive scar tissue.

Operative exploration was performed. The nerve was found constricted in scar tissue at the location identified by ultrasonography, and carefully released. Two days after successful neurolysis, the conduction block had partly resolved and the patient was able to walk again. At follow-up 3 months later muscle strength and knee jerk had normalized.

Comment: it is a frequent experience that conduction blocks promptly disappear after elimination of the causative compressive pathology.

8.2.3 Localization of Peripheral Nerve Lesions

A thorough clinical examination usually permits a crude locational categorization of nerve lesions. Locational precision is high in classic entrapment syndromes (e.g. CTS or TTS) and in segments of peripheral nerves at which numerous branches divide from the main trunk in a consistent order, but is comparatively low in most other instances.

EDX testing is particularly useful in assessing the exact site of a nerve lesion. Both a focal slowing of nerve conduction and emergence of conduction blocks have a high localizatory significance. In superficially located nerves suitable for short-segment stimulation such phenomena can be assessed with a precision of 5 to 10 mm (Figs. 8.14). This applies to most nerves of the upper extremities, the distal sensory branches of the sciatic nerve and the peroneal and tibial nerves at their course through the popliteal fossa or behind the fibular neck, respectively. In other nerves localizatory precision is much lower in the range of several centimeters.

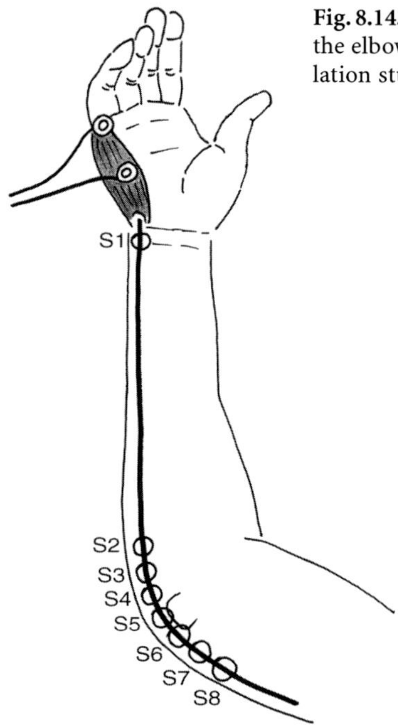

Fig. 8.14. Ulnar neuropathy at the elbow: short segment stimulation studies

In analogy to EDX studies, nerve ultrasound is capable of assessing the site of a peripheral nerve lesion in a majority of patients. Both diagnostic modalities are complementary in that conduction studies may reveal abnormalities in nerve segments with a normal sonographic appearance and, vice versa, ultrasound may document substantial pathologies in the absence of electrophysiological peculiarities. In this context it is worth mentioning that the nerve conduction velocity assessed by standard surface recording always reflects the speed of the fastest conducting axons. In compression syndromes propagation of the pressure within the nerve cross-section is often inhomogeneous and some fascicles may even be spared.

A special challenge is the localizatory differentiation between traumatic brachial plexus palsy and avulsion injury of nerve roots. In the latter disorder complex reflex studies utilizing cutaneous silent periods permit a reliable classification provided that there is at least minimal residual motor function in the affected arm and the patient is able to cooperate. In the more common case of a combination of both conditions, however, EDX testing mostly fails to give a clear diagnosis and myelography or magnetic resonance imaging are the diagnostic gold standard in this situation (Levin 2001).

8.2.4 Etiology of Peripheral Nerve Lesions

Nerve ultrasound and other radiological techniques are the method of choice for assessing the nature of compressive and intraneural pathologies (scar tissue, ganglia, anatomical variants, neoplasm, etc). In the case of external compression (e.g. classic pressure palsy), essential information on the eliciting event has to be obtained from a thorough exploration of the patient's medical history and clinical inspection of the lesion site.

The contribution of EDX testing to this particular issue is restricted to the exclusion of non-compressive mononeuropathies such as focal manifestations of systemic nerve disorders (e.g. multiplex and other asymmetric neuropathies, motor neuron disease, multiple neurofibroma in neurofibromatosis, etc) and immunological diseases of the peripheral nerve (motor neuropathy with conduction blocks). Sometimes entrapment syndromes emerge on the basis of predisposing polyneuropathies which can reliably be assessed by clinical and electrophysiological examinations.

8.2.5 Detection of Innervation Anomalies

Inconsistent anastomosis between nerves and true innervation anomalies are important sources of clinical misinterpretation and thus merit short consideration.

The most frequent anomaly is the Martin-Gruber anastomosis (Fig. 8.15) which occurs in up to 30% of healthy subjects (Kimura et al. 1976; Wilbourn and Lambert 1976). It entails a forearm crossover of nerve fibers from the median to the ulnar nerve. The shunted fibers usually supply the hypothenar and/or

Table 8.3. Commonly used terms in electrodiagnostic EDX testing

Neurapraxia
Least severe type of nerve lesion with the continuity of axons preserved and clinical deficits being attributable to local demyelination and manifestation of (reversible) conduction abnormalities (Fig. 8.12). *Electrophysiological characteristics:* slowing of nerve conduction and emergence of conduction blocks

Axonotmesis
More severe type of nerve lesion with disruption of axons and surrounding endoneurial sheets but maintenance of peri- and epineurium (Fig. 8.13). *Electrophysiological characteristics:* denervation activity and axonal damage on EMG

Neurotmesis
Most severe type of nerve lesion with complete disruption of axon, and endo-, peri- and epineurium. *Electrophysiological characteristics:* extensive denervation activity and no voluntary muscle activity

Nerve entrapment
Nerve compression at sites where it passes through a narrow space often termed a "tunnel"

Wallerian degeneration
Arises from severe nerve injury (axonotmesis or neurotmesis) and characterized by axonal enlargement and breakdown (fragmentation of axon and myelin) with subsequent phagocytosis of the entire axonal material distal to the site of injury (Fig. 8.13). This degenerative process takes up to 4 to 7 days and is immediately followed by slow axonal regeneration

Denervation activity
Consists of fibrillation potentials and positive waves – occurs on needle EMG after acute axonal nerve damage and represents a spontaneous depolarization of denervated muscle fibers. Fibrillations are brief spikes (duration 1 to 5 ms) and positive waves brief spikes followed by a slow negative phase. Both potentials manifest at rest (Fig. 8.8a)

F-wave
Late motor response triggered by an antidromic motor nerve action potential which results in a backfiring of a small subpopulation of anterior horn cells (Fig. 8.5)

Distal motor latency
Time (in milliseconds) between electric stimulation and initial deflection of the compound muscle action potential from baseline (Fig. 8.3a). It is composed of nerve conduction to the neuromuscular junction, the time delay across the neuromuscular junction and the synchronized depolarization of muscle fibers

CMAP
"Compound muscle action potential" – summation of the action potentials of all muscle fibers. CMAPs are recorded in motor nerve conduction studies (Fig. 8.3a). With the tendon-belly method of electrode placing the CMAP is biphasic with an initial steep negative deflection

MUAP
"Motor unit action potential" – is recorded while the patient is asked to slightly contract the muscle being sampled (needle EMG). MUAPs represent the electrical signal generated by all muscle fibers supplied by a single axon (motor unit) and are assessed for duration, amplitude, phases and recruitment pattern (Fig. 8.10). Analysis of MUAP morphology allows classification as normal, neuropathic or myopathic

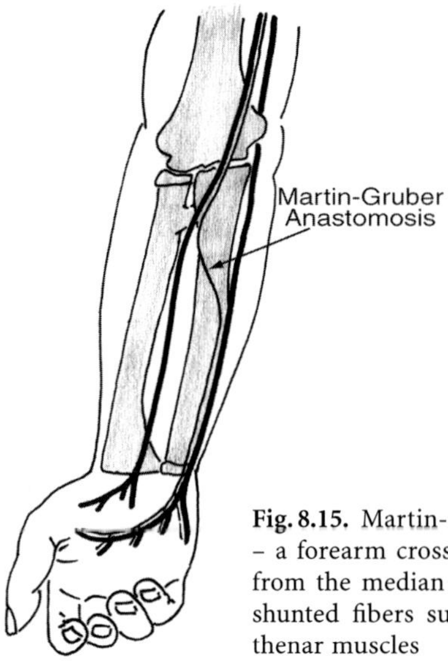

Fig. 8.15. Martin-Gruber anastomosis – a forearm crossover of nerve fibers from the median to ulnar nerve. The shunted fibers supply hypothenar or thenar muscles

thenar muscles. A further accessory communication between the two nerves may exist in the palm of the hand; this is known as the Riche-Cannieu anastomosis (RICHE 1897). From a clinical perspective, the presence of a nerve anastomosis may cause marked deviations of the innervation pattern from normal, and accordingly obscure the clinical presentation of entrapment syndromes. For example, severe carpal and cubital tunnel syndrome with advanced axon loss may exist in the absence of motor deficits. In general, innervation of intrinsic hand muscles is much less consistent than commonly assumed – ranging from an all-ulnar to all-median hand (ROWNTREE 1949).

Electronically, the presence of a Martin-Gruber anastomosis is indicated by a lower amplitude of the CMAP on distal than on proximal stimulation and by changes in the configuration of the motor response. Special focus should be on the initial deflection of the motor response from baseline and a potential composed of two components. If recognized, complex stimulation studies can determine the exact course of the anastomosis and the (motor) innervation afforded by the shunting fibers. Detection of innervation anomalies is equally important for diagnostic and therapeutic purposes.

8.2.6 Follow-up of Peripheral Nerve Lesions

Patients with axonal nerve damage may or may not be subjected to immediate surgery (Table 8.4). In the latter more common case short-term follow-up examinations aim at estimating the expected extent of spontaneous recovery as the basis for a decision on a possible later operative intervention. The longer the time elapsed since nerve injury, the more accurate is such a prognostic assessment. On the other hand, if surgery is delayed by more than 3 to 6 months endoneural tubes undergo shrinkage and obliteration and the probability of satisfactory remission gradually declines. Given these opposite requirements, optimal timing of follow-up examinations is a challenging task in each individual patient.

Clinical follow-up should include a detailed registration of the extent and course (onset and dynamics) of motor and sensory recovery, and testing for Tinel's sign along the nerve trunk, which gives a good impression of the velocity of axonal sprouting. Reinnervation starts in the muscles next to the nerve lesion and progresses distally. In addition to regeneration of the transected axons, recovery may arise from distal collateral sprouting of remaining intact axons (GUTIERREZ and ENGLAND 2001; MUMENTHALER et al. 1998) (Figs. 8.9, 8.12, 8.13).

EMG is particularly useful in the follow-up of patients because disappearance of denervation activity and emergence of early reinnervation potentials precede clinically visible motor recovery by up to 4 to 8 weeks (Fig. 8.8b). Accordingly, serial EMG

Table 8.4. Prognosis of peripheral nerve lesions

Neurapraxia
Prognosis is usually favorable with spontaneous recovery being expectable within 3 to 6 weeks after onset – or earlier if nerve compression is transient and mild. In a minority of patients, however, conduction abnormalities (especially conduction blocks) do not resolve or even worsen due to shrinking scar tissue. In some cases, surgical intervention may become necessary

Axonotmesis (partial/complete)
Prognosis is in part favorable but regeneration may take months or even years. An individual prognostic evaluation based on the extent of damage, regeneration distance and various other factors influencing the capacity of nerve regeneration (see Section 8.2.6) is mandatory for optimal therapeutic management. In some patients early operative intervention improves the probability of regular reinnervation; others, however, derive more benefit from withholding surgery. In the case of an initially conservative therapy, rigorous clinical and electrophysiological monitoring is recommended (for details see Section 8.2.6)

Neurotmesis
Because prognosis of spontaneous regeneration is definitely poor, surgical repair with adaptation of the nerve endings (end-to-end suture) or bridging of a potential gap with autogenous sural nerve grafts is warranted as early as practicable

examinations help to speed up the decision process. If no clinical and/or electromyographic evidence of functional reinnervation becomes evident patients are usually subjected to surgery. Further control evaluations at longer intervals are recommended and may serve as the basis for rehabilitation programmes and social reintegration.

8.2.7 Diagnostic Work-up in Patients with Peripheral Nerve Lesions

A thorough neurological examination by an experienced clinician is the mainstay in optimal management of peripheral nerve lesions and a necessary basis for the interpretation of all ancillary diagnostic procedures. A decision pathway for a cost-effective application of methodologically complex examinations is depicted in Fig. 8.16. Guidelines for an optimal timing of EDX studies are summarized in Table 8.5.

If surgical intervention is being considered, EDX testing and nerve ultrasound should be performed. The two examinations are not alternative procedures but highly complementary regarding strengths and limitations, and may substantially contribute to the final therapeutic decision and the choice of the surgical approach. A high level of diagnostic and localizatory security, as required in the preoperative setting, is achieved if the clinical appearance and the results of both the aforementioned diagnostic modalities fit well together.

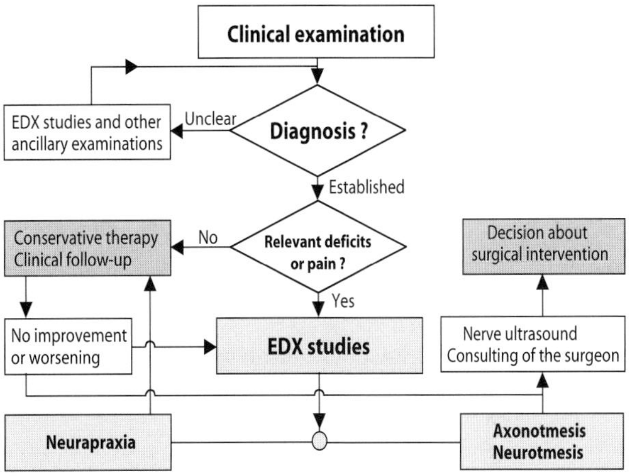

Fig. 8.16. Management of peripheral nerve lesions

Table 8.5. Timing of EDX studies (*days* denote days after nerve injury)

Days 1 to 6	Generally not useful	Nerve conduction studies and EMG provide no prognostic and little diagnostic information. Examinations in this time period should be reserved for solving a few well-defined clinical problems (e.g. differentiation between painful peroneal nerve lesion in vasculitis and L5 radiculopathy)
Days 7 to 14	Exceptionally indicated	Wallerian degeneration has now finished. Amplitudes of the compound muscle action potentials and sensory action potentials allow a crude estimation of the degree of axonal damage. However, since CMAPs can only be recorded from superficial (distal) muscles and the various fibers of a nerve are often not uniformly affected, accuracy of the prognostic evaluation has its limitations even in the hands of an experienced electrophysiologist. Therefore, EDX studies should only be scheduled in this time interval if early surgical intervention is being considered
Day >14	Adequate time for examination	In case of acute axonal damage, denervation activity has now developed. Detection and quantification of fibrillation potentials and positive waves on EMG and supplementary nerve conduction studies permit a precise assessment and localization of nerve damage in almost all patients. This information serves as a basis for a reliable prognostic evaluation
Follow-up examinations		Standard intervals for follow-up are 3 to 6 months. Shorter periods may be adequate if the therapeutic decision depends on the results of serial EMG examinations (monitoring of spontaneous regeneration) or if the lesion is distal and the regeneration distance short. Axonal sprouting at the site of injury (axon transection) along intact endoneural tubes occurs at an average of 1–2 mm per day provided that the growing axons find access to the distal nerve trunk. Expected nerve growth rates may be utilized for an individual adjustment of examination intervals. In patients with proximal nerve lesions, especially plexus palsy or severe damage to nerve roots, regenerative processes may be active for as long as 2 to 3 years

References

Eisen A, Schomer D, Melmed C (1977) The application of F-wave measurements in the differentiation of proximal and distal upper limb entrapments. Neurology 27:662–668

Gassel MM (1964) Sources of error in motor nerve conduction studies. Neurology 14:825

Guidelines in Electrodiagnostic Medicine (1999) American Association of Electrodiagnostic Medicine. Muscle Nerve, Rochester

Gutierrez A, England JD (2001) Peripheral nerve injury. In: Katirji B, Kaminski HJ, Preston DC, et al (eds) Neuromuscular disorders in clinical practice. Butterworth-Heinemann, Boston

Honet JC, Jebsen RH, Perrin EB (1968) Variability of nerve conduction velocity determinations in normal persons. Arch Phys Med Rehabil 49:650–654

Katirji B (2002) Electrodiagnostic approach to the patient with suspected mononeuropathy of the lower extremity. Neurol Clin 20:479–501

Kimura J, Murphy MJ, Varda DJ (1976) Electrophysiological study of anomalous innervation of intrinsic hand muscles. Arch Neurol 33:842

Levin KH (2001) Cervical radiculopathies. In: Katirji B, Kaminski HJ, Preston DC, et al (eds) Neuromuscular disorders in clinical practice. Butterworth-Heinemann, Boston

Liveson JA, Ma DM (1992) Laboratory reference for clinical neurophysiology. Davis, Philadelphia

Lubinska L (1977) Early course of Wallerian degeneration in myelinated fibres of the rat phrenic nerve. Brain Res 130: 47–63

Ma MD, Wilbourn AJ, Kraft GH (1984) Unusual sensory conduction studies. American Association of Electromyography and Electrodiagnosis, Rochester

Mumenthaler M, Schliack H, Stoehr M (1998) Läsionen peripherer Nerven und radikuläre Läsionen. Thieme, Stuttgart

Oh SJ, Kim DE, Kuruoglu HL (1994) What is the best diagnostic index of conduction block and temporal dispersion? Muscle Nerve 17:489–493

Rich P (1897) Le nerf cubital et les muscles de l'éminence thenar. Bull Mem Soc Anat Paris 5:251

Rosenbaum R (1999) Disputed radial tunnel syndrome. Muscle Nerve 22 :960–967

Rowntree T (1949) Anomalous innervation of the hand muscles. J Bone Joint Surg Br 31:505

Seddon HJ (1943) Three types of nerve injury. Brain 66: 237–239

Tinel J (1915) Le signe du «fourmillement» dans les lésions des nerfs périphériques. Presse Med 23:385–396

Wilbourn AJ, Lambert E (1976) The forearm median-to-ulnar nerve communication: electrodiagnostic aspects. Neurology 26:368

Subject Index

A
alcohol 95, 96, 109, 118
arcade of Frohse 47
arch of Frohse 24
artery
– median 9, 23, 53
axonotmesis 73, 109, 128, 129, 131

B
block
– axillary 100
– conduction 109
– interscalene 98
– psoas compartment 100
– pudendal nerve 103
– three-in-one 101
brachialgia paraesthetica nocturna 49

C
coaptation 115, 118
common peroneal *see* nerve common fibular
compound imaging 5
compound muscle action potential 122
conduction velocities 122

E
electromyography 73
– needle 125
elephantiasis neuromatosa 85
entrapment 37
entrapment neuropathy 38
epineurium 108
Erb's point 124
extended field of view imaging 10 see panoramic imaging

F
facial nerve 13
fibrillation 125
Froment's manoeuvre 39
F-wave 124, 128

G
Guyon's canal 38, 45

I
iatrogenic nerve lesion 61
interference pattern 127
intermetatarsal bursa 91
intermetatarsal space 89

L
Latency 122
ligament
– inguinal 29
– laciniate 56
lymph node biopsy 74

M
Martin-Gruber anastomosis 40, 131
median nerve compression 48
Morton's metatarsalgia 37
Morton's neuroma 83, 89
Mulder's sign 90
muscle
– anconeus epitrochlearis 39
– peroneus longus 54
– psoas 29
– supinator 23, 47
– trapezius 74

N
nerve
– accessory 14, 74
– axillary 21, 77
– common fibular 31
– common peroneal 80 *see* nerve common fibular
– conduction studies 121, 124
– cutaneous antebrachial 19
– digital palmar 27
– facial 13
– femoral 29, 77
– fibular 32
– grafting 115
– lateral femoral cutaneous 29
– long thoracic 17
– longitudinal motion 71
– median 19, 22, 25
– musculocutaneous 17
– palmar 25
– peroneal 54, 78 see nerve common fibular *see* nerve fibular
– phrenic 16
– plantar 34
– profound fibular 32
– pudendal 32
– radial 23, 28, 62
– regeneration 119

nerve *(continued)*
- saphenus 29
- sciatic 30, 77
- subcostal 35
- superficial fibular 32
- sural 115
- thoracodorsal 17
- tibial 31, 32, 78
- ulnar 19, 23, 80
- vagal 14
nerve sheath ganglion 88
neural fibrolipoma 83
neurapraxia 72, 109, 128
neurofibromatosis type 1 85
neurogenic tumors 83
neurolysis 112
- external 68, 112
- internal 69
neuroma 72, 83, 95, 114
- postsurgical 92
- traction 72
- traumatic 92
neurotmesis 73, 109

O
Osborne fascia 38

P
perineurium 108
peroneal see nerve fibular see nerve common fibular
phantom pain 93
phenol 95, 96
plexus
- brachial 16, 66, 67, 79, 97
- cervical 15
- palsy 128
postoperative scaring 71
pudendal block 32

R
radial 46
Recklinghausen's disease 85
regional anesthesia 96
Riche-Cannieu anastomosis 132

S
Schwannoma 84
sensory nerve action potential 123
sonographic guidance 96
steroids 95
sulcus
- nervi radialis 22
syndrome
- posterior interosseous nerve 47
- radial tunnel 46
- snapping triceps 44
- supinator 46, 47
- tarsal tunnel 55

T
Tinel's sign 40, 90
tissue harmonic imaging 5
total hip replacement 76
tunnel
- carpal 48
- cubital 38
- peroneal 54
- tarsal 55, 57

U
Ulnar nerve entrapment 38
ulnar sulcus *see* tunnel cubital

W
Wallerian degeneration 109
Wartenberg's sign 39
wrist drop 47

X
XRES imaging 7

List of Contributors

GERD BODNER, MD
Professor, Department of Radiology
Section for Diagnostic and
Interventional Sonography
University Hospital Innsbruck
Anichstrasse 35
6020 Innsbruck
Austria

HANNES GRUBER, MD
Department of Radiology
University Hospital Innsbruck
Anichstrasse 35
6020 Innsbruck
Austria

STEFAN KIECHL, MD
Professor, Department of Neurology
Section for Electrodiagnosis (EMG/NLG)
University Hospital Innsbruck
Anichstrasse 35
6020 Innsbruck
Austria

PETER KOVACS, MD
Department of Radiology
University Hospital Innsbruck
Anichstrasse 35
6020 Innsbruck
Austria

SIEGRIED PEER, MD
Professor, Department of Radiology
Section for Diagnostic and
Interventional Sonography
University Hospital Innsbruck
Anichstrasse 35
6020 Innsbruck
Austria

HILDEGUNDE PIZA-KATZER, MD
Professor and Chairman, Department of Plastic
and Reconstructive Surgery
and Ludwig Boltzmann Institute for Quality Control
in Plastic and Reconstructive Surgery
University Hospital Innsbruck
Anichstrasse 35
6020 Innsbruck
Austria

Medical Radiology Diagnostic Imaging and Radiation Oncology

Titles in the series already published

Diagnostic Imaging

Innovations in Diagnostic Imaging
Edited by J. H. Anderson

Radiology of the Upper Urinary Tract
Edited by E. K. Lang

The Thymus - Diagnostic Imaging, Functions, and Pathologic Anatomy
Edited by E. Walter, E. Willich, and W. R. Webb

Interventional Neuroradiology
Edited by A. Valavanis

Radiology of the Pancreas
Edited by A. L. Baert, co-edited by G. Delorme

Radiology of the Lower Urinary Tract
Edited by E. K. Lang

Magnetic Resonance Angiography
Edited by I. P. Arlart, G. M. Bongartz, and G. Marchal

Contrast-Enhanced MRI of the Breast
S. Heywang-Köbrunner and R. Beck

Spiral CT of the Chest
Edited by M. Rémy-Jardin and J. Rémy

Radiological Diagnosis of Breast Diseases
Edited by M. Friedrich and E.A. Sickles

Radiology of the Trauma
Edited by M. Heller and A. Fink

Biliary Tract Radiology
Edited by P. Rossi

Radiological Imaging of Sports Injuries
Edited by C. Masciocchi

Modern Imaging of the Alimentary Tube
Edited by A. R. Margulis

Diagnosis and Therapy of Spinal Tumors
Edited by P. R. Algra, J. Valk, and J. J. Heimans

Interventional Magnetic Resonance Imaging
Edited by J. F. Debatin and G. Adam

Abdominal and Pelvic MRI
Edited by A. Heuck and M. Reiser

Orthopedic Imaging
Techniques and Applications
Edited by A. M. Davies and H. Pettersson

Radiology of the Female Pelvic Organs
Edited by E. K.Lang

Magnetic Resonance of the Heart and Great Vessels
Clinical Applications
Edited by J. Bogaert, A. J. Duerinckx, and F. E. Rademakers

Modern Head and Neck Imaging
Edited by S. K. Mukherji and J. A. Castelijns

Radiological Imaging of Endocrine Diseases
Edited by J. N. Bruneton in collaboration with B. Padovani and M.-Y. Mourou

Trends in Contrast Media
Edited by H. S. Thomsen, R. N. Muller, and R. F. Mattrey

Functional MRI
Edited by C. T. W. Moonen and P. A. Bandettini

Radiology of the Pancreas
2nd Revised Edition
Edited by A. L. Baert
Co-edited by G. Delorme and L. Van Hoe

Emergency Pediatric Radiology
Edited by H. Carty

Spiral CT of the Abdomen
Edited by F. Terrier, M. Grossholz, and C. D. Becker

Liver Malignancies
Diagnostic and Interventional Radiology
Edited by C. Bartolozzi and R. Lencioni

Medical Imaging of the Spleen
Edited by A. M. De Schepper and F. Vanhoenacker

Radiology of Peripheral Vascular Diseases
Edited by E. Zeitler

Diagnostic Nuclear Medicine
Edited by C. Schiepers

Radiology of Blunt Trauma of the Chest
P. Schnyder and M. Wintermark

Portal Hypertension
Diagnostic Imaging-Guided Therapy
Edited by P. Rossi
Co-edited by P. Ricci and L. Broglia

Recent Advances in Diagnostic Neuroradiology
Edited by Ph. Demaerel

Virtual Endoscopy and Related 3D Techniques
Edited by P. Rogalla, J. Terwisscha Van Scheltinga, and B. Hamm

Multislice CT
Edited by M. F. Reiser, M. Takahashi, M. Modic, and R. Bruening

Pediatric Uroradiology
Edited by R. Fotter

Transfontanellar Doppler Imaging in Neonates
A. Couture and C. Veyrac

Radiology of AIDS
A Practical Approach
Edited by J.W.A.J. Reeders and P.C. Goodman

CT of the Peritoneum
Armando Rossi and Giorgio Rossi

Magnetic Resonance Angiography
2nd Revised Edition
Edited by I. P. Arlart, G. M. Bongratz, and G. Marchal

Pediatric Chest Imaging
Edited by Javier Lucaya and Janet L. Strife

Applications of Sonography in Head and Neck Pathology
Edited by J. N. Bruneton in collaboration with C. Raffaelli and O. Dassonville

Imaging of the Larynx
Edited by R. Hermans

3D Image Processing
Techniques and Clinical Applications
Edited by D. Caramella and C. Bartolozzi

Imaging of Orbital and Visual Pathway Pathology
Edited by W. S. Müller-Forell

Pediatric ENT Radiology
Edited by S. J. King and A. E. Boothroyd

Radiological Imaging of the Small Intestine
Edited by N. C. Gourtsoyiannis

Imaging of the Knee
Techniques and Applications
Edited by A. M. Davies and V. N. Cassar-Pullicino

Perinatal Imaging
From Ultrasound to MR Imaging
Edited by Fred E. Avni

Radiological Imaging of the Neonatal Chest
Edited by V. Donoghue

Diagnostic and Interventional Radiology in Liver Transplantation
Edited by E. Bücheler, V. Nicolas, C. E. Broelsch, X. Rogiers, and G. Krupski

Radiology of Osteoporosis
Edited by S. Grampp

Imaging and Intervention in Abdominal Trauma
Edited by R. F. Dondelinger

Imaging of the Foot and Ankle
Techniques and Applications
Edited by A. M. Davies, R. W. Whitehouse, and J. P. R. Jenkins

Interventional Radiology in Cancer
Edited by A. Adam, R. F. Dondelinger, and P. R. Mueller

Imaging of the Pancreas
Cystic and Rare Tumors
Edited by C. Procacci and A. J. Megibow

Intracranial Vascular Malformations and Aneurysms
From Diagnostic Work-Up to Endovascular Therapy
Edited by M. Forsting

Imaging Pelvic Floor Disorders
Edited by C. I. Bartram and J. O. L. DeLancey
Associate Editors: S. Halligan, F. M. Kelvin, and J. Stoker

High Resolution Sonography of the Peripheral Nervous System
Edited by S. Peer and G. Bodner

Radiology Imaging of the Ureter
Edited by F. Joffre, Ph. Otal, and M. Soulie

Printing and Binding: Stürtz AG, Würzburg